GERONTOLOGY IN HIGHER EDUCATION:
Developing Institutional and Community Strength

Editors:

Harvey L. Sterns
Edward F. Ansello
Betsy M. Sprouse
Ruth Layfield-Faux

Wadsworth Publishing Company
Belmont, California
A Division of Wadsworth, Inc.

Gerontology Editor: Curt Peoples
Production Editor: Jeanne Heise
Designer: Nancy Benedict
Cover Designer: Janet Wood
Copy Editor: Robert McNally

Printed in the United States of America
1   2   3   4   5   6   7   8   9   10—83 82 81 80 79

Library of Congress Cataloging in Publication Data

Main entry under title:

Gerontology in higher education.

    "Second in an annual review series by the Association for Gerontology in Higher Education."
       1. Gerontology—Study and teaching (Higher)—United States—Addresses, essays, lectures.   I.   Sterns, Harvey.   II.   Association for Gerontology in Higher Education.

HQ1061.G42   362.6'042'071173   79-9968
ISBN 0-534-00708-2

CONTENTS

iii

CONTRIBUTORS*

W. Andrew Achenbaum
Department of History, Canisius College, Buffalo, New York (108)

Edward F. Ansello
Center on Aging, University of Maryland, College Park, Maryland (116, 262)

James E. Birren
Ethel Percy Andrus Gerontology Center, University of Southern California, Los Angeles, California (2)

Nona Boren
The Gerontology Program, The George Washington University, Washington, D.C. (63)

Sherry L. Corbett
Department of Sociology, Miami University, Oxford, Ohio (28)

Donald O. Cowgill
Joint Centers for Aging Studies, University of Missouri-Columbia, Columbia, Missouri (21)

Dan Cowley
Geriatric Technician Training Program, Department of Human Services, Wayne Community College, Goldsboro, North Carolina (182)

Robert Deitchman
Department of Psychology and Institute for Life-Span Development and Gerontology, The University of Akron, Akron, Ohio (243)

David Demko
Older Population Programs, Delta College, University Center, Michigan (278)

Frederick G. Dorsey
President, American Geriatrics Society, Baylor College of Medicine, Houston, Texas (155)

*Numbers in parentheses refer to articles within the text.

Sister Mary Francilene
   President, Madonna College, Livonia, Michigan (44)

Donald E. Gelfand
   School of Social Work and Community Planning, University of Maryland-Baltimore, Baltimore, Maryland (56)

William C. Hays
   University Gerontology Center, Wichita State University, Wichita, Kansas (69)

Bert Hayslip, Jr.
   Department of Psychology, North Texas State University, Denton, Texas (262)

Tom Hickey
   School of Public Health and Institute of Gerontology, University of Michigan, Ann Arbor, Michigan (75, 130)

Ira S. Hirschfield
   Ethel Percy Andrus Gerontology Center, University of Southern California, Los Angeles, California (2)

Jerome Kaplan
   Department of Sociology, Ohio State University-Mansfield, Mansfield, Ohio (135)

Gerald A. Larue
   School of Religion, University of Southern California, Los Angeles, California (81)

Ruth Layfield-Faux
   Institute for Life-Span Development and Gerontology, The University of Akron, Akron, Ohio

Gari Lesnoff-Caravaglia
   Gerontology Program, Sangamon State University, Springfield, Illinois (101)

Aaron Lipman
   Department of Sociology, University of Miami, Miami, Florida (78)

Noel D. List
   Geriatrics Unit, School of Medicine, University of Maryland-Baltimore, Baltimore, Maryland (159)

Martin B. Loeb
   Faye McBeath Institute on Aging and Adult Life, University of Wisconsin-Madison, Madison, Wisconsin (34)

Jack Loman
   Training Officer, Wisconsin Bureau of Aging, Madison, Wisconsin (229)

Neil G. McCluskey
   The Center for Gerontological Studies, Center for Advanced Study in Education, The Graduate School and University Center, City University of New York, New York, New York (14)

Wanda McKee
   Training Officer, Indiana Commission on Aging and Aged, Indianapolis, Indiana (229)

Rick Miller
   Training Officer, Ohio Commission on Aging, Columbus, Ohio (229)

Shirley Mitchell
   Testing and Counseling Bureau, The University of Akron, Akron, Ohio (250)

Sister Colleen Morris
   Gerontology Department, Madonna College, Livonia, Michigan (44)

Wilbur N. Moulton
   Office of the President, Sangamon State University, Springfield, Illinois (42)

Jody K. Olsen
   Center on Aging, University of Maryland, College Park, Maryland (50)

Rosemary A. Orgren
Joint Centers for Aging Studies, University of Missouri-Columbia, Columbia, Missouri (21)

Michael D. Patrick
Department of Humanities, University of Missouri-Rolla, Rolla, Missouri (286)

John Peterson
Training Officer, Michigan Office on Services to the Aging, Lansing, Michigan (229)

Diane S. Piktialis
Massachusetts Department of Elder Affairs, Boston, Massachusetts (220)

Barbara Porter
Geriatric Technician Training Program, Department of Human Services, Wayne Community College, Goldsboro, North Carolina (182)

Eloise Rathbone-McCuan
George Warren Brown School of Social Work, Washington University, St. Louis, Missouri (195)

William A. Rogers
Continuing Education and Public Services, The University of Akron, Akron, Ohio (46)

Jeanette Secret
Training Officer, Minnesota Council on Aging, St. Paul, Minnesota (229)

Mildred M. Seltzer
Scripps Foundation Gerontology Center, Miami University, Oxford, Ohio (37)

Glorian Sorensen
Program on Aging, Augsburg College, Minneapolis, Minnesota (188)

Betsy M. Sprouse
Faye McBeath Institute on Aging and Adult Life, University of Wisconsin-Madison, Madison, Wisconsin (209, 238)

Harvey L. Sterns
Department of Psychology and Institute for Life-Span Development and Gerontology, The University of Akron, Akron, Ohio (238, 250)

Cyril P. Svoboda
Institute for Child Study, University of Maryland, College Park, Maryland (91)

James Tift
Aging and Human Development Program, St. Mary's Junior College, Minneapolis, Minnesota (188)

Sheldon S. Tobin
School of Social Service Administration, University of Chicago, Chicago, Illinois (166)

Sally Vaughan
Training Officer, Illinois Department on Aging, Springfield, Illinois (229)

Wilbur H. Watson
National Center on Black Aged, Washington, D.C. (145)

Thomas D. Watts
Graduate School of Social Work, The University of Texas at Arlington, Arlington, Texas (215)

Gamal Zaki
Sociology Department, Rhode Island College, Providence, Rhode Island (172)

Selma Zarakov
Gerontology/Programs for Older Adults, Palomar College, San Marcos, California (274)

Vicki A. Zoot
Center for Educational Development, University of Illinois-Medical Center, Chicago, Illinois (202)

INTRODUCTION

This volume is the second in an annual review series by the Association for Gerontology in Higher Education. The series focuses on key issues in academic gerontology and presents innovative approaches to the development of education, training, and research in aging.

What have often been artificially and unfortunately separated—the educational institution and the community—must be brought more closely together so that the field of gerontology will establish a responsive approach to education, research, and service. As we acknowledge, appreciate, and work with the links between theory and practice, the institution and the community draw upon each other's resources to establish gerontology as a permanent academic concern.

In addition to the community partnership, the development of institutional strength in gerontology also demands unusual levels of cooperation from faculty, administration, and students. Gerontology provides exciting opportunities for creative, multidisciplinary approaches, and at the same time it strengthens existing programs. Central to all academic endeavors in gerontology are efforts to establish a firm educational base for the field and to adequately prepare students who will undertake careers in gerontological research and practice.

The main theme of this work is developing the commitment of the institution and the community to gerontology education. The editors based their choice of the title of this volume and the papers to be included on the convictions that higher education and the community are inseparable partners in the shaping of gerontology education and that institutional development is based on multilevel cooperation.

The Association for Gerontology in Higher Education has developed during a period of rapid growth in academic gerontology programs. In representing its member institutions, the Association provides a forum for the exchange of ideas and knowledge, and shares the policy concerns of the membership at the national level. Through its annual meetings and publications, the Association explores national policy, institutional development, program design, faculty development, and services for older adults. The goal of the Association and of this volume is to strengthen the growth of educational commitment to gerontology.

Harvey L. Sterns
Edward F. Ansello
Betsy M. Sprouse
Ruth Layfield-Faux

PART ONE
BASIC ISSUES IN DEVELOPING INSTITUTIONAL STRENGTH

The following three papers discuss the evolutionary nature of gerontology in higher education. They describe academic gerontology in relation to professional education, to standards of quality, and to parallel developments in society.

The Emergence of Gerontology in Higher Education in America

James E. Birren
and
Ira S. Hirschfield
University of Southern California

Developing an adequate response to the emergent field of gerontology is one of the greatest unresolved issues in higher education today. It seems likely that the growing population of older adults and the needs of that population will present higher education with both a problem and an opportunity during the next two decades, or until such time as institutions incorporate the subject matter into regular curricula.

This paper has three parts: first, a report of some new research about professional education in gerontology; second, an examination of the current tenor of higher education, focusing on some preoccupations that may hamper the inclusion of gerontology; and third, a discussion about the extent to which gerontology's role should be increased, and suggestions about some of the questions meriting resolution.

The Role of Gerontology in Professional Education

What is the current role of higher education in gerontology? A partial answer to this question can be gathered from a study of professional education in California completed in 1977. The study has some important implications since it documents that there is little activity or anticipatory educational planning within the major professions that provide services to older adults. The results are discussed here not with the thought that their findings are definitive, rather, with the realization that their intention is to suggest trends and also to encourage gerontological educators to undertake similar analyses in other states so that a more comprehensive national picture can be drawn.

California is the highest-populated state of the Union. Although it has the largest aggregate of people over the age of 65 (over 2 million), the proportion of the aged is close to the national average. Thus, even though the size of the population of aged in California is greater than the total population of many states, the presence of this population is not so disproportionate that it would overwhelm the educational system.

In the fall of 1975, a committee of faculty and graduate students of the Leonard Davis School of Gerontology developed a plan for studying present and future activities in professional education in California related to the issues of aging. The following eight fields were selected for inclusion in the study: adult education, counselor education, dentistry, law, medicine, nursing, public administration, and social work. A grant from the Andrus Foundation supported the expenses of the study, entitled "An Analysis of Professional Education in the State of California for Services to Retired and Aged."

Two questionnaires were developed by the joint faculty and student group following an analysis of the published literature on the nature of professionalism in general and the professional development of each of the disciplines. The questionnaires were designed to record factual information as well as to record attitudes of the respondents in the schools and departments surveyed. Supplementing the questionnaires were course catalogues, bulletins, and announcements from the various academic units. Interviews were held with representatives of schools within a 100-mile radius of the University of Southern California. Telephone interviews were scheduled for individuals outside that area. The depth of information available from the different schools and areas varied considerably, but these methodological issues are not germane to this article. Overall, a total of 93 departments were surveyed to determine how their activities impinge on gerontology.

One of the more interesting points about the study is that the group responsible for it developed a doubt that the selection of school deans or department chairpersons represented the most informed individuals to interview about issues of gerontology. It became apparent that top-level administrators often had less access than other faculty members to the growth points in their programs, such as faculty affiliation with professional gerontological societies, numbers of placement agencies that have a focus on aging, and even information on course content that relates to gerontology. If academic administrators were not previously informed on these items, it is also unlikely that they would prepare themselves and become knowledgeable about these issues for the purposes of a survey.

Analysis of the data on many points cuts across the professional fields. What impressed us, or, we might say, depressed us, was that 70 percent of academic units surveyed claimed to have no required course offerings containing any gerontological content. An average of only two master's theses and less than one doctoral dissertation related to gerontology were approved in departments in these eight professions from 1971 to 1976. That is certainly a low level of activity related to gerontology.

Of all of the respondents surveyed, 85 percent felt that faculty members who teach courses about aging should have some specific training in gerontology. Seventy-five percent of all departments claimed that only 5 percent to 15 percent of their faculty who teach aging-related courses have such training. Three-fourths of the respondents also did not know whether their faculty members teaching courses were members of professional gerontological societies.

Of the eight professional areas, nursing and social work departments tended to have more course opportunities in aging than did the other fields; law tended to offer more overview courses with gerontological content, and social work and medicine offered more postgraduate courses.

It is also interesting to note that smaller departments tended to offer more aging-related courses than did the larger schools. This, of course, was influenced in the study by the fact that schools of social work and nursing have relatively smaller student bodies and, therefore, influenced the overall correlations.

Departments most active in continuing education are those requiring updating or recertification for practice in their field, such as medicine, nursing, and social work. Some gerontological education exists in continuing education programs in these fields, but there is very little evidence of it in the original or primary training of professionals. This would suggest that continuing education is more responsive to social needs than is the generic curriculum.

Public administration departments or schools show the least interest in gerontology of the eight areas surveyed and plan little or no action in the immediate future. Consequently, we are faced with a paradox. Given the rapid growth of Area Agencies on Aging and other governmental units, it is unfortunate and somewhat surprising that there has been no activity or contemplation of curriculum development in gerontology by schools of public administration. How long this situation will last is, indeed, a fundamental question.

Given the fact that health services to older people are becoming increasingly important, it is also significant that only one medical school claimed to have a required course with any gerontological content. There probably has been no concentrated attention to the issues of aging in medical school education in California up to 1978. Medicine and public administration may need some special mechanisms to encourage development.

In accounting for the overall low level of activity in teaching about aging, it is useful to consider future projections. Departments which are not planning to include aging content in their curricula cited as their major reasons: (1) lack of student interest, 60 percent; (2) lack of faculty interest, 58 percent; and (3) lack of trained faculty in gerontology, 52 percent. California is reputed to be a progressive state and often in the forefront of educational activity and professional involvement for the elderly. If California is considered to be in a good position, where does that place other states? On an average, less than one required course containing aging-related material was available per department, and as indicated previously, a low level of research was revealed at the master's and doctoral levels.

Looking at the study as a whole, we find it reveals that very little gerontological course content is offered for the training of professionals who will be providing services to older adults in California. Apparently schools are educating professionals who may spend most of their lives providing services to the aged, and yet these professionals may never have taken a course on aging nor been examined at the time of their certification or licensing on the content of aging. The low level of interest in curriculum development of courses containing information about aging portends a bleak immediate future. From this we may infer that we should not expect any dramatic increase in gerontological curriculum development unless the present pattern is altered by some direct and unexpected actions.

We should be concerned about the fact that the chairpersons and deans of professional schools show very little leadership in gerontology. We might have expected that administrators would be a step ahead of their profession, but in fact, most seem to be a step behind. Since university administrators are not interested in gerontology, we appear to have a leadership vacuum in higher education. Although there is public interest in professional education in gerontology, few within the educational structure are taking the initiative or planning to introduce the subject matter.

Studies similar to this should be carried out in other states, which can capitalize on the strengths and weaknesses of the study reported here and add to the total information available on trends in education related to aging. Perhaps, too, the Administration on Aging might collaborate with the Association for Gerontology in Higher Education (AGHE) and others in helping to promote such state surveys. In addition to curriculum analyses, we would recommend including some research on the licensing and certification requirements in various states with regard to content on gerontology. Beyond this specific information, we think studies of this nature are also needed to provide bench marks, so that within the next two to five years we can measure the degree of progress in each field.

Indeed, if one of the goals of AGHE is to gerontologize the professions, then one of the best ways of implementing this goal is to encourage surveys that arm us with useful data so that we may work toward more sophisticated and effective gerontological educational development.

The Tenor of Higher Education in America

Following the research findings of the previous California study, one cannot help but ask why the inclusion of gerontology in professional education has been so slow. By examining the current environment in many universities throughout the United States, we clearly understand why gerontology presents both a problem and an opportunity for higher education.

It is possible that some top-level university administrators will turn to the issues of gerontology as an area of educational innovation and an emergent field for research, education, and training. One reason that they may do so is the relative financial depression surrounding our academic institutions. At a time when society is undergoing an inflation of about 7 percent a year, academic salaries are increasing on the average only 5.2 percent (1977–78). There are limited funds for new programs, and for this reason, an entrepreneurial response might lead an academic administrator to stimulate programs in gerontology. However, our conjectural university president or other administrator has additional preoccupations. Being converted as he has been in recent years to an executive manager, he is more inclined to think about cost effectiveness of the existing activities of the university rather than move outside that arena to pursue new academic goals.

What are some of the major preoccupations of current academic life? Consider, for example, the University of California at Berkeley. It has been judged as having the outstanding graduate school in the country. In 1978, it was under investigation by the federal government's Office for Civil Rights to determine if there had been discrimination in hiring women and minority members. One department refused to let investigators see recommendation letters for unsuccessful candidates for positions. The chancellor and vice chancellor were involved in Washington hearings which challenged a $1.5 million federal contract with the university's Naval Bioscience Laboratory. The administrators were faced with an immediate layoff of 125 university employees if the contract was not approved because of the civil rights controversy. Obviously, with the senior administrators of that university flying back and forth to Washington under serious circumstances and the faculty senate debating whether a violation of confidentiality was inherent in the university's agreement to allow the civil rights agency to examine documents surrounding faculty appointments, little time or energy was available to think about the future of gerontological research.

A plethora of problems has plagued higher education. In one of the major publications reflecting higher education in America, *The Chronicle of Higher Education,* almost nothing has been included about the issues of aging. Perhaps one article has appeared over the recent two-year period. Although members of AGHE might claim that gerontology merits more attention, it obviously does not have a very prominent place in the arena or marketplace of higher education.

Other matters also vie for the preoccupation of university leadership, such as the increasing proportion of tenured faculty in some schools and the fear of stagnation and the need to discharge young faculty when programs retrench. Some schools are adapting to the economic uncertainties of the time by increasing the use of part-time faculty to the dismay of the full-time faculty and those who wish to obtain a tenure track position. Other issues dominating agendas of university meetings include: the drift of support away from basic research toward applied research, problems of repayment of student loans, the Bakke case and minority representation in the student body and on the faculty, admissions criteria, diminishing enrollments, lack of support for the humanities, the decline in liberal arts in contrast with the rise in preprofessional and professional education, the misuse of funds by comptrollers on a few campuses, comprehensive audits of federal support, the increasing need for security, the rise in unionization of staff and faculty, and the accusations of political favoritism in the awarding of grants to several institutions. These are only a few of the issues keeping academic administrations off balance.

These examples point out the fact that institutions of higher learning are under a great deal of pressure on a wide range of issues. It is understandable that administrators are not moving with alacrity to develop gerontology. However, there is a miscalculation of academic administrators in ignoring the potential role of gerontology in higher education. One of the most significant growth areas for academic institutions lies in research on aging and in serving the educational needs of the mature and older adult.

One would hope that more guidance would emerge from schools of education, but perhaps they are even more beleaguered than presidents, chancellors, provosts, and vice presidents of institutions of higher learning. Deans of schools of education are finding that their classical educational markets are drying up. Fewer teachers are needed for elementary and high school classes, and with schools closing and no new ones opening, fewer principals are needed. One adaptation a school of education can make to a contracting enrollment is to offer expanded continuing education programs, since teachers already in service need to take courses to retain their teaching certification. It is hoped also that some deans of education will soon discover new horizons in gerontology. Apart from education, other subjects and professions also show inertia. Educational administrators would rather maintain the status quo and serve an increasingly constricting area than undergo the pangs of renewal or reconstruction by considering the challenging educational issues involved in serving an aging population.

On the other hand, one can strike a rhetorical posture of being impressed by the rapid developments in the field of gerontology. First, there has been significant growth in the Association for Gerontology in Higher Education, the Gerontological Society, the Western Gerontological Society, not to mention the dramatic expansion of many other successful organizations. Concurrently, we continue to witness the creation of new courses, training, and degree programs. And still, in relation to identifiable need or what is yet to come, these are only the first "drops in the bucket." We are merely in the A-B-C stages of gerontology and higher education. It may be that we are fortunate that the growth of gerontological education is not occurring at a faster pace, since we have yet to develop viable, alternative models to accommodate the needs of the new mature-learner population. In fact, at present, serious concerns have been expressed by many gerontologists about the less than substantive and responsible gerontological education being offered.

It is perhaps understandable that the inability to dig deeply into the crucial issues of aging is due to the relative economic and leadership poverty of institutions of higher learning. It strikes us that professionals in the field need to prepare for what may resemble the 1849 gold rush, that is, when schools of education not only discover that they can contribute intellectually to the development of subject matter, but also sense the economic gain.

Although this picture may be slightly cynical, one of the reasons why there has been so little response in institutions of higher learning to the emergent problems in the field of aging is that academic administrators are more money minded and wage weary than they used to be. Frankly, many want something for nothing today, a small investment for a large return. Also they are faced with faculty who do not want to teach new and different courses instead of their favorite subjects, in which they have done research and have long-standing notes. There is, too, little seed money available to encourage an interested faculty member to prepare new courses and research. Yet, cagey administrators would probably become great gerontological advocates if they found a major benefactor with a large endowment or the eternal rich uncle, Uncle Sam, to initiate major programs.

Unfortunately, a response in some colleges has been to hire part-time instructors who have had little or no previous training in gerontology. It has not been uncommon to learn of an instructor who is one day ahead of the class in reading the assignments. Whereas hiring an uninformed instructor to teach may be better than not offering a course, serious mature learners tend to become much more involved in the subject matter than is sometimes expected and are often not amused when teachers cannot keep up with their pace.

Why did we get caught short in our planning as educators and academic administrators? Could we have better anticipated the needs of this emerging population since there were individuals who had forecast the present situation? In a publication of the United Nations organization of 1956, R. E. Tunbridge of England, a physician, points out: "The increasing population of the elderly and the diminishing proportion of children are creating a new form of society in the countries of western Europe and North America. By 1980, the over 60's in Sweden and Great Britain will constitute nearly one-third of the voting power. If intellectual, emotional and personality changes are a feature of increasing years, what is to be the pattern of society?" (Tunbridge, 1956, p. 84). He also wrote that: " . . . aging, therefore, has scientific, economic, social and political significance for the community as well as for the individual, and—with all of its ramifications—justifies consideration as a major biological problem of the second half of the twentieth century" (Tunbridge, 1956, p. 84).

Still earlier, in 1942, in Cowdry's *Problems of Aging*, Edward Steiglitz, also a physician, wrote a chapter on social urgency for research. He said: " . . . actual data are required for intelligent planning of attack on three important sociologic aspects of aging: (a) proper employment (placement) of older persons, (b) mental hygiene during senescence, particularly significant prophylaxis against devising infrequency of mental maladjustments at and after the climacteric, and (c) the problem of adult education."

Then in 1942, Steiglitz wrote: "Education has not kept pace with the dramatic increase in life expectancy and the shifting age distribution of the population. Scholastic curricula and objectives and educational processes are still geared to the day when life was some 15 years shorter. This places educational policies some 40 years behind the time. Then it sufficed that education prepared the boy or girl for the competitions for adult life, and no more. This seemed appropriate when life expectancy at birth was about 47 years, but it is hardly applicable today . . . " (Steiglitz, 1942, p. 904). Steiglitz goes on to say that: " . . . it has been completely assumed that the adult would learn how to grow old happily and usefully without prior training or guidance" (Steiglitz,

1942, p. 904). "Yet, facilities for, and encouragement of, continued . . . study after graduation are minimal, except for those following the scientific professions" (Steiglitz, 1942, p. 905). We could go back still further to G. S. Hall's book on senescence, *The Second Half of Life*, published in 1922. His writing contained a forecast of the emergence of organizations of retired people, " . . . the time is ripe for some kind of senescent league of national dimensions which should establish relations with all existing associations of the old, and slowly develop a somewhat elaborate organization of its own, with committees on finance, on the literature of senescence, including its psychology, physiology and hygiene, etc. If such an organization under any name were founded, it should have an organ or journal of its own that should be the medium of correspondence keeping its members informed to date upon all matters of interest or profit to them, perhaps keeping tab on instances of extreme longevity or unusual conservation of energy, with possibly a junior department with youngsters of 50. It should concern itself with the phenomena connected with the turning of tide of life, which so often occurs even in the fourth decade" (Hall, 1922, p. 194).

Certainly, this was prophetic, for today we have organizations with multimillion memberships of retired persons.

We could quote intellectual leaders from the early part of the century who were sagacious in identifying the issues and proposing actions. We can only conclude from the lack of response to the issues of gerontology that most current academic administrators may be good managers but they are not very good leaders. They may be intelligent, but they are not very wise. They may encourage cost effectiveness, but they are not very adverturesome. Indeed, it can be said about our academic administrators today that few are distinguished for their educational philosophy. They may have had distinguished academic backgrounds in their fields of origin and then moved into academic administration. Their time is now spent cajoling faculty, alumni, donors, and boards of trustees. They seek a balance in a field of strong conflicting forces in which the emergence of the older adult population has hardly registered a quiver on the academic seismograph.

Few, if any, senior administrators of major American institutions of higher learning are exercising significant leadership on behalf of the older population. Apparently, leadership in the field must come primarily from those like the members of AGHE, from the pioneers who have the vision, commitment, and energy to turn the heads of the academic administrators and to plot the directions for their institutions of higher learning. They cannot, of course, circle the walls of academia like the trumpeters circling Jericho and expect the walls to tumble down. Instead, they must first strive for simply securing the attention of those on the inside.

Does Gerontology Merit a Place in Higher Education?

The issues by now are so well described that they are almost redundant: the growing numbers of older adults in society; rapid antiquation of skills requiring adult reeducation; shorter career lives, or if you will, shorter occupational half-life in the population; a need for continuing education in all professions to keep them up to date; the return of middle age men and women seeking advanced degrees for the first time or changing their basic professional orientation; and the training of professionals specifically in gerontology. There are lawyers who seek degrees in psychology; there are engineers who seek degrees in the humanities; there are physicians who seek degrees in law; and then there are retired individuals who have a sincere interest either in pursuing a first degree or extending the range of their cultural knowledge by pursuing personal growth through education. Where are the gerontological educational counselors who attempt to fit each population and individual into our institutions of higher learning? Where can people within the disciplines and professions greet mature and older people and facilitate their entry or reentry into higher education?

Questions to be Resolved

We have given a picture of the scarce state of art for gerontological education within eight professional disciplines. Then we analyzed the societal context within which universities are struggling to retain their existence, at the cost of having any energy, resources, or leadership left to develop gerontology programs. The emergence of gerontology in higher education must be viewed from a variety of perspectives. The last one included in this paper is the raising of a series of difficult issues with which we, as leaders within the field, must concern ourselves during the next two decades. These issues have emerged from students engaged in academic programs awarding master's degrees in gerontology, from faculty with single and joint appointments, from researchers seeking to determine how aspects of the field should evolve, and from administrators of agencies on aging.

The questions fall into four areas: (1) the creation of a master's of science in gerontology; (2) the issue of other advanced degrees in aging; (3) the administration and organization of the field; and (4) the assessment of gerontology as a semi- or full-fledged profession.

1. Questions regarding the master's degree in gerontology.
    a. Is the body of knowledge clearly defined? By whom? What is its degree of acceptance? Where can it be found?
    b. Is there a need for a generalist or specialized track preparation?
    c. What should be the balance of emphasis between liberal arts education vs. direct vocational preparation?
    d. Is it essential to have a two-year master's degree program? Can one receive appropriate training in one year?
    e. What are the responsibilities of the granting institution regarding job placement, or explaining the risks when one enters into a new program?
2. Questions pertaining to advanced-degree training and education in gerontology.
    a. Do we need to develop a doctorate in gerontology? Within which dis-

cipline would it be placed? What subjects would it teach? Is there a trend in this direction? Do we need to be responsive to educational trends? In aging, has that caused us difficulty?

b. Are there advanced paths of education and training that we can outline (i.e., a MSG and then a broad-based doctorate in education or public administration)?

c. What need we prepare if there emerge 100 MSG programs in institutions of higher learning? Who will direct and teach in these programs? What are the optimum combinations of skills and expertise needed for the leadership of these programs?

d. What are the problems of young professionals and their identity conflicts in gerontology? Will institutional settings tolerate dual identities for the young professional securing tenure?

e. In what departments should gerontologists receive their faculty appointments?

3. Questions regarding the administration and organization of the field.

a. Issues of power and decision making in the field. Professionals are asking for guidelines for education. Some are even suggesting stricter criteria in the form of standards. A myriad of different kinds of education programs are cropping up. Who will seize decision-making power about the field's direction? Who will try to bring the factions of the field together? At this juncture, we see more splitting off than joining together of thought and effort. There is a great deal of mini-institution-building occurring, but little collective action is evolving. Who holds the purse of power? Who has given the power to this group?

b. Qualitative issues and their measurement. Who is or should be concerned with the qualitative development of the field, and in specific, educational programming offered to our students? What models are we providing them? (E.g., How can we allow a sociology of aging course to be taught by someone who has never read in the field, or a faculty to develop a program without having any previous experience or knowledge in program development in gerontology?) How do we begin to measure the qualitative issues? Who monitors them?

c. Where does the cadre of MSG's we are training fit into the hierarchy of the field? Where will they receive the best representation? In which professional society should they be making their investment? Is it logical to think that with their development, they may splinter off and form yet another aging group?

d. Ambiguity, in the past, has sometimes worked to advantage. Can this continue, or is the field asking for more structure, definition, and guidelines?

e. Role of the purse. What role does federal money play in directing the field? Has its decision making reflected the needed growth? What kind of quality monitoring can it do over the programs in which it (the Administration on Aging as an example) is funding? Is federal money leading us down the yellow brick road to a fortuneless horizon?

f. Our image. What kind of reliable or uniform face does the field of gerontology present to its many publics, such as other professional groups, industry, the media, labor, the citizenry?

g. Professional spirit/mission flavor. This is one of our strengths. How can we make it work even more for us as a field?

h. Demography of the current players. Who's in the field? Do we know enough about the backgrounds of the major players? And which areas are not represented so we can more carefully plan future development?

4. Questions concentrating on gerontology as a profession or semiprofession.

a. Is there a new model needed to conceptualize the growth of a multi-discipline or multiprofession?

b. According to classic criteria, gerontology is not yet a profession. In spite of the literature, will it move in that direction because of the emergence of greater need, more people trained with a unidimensional affiliation, and a population that expresses needs which go unmet?

c. If we believe that the task is to prepare and catalyze other professional groups to design sophisticated components in theory and practice as it relates to aging, then what becomes of the MSG cadre developed when that goal is accomplished?

d. Is it important to attach labels to the field, or do they give us unnecessary baggage?

Many questions will take several decades to resolve. But some research is already being conducted. Ira Hirschfield has surveyed the professional growth of the field in a random sample of the membership of the Gerontological Society and the Western Gerontological Society (a sample of 630 subjects). He mailed a questionnaire to determine the demographic profile of the memberships of the societies; what the characteristics of the membership are regarding personal commitment, attitudes about educational career development, political participation, the establishment of traditional professional criteria in gerontology; and to what extent gerontology meets these criteria for becoming a profession.

The returned response to his survey of 93 percent of the sample indicates the high degree of interest in and possible frustration about the issues he addresses. Hirschfield predicts that the attitudes about the growth of the field, its educational curricula, and the commitment that individuals bring to it will vary greatly between the two gerontological societies. A study such as his will be useful not only because it will describe the current state of thinking by practitioners, educators, and scientists in the field, but also because it will provide a bench mark from which to measure the growth and changes in the field with greater insights and a frame of reference.
insights and a frame of reference.

If one idea becomes clear about the emergence of gerontology in higher education, it is that we will have to look to ourselves for the appropriate leadership, support, diligence, and creativity.

On one hand, we have urged gerontologists to analyze and then pursue the design of gerontological curricula in each of the fields that interrelate with this multidiscipline. On the other hand, we have raised the red flag of concern about the quality of education in which we involve ourselves and the degree of investment we are willing to make to accomplish our goals.

We must be our own missionaries as well as our own best critics. And most important, we must design responsive educational programs for the new populations of mature learners who seek to make their education more personally accountable than ever before.

It is said that there is no denying an idea whose time has come. The emergence of gerontology in colleges and universities has never been more timely, but its entry has to be based on creative programming, persuasive advocacy, careful evaluation and analysis, sensible economics, and a demanding spirit.

However, it is not just the potential of higher education to respond to gerontology that is of interest, but also the emergence of the mature and older adults and their potential to increase their roles in serving institutions of higher learning. The environment of higher education is prime, not only for developing curricula, but also for welcoming the resources and providing a structure within which mature learners can flourish.

References

Hall, G. S. *Senescence.* New York: D. Appleton and Co., 1922.

Steiglitz, E. D. Social urgency for research. In E. V. Cowdry (Ed.), *Problems of aging.* Baltimore: Williams and Wilkins, 1942.

Tunbridge, R. E. Medical and social problems of aging. *Impact of Science on Society,* UNESCO, 1956, 7, 65–84.

New Dimensions of Academic Gerontology Programs

Neil G. McCluskey
The City University of New York

An observer of the contemporary scene can discern several new dimensions of gerontology programs under university and college sponsorship. They are new only in the sense of fairly general acceptance, not in the sense of intrinsic originality. Everyone now accepts them—or should accept them—as gospel even though the level of fidelity to their implementation continues to vary from institution to institution. Three dimensions seem to stand out: a dimension of *excellence*, which speaks to the problems of academic and scholarly integrity; a dimension of *efficiency*, which implies the multidisciplinary approach; and a dimension of *practicality*, which involves the bringing together of academicians and practitioners. Although somewhat arbitrarily chosen, these words are each broad enough to conveniently package several related trends.

Dimension of Excellence

It is an axiom that respect cannot be legislated; respect must be earned, for it is simply recognition of quality. Today's gerontologists are looking for respect from their academic colleagues. Accordingly, there seems to be a growing awareness of the need to base the gerontological enterprise solidly, just as the older, respected disciplines are based. Gerontologists are becoming more sensitive about offering any grounds for criticism to colleagues, in whom the new and successful often arouse suspicion and fear. Perhaps academic gerontologists are unconsciously trying to avoid repeating what happened to the early professional educators who, in the process of trying to make a discipline out of "education," failed to anchor it firmly to acceptable standards.

Today the gerontology market is bullish. The ballooning of membership in the Association for Gerontology in Higher Education accurately indicates the upsurge of gerontological interest in higher education. We can feel satisfied that schools are at long last facing up to their responsibility and beginning to define a sphere of influence. Nevertheless, our phenomenal growth has evoked repeated notes of caution from AGHE leadership. In fact, this concern has given rise to the Foundations for Establishing Educational Program Standards in Gerontology project of the Association now under way in collaboration with the Gerontological Society.

For anyone who is nervously caught between the horns of uncontrolled expansion of selective criteria and their premature imposition, history may be an encouraging instructor. Some sort of inexorable law of development seems to be at work here. The pattern can be seen in the history of other academic fields that emerged from the social and behavioral sciences and served as foundations of new professions. A new field opens up, and like those who swarmed the land to the Far West in the last century, hordes of the eager and ambitious rush in. After some initial disorder, social pressure and prudent leadership usually bring order to the chaos.

As an excellent example, let us take medicine. Between 1810 and 1910, some 450 medical schools were established, many of them unabashed money-making ventures. The sweet smell of the green attracted an army of entrepreneurs, who quickly saw, as one historian (Kissick, Note 1) recorded, "the economic rewards of organizing proprietary medical schools to sell medical degrees uninhibited by the academic constraints and standards of the university."

In 1847 the American Medical Association was founded expressly to improve medical education. It took time, however, for its impact to be felt. The association had been in existence for 20 years when its president William O. Baldwin (Note 2) lamented, "The plan of action . . . of endeavoring to induce 40 or 50 medical colleges . . . to agree voluntarily upon a uniform and elevated standard of requirement for the degree of M.D. . . . has become almost a utopian idea, a forlorn hope." Seven years later, the American Medical College Association was organized and promptly introduced uniform standards for the curriculum in medicine. However, neither the proprietary schools, which saw the move as a threat to their own profits, nor the university schools, which regarded it as interference with their academic autonomy and flexibility, were about to change overnight. The demand for reform resulted primarily from an alliance of professionals and laymen. Nevertheless, Kissick (Note 1) records, "Decades were required to generate social pressure to overcome the proprietary excess of the diploma mills, whose graduates learned the practice of medicine by trial and error on their unsuspecting patients."

However, the momentum of education reform could not be stopped. The American Medical College Association was revived in 1890 as the Association of American Medical Colleges. In partnership with the American Medical

Association, it continued the movement by establishing standards for premedical and medical education, yearly inspection of medical schools, and the creation of licensing boards. Scientific and academic standards continued to rise slowly, with the greatest impetus coming from the publication of the Flexner report in 1910. This devastating report on the poor state of medical education (Note 3) was named for its author, Abraham Flexner (1866–1959), who was a member of the research staff of the Carnegie Foundation for the Advancement of Teaching. Between 1900 and 1950, 158 medical schools closed. During this same period another 70 were founded, but by 1930 the last substandard medical school had been closed, and only 25 of the 70 are still in operation. Accrediting associations are never, of course, the complete answer, despite the importance of their place in the scheme of things. Alas, their procedures for establishing quality and control are not foolproof. Despite the Association of American Medical Colleges and the American Medical Association, there are still mediocre medical schools and incompetent doctors. Perhaps this is only another way of acknowledging basic limitations to anything in the finite human order. It is predictable that the field of gerontology will continue to pass through a phase of rapid and uncontrollable expansion during which numbers may be more in evidence than quality.

Nevertheless, parallels with medical education should not be overdrawn, nor should any impression be left that gerontology is becoming a refuge for the academically lame, halt, and blind. Scholars and teachers with impeccable credentials earned in cognate disciplines are moving into the field. Some of the brightest and most ambitious students are choosing gerontology as a career. A sincere, unremitting effort to ensure quality in our gerontological programs will be the best guarantor of academic excellence and their acceptance in the scientific communities.

Dimension of Efficiency

The leading gerontology programs in America today are built upon the multidisciplinary nature of the field. Their success invites reflections upon the necessity of a multidisciplinary approach.

Academic disciplines are as subject to change as the flora and fauna. It comes as a surprise to many people to find out that, until the end of the seventeenth century, science was considered a part of philosophy. Similarly, psychology, which was classified as a branch of philosophy until about 1900, became a separate discipline only in the early twentieth century. At the time, though, no one could have imagined that it would split into today's specialties of developmental psychology, clinical psychology, experimental psychology, cognitive psychology, environmental psychology, educational psychology, social psychology, personality psychology, biopsychology, neuropsychology, and so forth.

If there is a problem, it is an embarrassment of riches—the ever-expanding knowledge base that continually forces us to devise new labels and categories. One of these new divisions is *gerontology*, a word that, until a few years ago, most people had to look up. Many still use it interchangeably with *geriatrics.* In fact, the new *Britannica* calls gerontology "the scientific study of the phenomena of aging, including the sociological, historical, and biological aspects as well as the medical phases (geriatrics)."

Obviously gerontology is a hybrid, or a composite, that borrows from older sciences or disciplines—anthropology, sociology, psychology, biology, philosophy, social work, and many others. How then does one become a "gerontologist"? There is no doctoral program in gerontology as such at any university today, and there is no considerable movement to create one. At the master's level, there is an increasing number of programs with a specific major in gerontology emerging from programs in the social sciences, and many schools continue to offer a master of social work degree with an optional concentration in gerontology.

Until recently anybody who identified himself or herself as a "gerontologist," of necessity, came from a background in social science, humanities, or biomedical science. Most of these people developed an interest in some phase of aging that led them into the new composite, and so they became "gerontologists."

A few simple conclusions emerge: No one discipline owns the field; no single discipline can claim to be the best or the only preparation for entry into the field; many disciplines have enriched and will continue to enrich gerontology. Its many facets will continue to attract different people for different reasons to do different things.

Gerontology, then, is both interdisciplinary and multidisciplinary by nature. For convenience we can speak of a *multidisciplinary* course as an offering within the formality, methodology, and jurisdiction of a particular academic discipline, but one whose content is complementary or equally relevant to material in another discipline. For example, a course on adulthood and aging could be offered by a psychology department, but the same material substantially could be presented by a sociology department as one of its courses. An *interdisciplinary* course would be one jointly taught by the two departments.

Gerontology's health as an academic and scientific discipline, as well as its acceptance within the academic community, will depend greatly on how faithful it remains to its multidisciplinary nature. Again, there is a classic example of what happens when a discipline forgets its multidisciplinary origin and acts as if it were alone on the planet.

Since at least 1900, education as an academic branch has been characterized by its isolation from other disciplines. The field has pretty much remained outside the mainstream of scholarly research, writing, and even teaching. Its historians were historians of education; its sociologists were sociologists of education; its psychologists were psychologists of education. As specializations within older and more encompassing disciplines, the distinctions were fully valid. But alas, what actually happened was quite different. Bernard Bailyn (1960) writes of the history of education: "The development of this historical field took place, consequently, in a special atmosphere of professional purpose. It grew in almost total isolation from the major influences and shaping minds of twentieth-century historiography; and its isolation proved to be self-intensifying: the more parochial the subject became, the less capable it was of attracting the kinds of scholars who could give it broad relevance and bring it back into the public domain. It soon displayed the exaggeration of weakness and extravagance of emphasis that are the typical results of sustained inbreeding." Bailyn, himself a distinguished Harvard historian, argues effectively that "the main emphasis and ultimately the main weakness of the history written by the educational missionaries of the turn of the century" arose directly from their professional interests.

The message needs no further elaboration. Gerontology will wax a healthy academic discipline as it continues to draw nourishment from its sources within the social and behavioral sciences, as well as from the humanities.

The Research Training Program in Urban Gerontology at the Graduate School of the City University of New York provides an example of both the interdisciplinary and multidisciplinary approaches to gerontology. The program, involving seven academic disciplines, is designed to develop professionals who can apply their knowledge in the field of gerontology. Doctoral students in anthropology, economics, educational psychology, political science, psychology, sociology, and speech and hearing sciences receive systematic training in various aspects, both theoretical and practical, of gerontology. They relate this training to their own discipline and, conversely, relate their own discipline to the area of gerontology. The planned outcome is a select group of Ph.D.'s who are competent both in their own disciplines and in gerontology. They are trained to carry out research, to work in social agencies, to develop programs in governmental bodies, to act as professionals in health-related agencies, to take faculty positions in colleges and universities offering gerontology courses, and to assume other professional work in gerontology-related activities.

Each of the seven participating disciplines has its own methods, theories, and substance. This training program makes no effort to reorient the methods or theories of, for example, economics. Instead, it focuses on urban gerontology as a specialization within the seven fields. The participating disciplines offer both background courses and seminars and specific work on urban gerontology. The Center for Gerontological Studies works closely with the Graduate School's Committee on Interdisciplinary Study and Research to coordinate and support the program (Note 4).

Dimension of Practicality

Practicality entails the bringing together of the academic and the practical. Again, this characteristic of model gerontology programs is not really something new. Our pragmatic times pay little heed to the old question that for centuries intrigued our more philosophical forebears: What should be superior in life—action or contemplation, activity or thought, practice or theory, the marketplace or the ivory tower? The argument can never be satisfactorily settled because its terms are unreal. The dichotomy is false because circumstances never allow one function to operate without depending at least somewhat upon the other. The two spheres cannot be separated.

Gerontology is a striking example of intermingling and mutual interdependence of the academic and the practical. It should be a crossroads where researcher meets practitioner, planner meets deliverer. A majority of the early gerontologists were practitioners, most often individuals trained in the delivery of social services. They were the professionals. They had the experience and the know-how. It is understandable that they felt a certain amount of resentment when the universities began to move heavily into the training field, motivated as much by the lure of new federal largess to support programs as by any love of learning (or of the elderly). The criticism is still heard that many college faculty charged with training those students who will go out into the field are themselves spinning theories from thin air and are quite innocent of the realities of the world of the elderly. Understandable as such bickering may be in its origins, it remains mischievous and sterile.

For their work, the researchers and scholars of the university need the experience of the professionals in the field. Likewise, health care and other social services would suffer without input from the academic world. In explaining why Congress established the research-oriented National Institute on Aging (NIA) when services to the elderly are still woefully inadequate and increasingly expensive, Director Robert N. Butler (1977) wrote: "It is only through the judicious application of new knowledge acquired through research that existing services and health care can improve. Research is the ultimate service and the ultimate cost-container."

These thoughts are not really new, but we do need to remind ourselves of eternal verities from time to time. The alternative is to keep rediscovering the wheel or, as more often happens, the flat tire. Every successful university program has built up a network of close relationships with organizations and groups in the community. Usually the closer the relationships, the more successful the program.

One example is the Syracuse All-University Gerontology Center. It is located in Brockway Hall, the centerpiece of a university complex that contains housing for both students and the elderly on the edge of the campus. Another example is San Diego State University's Center on Aging, which is located in the Catholic Community Services building in central downtown San Diego. Within the building are other agencies such as the Catholic Family Services, Youth Services, the Diocesan Department of Aging, and the interfaith Cedar Community Center for older persons. Adjacent are Luther Towers, Westminster Towers, and Cathedral Towers—immense high-rise residence complexes for older people. These and other residential facilities make the elderly residing in downtown San Diego close neighbors of the university center.

Few centers can exist side-by-side with partners in the community, but the opportunities for close collaboration with them in the field are legion. An example is the cooperation between the Edgewood Community Services Center and The University of Akron's Institute for Life-Span Development and

Gerontology, of which it is an important part (see Deitchman, this volume). Edgewood provides activities and services on a daily basis both for pre-schoolers and older adults. As a working model of public service, Edgewood is a training and research facility for faculty and students of the university as well as the professional people of the Akron community. Support for these programs comes from community resources with a great deal of voluntary effort from faculty and students.

Finally, the City University of New York Gerontological Center rallied the collaborative activity of an unusual consortium around a research topic of wide and keen interest. From the usual horror anecdotes of unprepared retirement and from conversations with concerned school leaders, the need for an effective program of retirement planning for New York City school personnel surfaced as a top priority. The center accepted "first-among-equals" leadership in the project, which became a joint undertaking of the Personnel Office of the New York City Board of Education and of the staff unions—the United Federation of Teachers and the Council of Supervisors and Administrators, along with their retired chapters. After only a few planning sessions of the steering committee, there was a lessening of suspicion among often hostile neighbors. Each partner contributed ideas, money, and time in fairly equal measure. By now, the project is well along, but a special dividend for everyone involved was the accomplishment of a successful common enterprise by groups that often seem separated. Theory and practice, the ivory tower and the marketplace, can join fruitfully.

Notes

1. Kissick, W. L. Medical education. *Encyclopedia of Education* (6th ed.).

2. Baldwin, W. O. 1869 address of William O. Baldwin, M.D., president of the association. *American Medical Association Transactions, 20,* 53–80.

3. Medical education in the United States and Canada: A report to the Carnegie Foundation for the Advancement of Teaching. Bulletin No. 4, New York: The Foundation, 1910. Reprinted in 1960 by Updyke.

4. The Center for Gerontological Studies is a unit within the Center for Advanced Study in Education (CASE) of the Graduate School and University Center, the City University of New York.

References

Bailyn, B. *Education in the forming of American society.* Chapel Hill, N.C.: University of North Carolina Press, 1960.

Butler, R. N. Will research in aging help today's elders? *Retirement Life,* October 1977, 16–17.

The International Development of Academic Gerontology

Donald O. Cowgill
and
Rosemary A. Orgren
University of Missouri-Columbia

When we began to think about the international development of academic gerontology, we found the issue posed an interesting challenge. It appeared likely that the development of gerontology as a self-conscious discipline was linked with other types of developments that had concerned Cowgill in the past and could prove to be merely an extension of his previous involvement.

A close examination of earlier works (Cowgill and Holmes, 1972, and Cowgill, 1974) revealed, however, that they contained practically nothing about the development of gerontology as a discipline or about the inclusion of gerontology in higher education. These works were about the phenomenon of aging as a sociocultural process: the condition of older people within specific social settings or the theory of interrelationships between the general social structure and the status or condition of older people. Although these works may be considered a part of the growing corpus of gerontology, they did not usually include gerontology as a system of thought and a discipline. They failed to look at the development of gerontology as an intellectual reaction to demographic and social conditions, conditions that have been the subject matter of much of Cowgill's earlier study and writing.

Therefore, this paper is devoted to examining the emergence of gerontology as a system of thought, and it includes the varying stages of the development of gerontology in relation to the types of societies and social conditions. A direct statement of the theory is: Gerontology as an intellectual corpus and scientific discipline emerges only in certain social and historical contexts, and its development is conditioned by further social and historical changes. Concretely, we may posit that societies with a small proportion of their population in advanced ages (and whose institutions have evolved in such a way as to absorb and care for the needs of older people) will not develop a self-conscious analysis of old age, nor will they be concerned with the problems and conditions of aging. With increasing numbers and proportions of older people in modernizing societies and the concomitant institutional changes that render traditional forms either obsolete or inadequate for management of problems of aging, a development of study, analysis, and teaching about aging—that is, gerontology—will emerge.

No doubt the best way of testing this proposition, from a methodological point of view, would be through longitudinal, historical studies in specific societies where such development has occurred. Little systematic work of this kind has yet been done, and none of it, to our knowledge, has assumed a sociology of knowledge perspective. In this paper, we have paid attention to descriptive, historical materials from several of the more advanced societies, such as Norway (Berverfelt, Note 1), West Germany (Fulgraff, 1978), and the United States. These data have been compared with and interrelated with cross-sectional materials on the current status of gerontology in a variety of countries. These were assembled largely on the basis of personal contacts, and we are indebted to about two dozen people scattered around the world for their prompt and sometimes costly responses. In at least two cases our informants were the same as those Palmore used in his forthcoming handbook (Note 2).

We have hurriedly assembled information for some 20 societies on: the volume and types of research being conducted; the number of academic specialists devoting major attention to some aspect of gerontology; the number and kind of courses being taught; whether there are institutes or centers devoted primarily to gerontology; whether there are national associations or professional organizations of gerontology; whether there are professional journals in the area; and to some extent the nature of the sponsorship of both research and teaching in those societies. On the basis of this information, we wish tentatively to suggest that there appear to be about five stages of development of academic gerontology which are closely associated with different levels of demographic and social modernization.

In the first stage, there is no gerontology of any form—no research, no teaching, and usually no specialized service programs. Without exception this stage characterizes societies we now label as developing. Demographic aging has not yet occurred to any measurable degree, and older persons are cared for and integrated into familial and kinship institutions that have traditionally performed this social function. Indeed, in countries that show no sign of gerontological development, only 3 percent or less of the population is 65 and over. In many of the societies in this stage of development, modernization has had the demographic effect of "younging" their populations, that is, of increasing the emphasis on youth rather than developing emphasis on aging. One of the informants illustrates this by the statement, "The present concerns of this country are with youth and economic dependency of the young rather than of the aged." Thus, in these societies it is not so much that the aged have not yet been defined as a social problem; it is more that the present social problems are overwhelmingly concerned with youth. Therefore, we cannot expect much intellectual attention to be given to older people, and we cannot expect much programmatic response or innovation in the direction of aging. Some of the sample countries in this stage of development include Brazil, Peru, Iran, Jordan, Nigeria, and American Samoa.

The second stage of development appears in several countries where there is no greater demographic aging, but there are indications of some beginning interest in research relative to aging. In each case, this is either a transplanted interest stimulated by contact with gerontology elsewhere or a response to some specific problem. For example, in Thailand, a former student of Cowgill's is planning to study the inmates of several of the old folks' residential homes. In Egypt, there has been a study of widows and some attention to poverty, including poverty among the aged. In Taiwan, a survey of old people in institutions for the aged is currently being completed, and some attention is being given to the problems of differential service (not to say discrimination) between mainlanders and native Taiwanese aged. A recent migrant to Kuwait is a demographer with considerable interest in and commitment to gerontology. In Kenya, Cox and Mberia (1977) report on an old folks' home established by missionaries. Thus, research interests and expertise are being diffused from developed areas to less developed ones. And it is evident that many of the limited services available to the elderly in these societies are also imitative responses to Western patterns.

The kind of research under way or being planned in second-stage societies is primarily demographic or sociological in nature. Apparently, a cross-sectional method provides a kind of observation that does not fit the sequences of development shown in longitudinal studies carried out in more advanced societies. However, it may be that biological and medical research is under way in these countries that our informants, mostly social scientists, did not know about. In Europe and the United States, biological and medical research in aging preceded sociological and psychological research by several decades. However, currently developing countries, now beginning to face some social problems related to age, seem to be leaving the basic research on biological and medical aging to the more advanced societies and devoting their research attention to the demographic and sociological problems specific to their societies.

The third stage of gerontological development is to be found in such places as Australia and Japan, where both biomedical and sociological research are under way. Furthermore, much of this research is taking place within organized structures, the results are published in formal journals, and the researchers are affiliated with formal professional associations. However, courses in aging or gerontology are few, and few if any faculty describe themselves as gerontologists. It is probably significant that in both of these societies about 8 percent of the population is 65 or over, and in both, the proportion is increasing quite rapidly. Some of the research interest is undoubtedly an anticipatory response.

The fourth stage of development is represented by societies that have developed a full range of academic programs in gerontology. These include research institutes, associations, journals, gerontology courses, and faculty who identify themselves with the field of gerontology for research and instructional purposes. This seems to have happened in many of the countries, such as Sweden, Norway, Austria, West Germany, Holland, and France. All have populations with 14 percent or 15 percent 65 and over. However, there are some countries where similar phenomena have occurred at an earlier stage of demographic development. One of these is Israel, where large numbers of the population are migrants from Europe, who carried their skills and interests with them and developed programs very much on the European model. Another case is Canada, with only 8 percent of its population 65 and over. Here we see gerontology developing parallel to its neighbor to the south and interacting closely with programs and developments within the United States.

The fifth stage involves national policy as well as demographic changes. The national government formally sponsors gerontological research, training, and institutes. This appears to be an advanced and late stage of gerontological growth. Here in the United States, the entry of national government into this role has been painful and unsteady.

If these stages fairly approximate the order of development of gerontology in general, some subordinate principles should also be mentioned. One is the sequence of institutional response to demographic aging reflected in research interests.

The earliest area of concern appears to be sheer economic security and the means of survival. Thus, we find the establishment of almshouses, old folks' homes, social security and pension schemes, followed by related research. So we have studies such as Charles Booth's (1894) classic study of *The Aged Poor in England and Wales* and a parallel contemporary concern with poverty among the aged in Egypt today.

The next general interest is health. Even here, there is a sequence in which the first line of attention is an extension of curative medicine. Doctors and hospitals continue to apply the views and skills appropriate to younger populations; that is, to cure people of acute and reversible conditions. It takes considerable time for our institutions to adjust themselves to the reality of a changed population and to realize that health care in an aged population must stress preventive medicine and the treatment of chronic conditions. Beverfelt (Note 1) reports that medical schools in Norway provide for specialization in geriatrics, but that the training of other specialists includes nothing on aging. Still later comes the acknowledgement that old people are total human beings with all of the psychological and sociological needs of any person. The adaptation of our mass urban institutions to this need is a continuing challenge at which no one has yet succeeded very well.

A second subordinate sequence has to do with the emphasis and interpretation of research—what we research and how we interpret it. As we first become conscious of the reality of an aging population and its evident needs, our research tends to concentrate on problematic aspects of aging. One explanation is that researchers often concentrate on captive audiences in clinics and in hospitals. Another is that the motivation for the research often is to convince decision makers that something needs to be done about perceived problems. Therefore, the result is an effort to count problem cases and a tendency to exaggerate the seriousness of the problem. Much of the research in the United States before about 1960 was of this kind, and it tended to reinforce the stereotype of old age as a period of decline, weakness, senility, poor health, and poverty.

Apparently it takes some time for science to escape from the intellectual confinement and stereotypes of its clinical and hospital cases to undertake the more difficult and costly research of looking at normal and representative people. Gerontology in the advanced areas of the world is just now attempting to readjust both its method and its interpretation to these imperatives. Ageism is still rampant, and the stereotypes are still abundant, even among gerontologists. The reason for these vestiges in the literature is not merely inertia, biased samples, and cross-sectional research designs. Rather, many continue to feel the need for the "poor old dear" approach as a means of tugging at the heart strings to justify appeals for money for services and research. How do we justify our appeals for funds except in terms of serious and prevalent problems to be solved? Many do not find the Louis Harris (1975) survey (which showed most old people as reasonably happy, healthy, comfortable, and active) very helpful for promoting aging programs or grants. In these later stages of development, the appeals must be much more sophisticated and precise. No longer can we ascribe to the old in general a prevalent failing to which our particular project will supply the ultimate answer. Now we must say precisely where the specific problem is, how extensive it is, and how our project will have significant impact upon the target population.

In conclusion, it appears that the development of academic gerontology does occur in response to demographic and institutional changes in society. There are somewhat regular stages of its development, beginning with individually initiated and scattered research, gradually maturing into organized activities in institutes and professional associations, ultimately culminating in a full range of research and teaching. Biological and medical research seems to have preceded social and psychological research in the developed parts of the world, but in the developing areas this sequence is less clear. In most places, the early concern is sheer economic survival, followed by the availability and practice of curative medicine, then by attention to health maintenance programs, and ultimately by a realization that older people must be treated as whole persons in all institutional settings. In early stages, our research tends to concentrate on problematic aspects of aging and only later, with representative samples and longitudinal designs, do we arrive at a balanced and sanguine view of the aging process. We in the United States have not yet fully arrived in this latter stage, and it remains to be seen whether the developing societies must pass through all of the painful stages of development that the more advanced societies have undergone.

Notes

1. Beverfelt, D. Research and education: A historical note. In E. Palmore (Ed.), *International handbook on aging*. Westport, Conn.: Greenwood Press, Inc., in press.

2. Palmore, E. *International handbook on aging*. Westport, Conn.: Greenwood Press, Inc., in press.

References

Booth, C. *The aged poor in England and Wales*. London: Macmillan, 1894.

Coser, L. A. Sociology of knowledge. *International encyclopedia of the social sciences*, 1968, *8*, 428–435.

Cowgill, D. O. Aging and modernization: A revision of the theory. In Jaber F. Gubrium (Ed.), *Late life*. Springfield, Ill.: Charles C. Thomas, 1974.

Cowgill, D. O. & Holmes, L. D. (Eds.). *Aging and modernization*. New York: Appleton-Century-Crofts, 1972.

Cox, M. & Mberia, N. *Aging in a changing village society: A Kenyan experience*. Washington, D.C.: International Federation on Aging, 1977.

Fulgraff, B. Social gerontology in West Germany: A review of recent and current research. *The Gerontologist*, 1978, *18*, 42–58.

Harris, L., & Associates. *The myth and reality of aging in America*. Washington, D.C.: National Council on the Aging, 1975.

Mannheim, K. *Ideology and utopia: An introduction to the sociology of knowledge*. New York: Harcourt, 1954.

PART TWO
THE INSTANT GERONTOLOGIST

What qualifies one as a gerontologist? Is it sensitivity? Interest? Declaration? Academic training? These basic questions, posing whether or not gerontology is a discipline and a profession, have challenged educators since aging emerged as an academic concern. The various education and training programs in gerontology across the country indicate the ways educators have tried to answer these questions. The basic issues, though, remain unresolved. The following three papers illustrate that the ultimate answers will be found by examining the long-range consequences of our educational and training efforts.

The Phenomenon of the Instant Gerontologist: How to Maintain Quality Education in Gerontology

Sherry L. Corbett
Miami University

Just as childhood and adolescence have become categories for investigation and research, so middle age and old age are now seen as life stages with unique features worthy of study. The 1970s have brought about the emergence of aging as a legitimate and significant topic for social science research (Shanas, 1975, p. 499). Along with the legitimation of gerontology has come a proliferation of gerontology courses and "quasi-professionals."

Academia has discovered gerontology. Government grants are encouraging interest in the study of aging—in terms of research, services, and education. Publishers are filling the market with books on aging directed toward both lay people and professionals. Students, hearing that there are job opportunities, enroll in newly created gerontology courses. All this contributes to the phenomenon known as the "instant gerontologist."

The question most often asked of the college advisor is What jobs can I get with this degree? Aware of demographic data that predict continued and increasing attention on older people, students are beginning to consider gerontology as a vocational choice. Overall estimates based on the projections of the 1970s indicate two or three times more jobs in aging than existed at the beginning of the decade (Hendricks & Hendricks, 1977, p. 408). Atchley and Seltzer (1977, p. 2) view gerontology as a field appealing to students for several reasons: (1) students now have more contact with older people (more people live longer) and have become interested in understanding them; (2) gerontology is a growing area of employment; and (3) students feel that the multidisciplinary approach of most gerontology programs leads to a better understanding of "the whole person."

Responding, at least partially, to student interest, universities, colleges, and even junior colleges are suddenly setting up new courses in the study of aging. Educators are addressing the question of student goals in gerontology—in liberal arts environs, community colleges, and continuing-education programs (Whitbourne, 1977, p. 131). A variety of degrees in aging have become available (Peterson, 1976, p. 66). The academic community has even become involved in the "aging phenomenon" by offering courses in adult education (Spinetta & Hickey, 1975). Educational gerontology has become a subarea, complete with its own journal, *Educational Gerontology: An International Quarterly*.

The crucial question in the field of gerontology, however, becomes: Who will teach the courses? College teachers, many of whom have no academic or research background in gerontology, are forced into the position of "instant gerontologist." Professionals have noted the gap in educational training of academicians and practitioners in the field (Weg, 1973, p. 449). The White House Conference on Aging in December 1971 documented the inadequacy of available programs and personnel. "The main feature about training and education on problems of aging is that there is so little of it" (Birren, Gribbin, & Woodruff, 1971). Many of these "situationally created gerontologists" mistakenly reinforce existing stereotypes about the aged.

The struggling newcomer in gerontology may also be handicapped in choosing accurate literature. The quantity of gerontological writing has multiplied rapidly, but quality has not always matched quantity. Woodruff and Birren (1975) write: "At the turn of the century there were five or six books published [in the area of aging], and this rate continued until 1949, with some interruption due to World War II. The literature generated between 1950 and 1960 equaled the production of the literature published in the entire preceding 115 years. It appears, then, that research and interest in aging are showing an exponential curve of growth. If this continues, it is expected that between 1970 and 1980 the publication rate will double again" (Woodruff & Birren, 1975, p. 24). Since there is a market and a demand for gerontological writings, pseudoprofessionals have contributed poor, misleading, or useless research.

Gerontology has had more than its share of poor research, including lack of reliability and validity tests and incomparable samples (Seltzer, 1975, p. 506). Butler notes that "while perhaps 4% of federal life-sciences funds will go into the gerontological sciences by 1982, fewer than 1% of scientists will have been formally trained to work in this area" (Butler, 1977, p. 113). Butler also shows (1977, p. 111) that a significant increase in funding for research in gerontology has occurred since the founding of the National Institute on Aging in 1974. The NIA budget has gone from $16 million in fiscal year 1975 to $19 million in fiscal 1976 to $30 million in fiscal 1977. The concern is that researchers attracted into the aging field by the available funds should know sound research strategies and should be sensitive to gerontological literature.

Lack of sufficient education and training is not limited to academic settings; practitioners have been equally handicapped. Merrill Elias (1974, p. 526), in a discussion of service delivery programs for the elderly, notes that "never before has the responsibility for delivery of service to elderly persons been in the hands of so many who know so little about aging." Jerome Kaplan (1975, p. 2) discusses the problems of federal funds flowing into area agencies on aging where the gerontological planner, an individual expert in both planning and gerontology, is unlikely to exist. Hendricks and Hendricks (1977, p. 406) estimate that less than 10 to 20 percent of those directly working with an older clientele have received formal training for their jobs.

The medical profession has likewise felt the deficit in gerontological training. A study by Freeman (1971) indicates that less than half of the medical schools surveyed had formal courses on aging and that only 15 faculty members out of 20,000 felt they were qualified in geriatrics. Medical journals strongly advocate geriatric courses and geriatricians at medical schools and hospitals (Freeman, 1976, p. 115; Libow, 1977, p. 102).

The multidisciplinary nature of gerontology creates both advantages and limitations. Multidisciplinary research has been described as a "type of group research involving investigators from several distinct scientific disciplines working in parallel with one another" (Busse & Pfeiffer, 1977, p. 1). With a cooperative effort, researchers can maximize the breadth and potential of their work. Rather than "dissecting" the older person, studies of aging can use a holistic approach.

By nature, however, multidisciplinary programs often lack a departmental home in the university structure. Since organization, salaries, and administrative support are built into departmental systems, a nondepartmental multidisciplinary center can be at a great disadvantage. Gerontology in higher education has often ranked low in status and rewards. Beattie (1974, p. 547) notes the importance of administrative strategies and understanding with regard to the multidisciplinary setting for interdisciplinary linkages if we are to go "beyond isolated unidimensional course offerings to substantial commitments of resources—faculty, facilities, and fiscal—for the development of gerontological programs relevant to academic and societal needs." Birren, Gribbin, and Woodruff (1972, p. 78) describe attempts in some universities to create a cooperative interdisciplinary degree program involving collaboration of existing departments. Whereas this eliminates the need to create still another department, it has administrative complications. Gerontologists may need to become familiar with the inner workings of university administration in order to survive in a traditionally department-oriented system.

Researchers may find bibliographic searches cumbersome owing to the multidisciplinary nature of the subject and the dispersion of relevant bibliographic materials. Miller and Cutler (1976, pp. 198–205) review the problems and concerns of gerontological researchers, including the quality of information and its dispersion due to the involvement of many different disciplines.

What are the implications for gerontology in light of the problems posed in this paper? How shall we fill the necessary academic and service positions with qualified professionals? Who shall train the trainers? In addressing the question of training needs, Weg (1973, p. 451) advocates traditional and nontraditional degree programs, which include undergraduate degrees, certificates, two-year postbachelors, masters, work-study plans, long-term continuing education, short-term institutes (from two days to two months), and exchange and intern programs. To counter the phenomenon of the "instant gerontologist," attempts are being made to orient professionals into the study of aging. Schaie (1974, p. 533) discusses the "training of trainers to train trainers." He views the ideal trainer as having knowledge and skills in the interpersonal, social organization, and educational technology areas, as well as having a broad enough gerontological base to know where to go for needed information.

Some notable attempts to orient professionals in the study of aging (which should be continued and expanded) include: National Science Foundation programs such as the Chautauqua-type short courses for college teachers; orientation sessions held within specific institutions to educate interested professionals; special sessions within professional meetings, such as the preliminary sessions held on education at the 1977 meeting of the Association for Gerontology in Higher Education; and the Gerontological Society meeting sessions that have dealt specifically with educational objectives.

Universities must develop content and methodology appropriate for practitioners as well as academicians. Programs for practitioners (Ehrlich & Ehrlich, 1976, p. 245) should include departmental and interdepartmental courses, continuing education, and short-term training, such as workshops on the needs of the aged or on the aging processes.

Taylor (1977, pp. 162–166) notes that programs developed to increase the number of trained personnel, as well as to improve the quality in the field of aging, will have to deal with the following questions:

1. To what extent should training efforts be channeled to "aging" instead of making greater efforts to alert and assist disciplines to meet their responsibilities for aging?

2. How are we going to allocate resources among the various needs and the particular institutions to prepare the people to meet those needs?

3. Is it better to develop a person who fits present job descriptions or one who is capable of meeting a range of needs and of proceeding not only to new challenges but even to new levels of responsibility?

4. Should each community, state, or region be responsible for developing its own source of manpower, or should a general pool be developed to serve all areas of need?

More than anything else, departments and universities should be encouraged to evaluate their basis for initiating gerontology programs. One or two faculty committed to the area of gerontology do not constitute a gerontology program (Beattie, 1974, p. 546). Lack of administrative support or basic support systems within the university, such as library help and research potential, may indicate real problem areas. If the sole reason for the development of a new gerontology program is the availability of "soft" money, the program may be self-destructive (Atchley & Seltzer, 1977).

In summary, if gerontology is to expand without sacrificing qualitative concerns, institutions and individuals must evaluate their motivations and need for further education and training.

References

Atchley, R., & Seltzer, M. *Developing educational programs in the field of aging.* Oxford, Ohio: Scripps Foundation Gerontology Center, 1977.

Beattie, W. M. Gerontology curricula: Multidisciplinary frameworks, interdisciplinary structures, and disciplinary depth. *The Gerontologist*, 1974, *14*(6), 545–549.

Birren, J. E., Gribbin, K. J., & Woodruff, D. S. *Training: Background.* Washington, D.C.: White House Conference on Aging, 1971.

Birren, J., et al. Research, demonstration, and training: Issues and methodology in social gerontology. *The Gerontologist*, 1972, *12*(2, Pt. 2, Summer), 49–82.

Busse, E., & Pfeiffer, E. *Behavior and adaptation in late life.* Boston: Little, Brown, 1977.

Butler, R. Trends in training in research gerontology. *Educational Gerontology: An International Quarterly*, 1977, *2*, 111–113.

Ehrlich, I., & Ehrlich, P. A four-part framework to meet the responsibilities of higher education to gerontology. *Educational Gerontology: An International Quarterly*, 1976, *1*, 251–260.

Elias, M. Symposium—the real world and the ivory tower. *The Gerontologist*, 1974, *14*(6), 525–526.

Freeman, J. T. A survey of geriatric education: Catalogue of the United States medical schools. *Journal of the American Geriatrics Society*, 1971, *19*, 746–762.

Freeman, J. T. Gerontology's educational profile. *Geriatrics*, 1976, *31*(10), 115–116.

Hendricks, J., & Hendricks, C. D. *Aging in mass society: Myths and realities.* Cambridge, Mass.: Winthrop Publishers, 1977.

Kaplan, J. The area agency on aging: Instant planning. *The Gerontologist*, 1975, *15*(1), 2.

Libow, L. S. Issues in geriatric medical education and postgraduate training—old problems in a new field. *Geriatrics*, 1977, *32*(2), 99–102.

Miller, E., & Cutler, N. Toward a comprehensive information system in gerontology: A survey of problems, resources, and potential solutions. *The Gerontologist*, 1976, *16*(3), 198–206.

Peterson, D. Educational gerontology: The state of the art. *Educational Gerontology: An International Quarterly*, 1976, *1*, 61–73.

Schaie, K. Training of trainers to train trainers. *The Gerontologist*, 1974, *14*(6), 533–535.

Seltzer, M. The quality of research is strained. *The Gerontologist*, 1975, *15*(6), 503–507.

Shanas, E. Gerontology and the social and behavioral sciences: Where do we go from here? *The Gerontologist*, 1975, *15*(6), 499–502.

Spinetta, J., & Hickey, T. Aging and higher education: The institutional response. *The Gerontologist*, 1975, *15*(5), 431–435.

Taylor, C. Evaluation of manpower training programs in aging. In O'Brien and Streib (Eds.), *Evaluation research on social programs for the el-*

derly. Washington D.C.: Administration on Aging, U.S. Government Printing Office, 1977.

Weg, R. Concepts in education and training for gerontology: New career patterns. *The Gerontologist,* 1973, *13*(4), 449–452.

Whitbourne, S. K. Goals of undergraduate education in gerontology. *Educational Gerontology: An International Quarterly,* 1977, *2,* 131–139.

Woodruff, D., & Birren, J. *Aging: Scientific perspectives and social issues.* New York: D. Van Nostrand, 1975.

Gerontology Is Not a Profession—the Oldest or the Youngest

Martin B. Loeb
University of Wisconsin-Madison

No matter how you slice it, grind it, squeeze it, or knead it, there is no such thing as the profession of gerontology. One can, however, be a gerontologist within most disciplines or professions. Those who call themselves gerontologists in this context are assumed to have a basic if not larger competence. The problem is the "instant gerontologist," who takes sound, discipline-grounded knowledge and puts it into an inappropriate context that renders it useless.

The self-proclaimed gerontologist who has no basic discipline or profession may have many of the attributes of a fraud if he claims to be able to read the *Journal of Gerontology* from cover to cover with full comprehension. Those people who can understand a "Spectrophotofluorometric and Electron Microscopic Study of Lipofuscin Accumulation in the Testis of Aging Mice" as well as "The Relative Importance of Physical, Psychological, and Social Variables to Locus of Control Orientation in Middle Age" are rare indeed. If our instant gerontologist reads (and believes he comprehends) only one of the *Journal's* sections such as "Social Gerontology," this indicates that he lacks the convictions that are part of the discipline and skills developed in professions such as social work, public administration, and planning.

Therein lies the problem of the instant gerontologist. If it were required to have a grounding in some well-known discipline first (or simultaneously), then it would be less likely for gerontology to be proclaimed a discipline or even a profession. At the present time there are no barriers to the self-proclaimed gerontologists, nor will there be in the future. One might say that the best qualification for being a gerontologist is to be old! This is analogous to saying that being mentally ill or retarded qualifies one as an expert in those fields. Or, perhaps a gerontologist is one who is interested in old things such as pre-Columbian pots or Pompeii.

Concern about the elderly—in commerce, the economy, professions, politics, and science—is hot stuff these days. Every university administration looks for possible research and teaching income from federal agencies and foundations concerned with aging. The administration also looks increasingly to the older student to compensate for falling enrollment. Occasionally, the administration looks for places to put tenured professors without much other current use. The internal pressure in colleges and universities is sufficient to produce some instant gerontologists in relatively high places. If we allow gerontology programs to be established as automatic professional programs, there will be many offspring of this immaculate conception who will proclaim that they alone have the true word. Heathens, such as nurses, social workers, and public administrators who have become true gerontologists in their own professions through study and practice, will be termed the dilettantes.

It is the professional areas where the instant as well as the three-minute gerontologist is most dangerous. In the scientific disciplines there are not likely to be gerontologists who displace or even demean physiologists, biochemists, geneticists, or zoologists. Perhaps I and my many colleagues with doctorates in human development come as close as possible to establishing a scientific discipline in gerontology. Even so, we are still oriented to either anthropology, sociology, psychology, or biology, and most of us (if not all) know our limitations. The interdisciplinary approach of human development allows one to have a major focus as well as some acquaintance with correlative disciplines.

For me, gerontology as a new practice profession is a horrifying prospect. I can see a kind of knowledge base, but I cannot see what skills would be unique to a gerontologist. Would such a person be an expert in housing design, nutrition, retirement, counseling (both economic and socio-psychological), health service delivery, senior center programming, social planning, or legal services?

Of course not, but such a person could be knowledgeable about resources for the elderly and could make referrals to those who do know what they are doing. Such a gerontologist is a case manager, and case managers can be "trained" almost instantly. This is what the Office of Economic Opportunity did with so-called indigenous workers in poverty-stricken neighborhoods.

What we need to do is focus our attention on incorporating gerontological knowledge and skills into the various professions so that they can be helpful to the aged. This means basic research, research on the applications of new knowledge, and research on the skills necessary for work with the aged. We did it for children, we can now do it for the aged.

References

Kivett, V. R., Watson, J. A., & Busch, J. C. The relative importance of physical, psychological, and social variables to locus of control orientation in middle age. *Journal of Gerontology,* 1977, *32,* 203–210.

Miquel, J., Lundgren, P. R., & Johnson, J. R., Jr. Spectrophotofluorometric and electron microscopic study of lipofuscin accumulation in the testis of aging mice. *Journal of Gerontology,* 1978, *33,* 5–9.

Reflections on the Phenomenon of the Instant Gerontologist

Mildred M. Seltzer
Miami University

To react to Loeb's kneading, grinding, and other physical actions is the equivalent of the burlesque dancer bumping and grinding after Nureyev has performed. It hardly seems necessary to say that Loeb expresses himself with wisdom and with the perspective of one who has been involved in the creation and development of whatever it is we are discussing. I am still wavering on the brink between deciding whether I agree with him or whether we are in the midst of an emerging discipline—that of gerontology. As I have thought about the issues we are faced with, I have had a series of associations—the riddle of the sphynx, the complications of peer reviews, and the crisis of ego identity versus role diffusion.

As Troll reviews this crisis, she notes that its successful resolution results in strongly defined social roles. The individual who has resolved this issue is comfortable at home, in work, with family, and in his/her sex role. That individual enjoys carrying out role behavior, has a sense of (sensible) longing, enjoys his or her style of life and daily activities. That individual is equally definite about his/her sense of self and identity. He or she has continuity with past and present (and thus presumably can march forward into the future clear-eyed, pure-hearted, sterling of soul). An unsuccessful resolution results in discomfort with roles, a sense of being lost in groups and affiliations. The individual lacks conviction in role behavior and may indulge in purposeless and meaningless changes in work and residence (Troll, 1977, pp. 6–7).

This is one of the issues facing those engaged in the study of aging. Who or what is a gerontologist? This question must be answered before one can discuss the phenomenon of the instant gerontologist. What are the external definitions and internal validations of gerontologists? Are there accepted criteria for the position known as gerontologist and for its appropriate role behavior? How is a gerontologist legitimized? As usual, my approach to these kinds of issues raises more questions that it answers. In political organizations, this has been referred to as being a provocateur. In parental relationships, it is called the "do-you-know-what-you-are-doing?" syndrome.

Loeb's position is that somebody must be something else before he or she can be a gerontologist. An individual must be a psychologist before becoming a specialist about the psychology of adult development and aging. Loeb's model is additive and, for the most part, traditional and conventional. For the most part, also, it is the position with which I tend to identify. At the same time, I think it is an increasingly questionable position because there is a body of cross-disciplinary knowledge as well as a core of professional beliefs characteristically found among those who purport to be gerontologists whether biological, social, or psychological. In part, this is a shared ideology. In fact, one sometimes wonders whether being a gerontologist is the overt behavior and professionalization of a social ideology. There is a belief that it is important to understand something about the nature of aging. That is not a unique kind of orientation to any "ology." What is unique, however, is the implicit activism in the assumption that such knowledge should be used to improve the quality of life for a subpopulation in our society—older people. Equally implicit is the assumption that the aged, for the most part, are mistreated in our society and that the quality of their life is, across the board, poor. A third assumption, although not a final one, is that there is often more to be learned from older people as subjects and from those practitioners engaged in providing services to older people than from other methods. It is a form of romanticism that elevates the affective over the cognitive.

Until we can recognize and deal with some of these concerns, it will be difficult to deal with the phenomenon of the instant gerontologist. Of course, from the practical viewpoint, these questions are being answered by our actions. There are people who define themselves as gerontologists. There are degree programs in gerontology. There is a Gerontological Society, a Western Gerontological Society, and the Association for Gerontology in Higher Education. We may not know *what* a gerontologist is but we know *that* a gerontologist is. These are issues, however, which relate to but do not focus on the phenomenon of the instant gerontologist.

Given Loeb's definition, most of us, I am sure, can come to some consensus about the nature and characteristics of instant gerontologists. They are people whose professional identification is in a discipline or applied profession, and who are, for one reason or another, going to be teaching courses relating to aging. Motivated by the push of failure or pull of success, or by creative flexibility, into a new and, as yet, undefined academic activity, instant gerontologists move across disciplinary boundaries. Although Loeb stresses those who see the bright future, there are also those who have been assigned the responsibilities for developing and teaching in gerontology programs. These are the "many called but few chosen" candidates, often sans commitment, knowledge, sans some other things. Their task, among others, is to build up faltering FTE's and budgets. Others accidentally wander in, some drawn by the humanist elements they sense, others by their desires to redress social grievances. Because of the diffusion of disciplinary boundaries, still others, capitalizing on the intellectual uncertainty of identity, find a new home, as did our early and sometimes less than savory settlers.

The connotation of the expression *instant gerontologist* emphasizes the instantaneous nature of becoming. It implies that, by reading some books, attending a workshop or two, and being concerned about old people, one is qualified to call oneself a gerontologist and thus to teach, train, consult in gerontology. My concern is not whether there is someone or something known as an instant gerontologist, but rather, since there is, how are we to maintain a degree of quality control? This is, at best, a touchy issue. The ethos of academia stresses academic honesty, integrity, and freedom, virtues not always evident. Dealing, therefore, with colleagues on matters regarding maintenance and protection of quality education is both difficult and ambiguous. A major concern is with professional courtesy and respect for colleagues. It is assumed, in the hallowed halls of academe, that possession of an advanced terminal degree in an area, any area, is prima facie evidence of competence and legitimacy. Thus, to criticize a colleague for exploring new fields, developing new expertise, and teaching the newly developed area of expertise is, at best, discourteous and, at worst, a violation of professional ethics. How can you deny someone the opportunity to enter into a new area of teaching? How can you criticize the competence of the incompetent? How can you throw the first stone? What doctor would dare to criticize another for poor medical practices? What attorney, another attorney? And, what academician, another academician? How can you, for example, tell a colleague who is discipline-based and adequate in that discipline that he or she is totally inadequate in his/her knowledge about and of aging. You can, of course (although it's not nice), but in so doing you throw out the cherished belief in lifelong development and learning and, of course, those highly touted administrative programs of faculty development. On an informal level, however, criticism runs rampant in a coat of hyperbole.

The questions I have raised have always been around—they are not unique to those concerned with the study of aging and with teaching the results of the study. They exist in all disciplines and quasi-disciplines, although they may occur more frequently in newly emerging academic disciplines and combinations of disciplines. We know that there are people poorly equipped to teach courses about aging; yet we also know that such people are doing precisely that—teaching about the nature of aging as they see it, often perpetuating the myths and stereotypes our data are destroying. From a formal point of view, there is very little we can do about instant gerontologists unless we move in the direction of accrediting programs and legitimizing individuals through some formality of credentials. Whether we do this and who would (or, more important, who should) do this is another of those major issues that, à la Scarlett O'Hara, we can face at another time. In the meantime, peer-review activities provide some quality control. Our professional organizations—conferences, workshops, consultants—all provide general roadmaps for people whose background is in other areas and whose intellectual stance permits them to continue to learn without threat. (It is the intellectually arrogant who are most assured of their expertise, and these we cannot reach.) On a more informal basis, we advise our students and colleagues about courses to take, which ones to avoid, and other such folklore and folkways. We stress the importance of commitment and point out that grants do not a commitment make. Although cash and commitment are a fortuitous combination, it is obvious that grants alone do not "make" gerontology programs any more than a single course "makes" a gerontologist.

Some of you may have read Gilbert Millstein's article in the February 5, 1978, issue of *The New York Times Magazine*, "Grey-Power Blues." You may also recall that, according to the Harris Poll, a large proportion of the American population dates the onset of old age to a specific event rather than to a chronological age. Millstein's moment of truth came when he found an issue of *Retirement Living* in his mailbox addressed to him. He was "old." It is an interesting article, and it is obvious from the article that he has read "the social gerontological literature." He comments on it scathingly. Where he found his solace and knowledge about aging was not in the gerontological literature as such but in T. S. Eliot and in a comedy sketch by a now deceased comedian Milt Kamen. His last paragraph says, "Above all, I know now, it was not that 'social scientist' who instructed me in what it means to be old. It was Eliot and Kamen, and while I may not like what they told me, they did tell me the truth" (Millstein, 1978, pp. 31–33). I am not sure I agree with him, but like Millstein, I, too, am seeking instruction in what, if anything, it means to be a gerontologist.

References

Harris, L., & Associates. *The myth and reality of aging in America.* Washington, D.C.: National Council on the Aging, 1975.

Millstein, G. Grey-power blues. *New York Times Magazine*, February 5, 1978.

Troll, L. E. *Early and middle adulthood: The best is yet to be—maybe.* Monterey, Calif.: Brooks/Cole, 1975.

PART THREE
ADMINISTRATIVE INVOLVEMENTS

The growth of academic gerontology requires imaginative and goal-oriented administration for the development of faculty and institutional resources. The challenge to the administrator is to facilitate logical, cooperative programming.

The papers in this section investigate the problems and prospects of creating multidisciplinary frameworks for gerontology within colleges and universities. Perspectives on the administration of gerontology programs are provided by college officials and by educators who direct these programs. The final paper takes a different approach and shows how, in one instance, a consultant team from the Association for Gerontology in Higher Education helped analyze and resolve administrative problems.

Administrative Support for Gerontology

Wilbur N. Moulton
Sangamon State University
Sister Mary Francilene and
Sister Colleen Morris
Madonna College
and
William A. Rogers
The University of Akron

The Gerontology Program
at Sangamon State University
Wilbur N. Moulton

Sangamon State University is an upper-division institution with work at junior, senior, and master's levels only. The university was established in 1969. At that time, in an attempt to be innovative and to respond to the abuses of departmentalism in the universities in the 1960s, academic studies at Sangamon State were organized around units called programs. Some of these programs are disciplinary in character and carry traditional names such as history, biology, and economics. Others are organized around themes or professions and carry such names as social justice professions; child, family, and community services; environments and people; and gerontology. Planning for gerontology involved faculty from biology; sociology; nursing; administration; child, family, and community services; and several other programs. In a traditional institution, such a group of faculty might have only formed a committee and organized an academic specialization that would amount to little more than a list of related courses offered by a variety of departments. In the flexible and innovative environment at Sangamon State University, though, a coherent academic and administrative unit developed relatively smoothly.

First, a minor in gerontology at the baccalaureate level was introduced through the university's relatively unique individual option program. Students in the program contract for a major or a minor at a baccalaureate or a master's level. They receive direct assistance in the development of their degree proposals from the Individual Option faculty and then move out into the university and the community to find the appropriate learning opportunities, which may or may not be formal courses. At present, the individual-option minor is the only opportunity in gerontology for undergraduate students, but the university has declared its intention to submit an undergraduate degree proposal to our governing bodies for approval next year.

The development of a major concentration in gerontology at the master's level first has worked well. Interest in the program and demand for its graduates are primarily professional. In addition, introducing the program at the master's level allowed students with a wide variety of backgrounds to enter it. That not only expanded the potential clientele, but it also brought into the program students with wide educational and work experiences that enriched the educational experience of their peers. This educational mix characterizes a great many of the programs at Sangamon State University; only a minority of our graduate students pursue the same discipline or specific program in which they got their undergraduate degrees. These differences in backgrounds, as well as differences in age and work experience, make teaching at Sangamon State University both frustrating and rewarding for our faculty, particularly those whose prior teaching experience has been in traditional colleges and universities.

One of the major contributions of the gerontology program to Sangamon State is that it serves as a catalyst in bringing together persons and organizations outside the university who share interest in the elderly but who, for a variety of reasons—institutional, bureaucratic, and personal—had not previously met to share those interests and to solve common problems. The advisory committee that guided the development of the gerontology program was chaired by the director of the Illinois Department on Aging and included among its members the dean of the Southern Illinois University School of Medicine, the director of the Illinois Department of Mental Health and Developmental Disabilities, the director of the Illinois Department of Children and Family Services, two hospital administrators, the vice-president for academic programs at Lincoln Land Community College, and the directors of several local service agencies.

As the gerontology program developed, lectures and seminars held occasionally for the public grew into an annual gerontology institute. The institute, held on three successive weekends in the spring of each year, brings degree students in the university together with practitioners and interested persons in the community and in state government, giving these groups an opportunity not only to hear distinguished scholars and leaders from across the country but also to get to know each other better.

The development of the gerontology program is a continuing effort. In addition to the preparation of a proposal for a baccalaureate degree program in gerontology, a number of other activities are in progress. The university and the Illinois Department on Aging are providing leadership for a new Illinois Gerontology Consortium. This organization, to be made up of public and private colleges and universities, state agencies, and professional organizations, will serve as a clearinghouse for information about gerontology programs being offered and developed in higher education and will coordinate research activities, conduct educational-needs assessments, and generally work to improve gerontological education and services in the state. At the university work is going forward on a gerontology center, which will serve as a focal point for educational programs and community services, thus providing a laboratory setting for instruction and research.

Lest this all sound blindly optimistic, let me add that the development of the program has created some institutional problems. The primary one has been the allocation of scarce resources. In the financially happy years of the 1960s, no serious program proposal received a decision more negative than a postponement. In the current steady state of the economy in higher education, any decision to do one thing is a decision not to do something else, and an easy promise to wait until next year is neither honest nor believable. The development of a coherent gerontology program as an academic and administrative unit not only deprives other university programs of badly needed human and financial resources, but it also limits the extent to which they can claim the current social and governmental concern for the elderly as part of their programmatic responsibilities. However, the problem can be solved, if the gerontology faculty work closely with their colleagues and if those with broader administrative responsibilities react thoughtfully and considerately to those who feel that the gerontology program has developed at their expense.

Actually the gerontology program has developed very much like any other interdisciplinary program. These programs are not deeply rooted in the academic tradition, and the decision to establish a new interdisciplinary program is essentially an act of faith. In good times, when the mood of higher education is expansionistic, such acts come easily. At other times, when resources are scarce and the fires of enthusiasm burn more lowly, the decisions are difficult. In such times, broad public acceptance of the importance of the substance of the program is critical in securing both support for the hard internal institutional decisions and approval of external governing boards and state agencies. Once established, interdisciplinary programs are successful only if they can draw students and can meet the needs of our society with high-quality performance. Unlike traditional disciplinary programs, interdisciplinary programs are not good candidates for life insurance. But we at Sangamon State believe our gerontology program is here to stay.

The Liberal Arts: Gerontology as a Catalyst for Interdisciplinary Research, Program Development, and Services
Sister Mary Francilene and Sister Colleen Morris

Four years ago, when the Association for Gerontology in Higher Education met for the first time, some administrators of small colleges, particularly liberal arts schools, may have asked the question, Why should we support the growth of gerontology programs? Others wondered, How do we start? As administrators at Madonna College, we can respond very positively to these questions without hesitation and with a firm commitment to gerontology as a major area of study and a provider of services to elderly persons and to those who are working in or preparing for this field.

Madonna College is a small liberal arts college in southeastern Michigan. The region has a concentration of elderly, including a large percentage of poor, minority elderly. According to the 1973 census, approximately 750,000 elderly live within a 50-mile radius of the college.

Madonna College's approach to gerontology is both interdisciplinary and multidisciplinary. It is interdisciplinary in that curriculum development has extended into the departments of biology, criminal justice, interpreter for communication with deaf persons (ITC), home economics, psychology, religious studies, emergency medical technology, legal assistant program, social work, and education. It is multidisciplinary in that Madonna College hosts a wide variety of workshops and implements unique training and service programs in gerontology. This includes a special project for the deaf and hearing-impaired older adult.

In 1974 the college originated its first project in gerontology. The project, entitled Volunteers to Assist the Aging, was to recruit, screen, and train 200 volunteers either to assist the homebound elderly or to act as advocates and friendly visitors for residents of long-term care facilities who seldom, if ever, have personal visitors.

The success of the volunteer program prompted a second project for the elderly. This effort, called Paraprofessional Training in Gerontology, was a direct response to the need to train competent personnel to care for aging citizens in Wayne, Oakland, and Macomb counties.

The Madonna College training program in gerontology was designed and implemented to provide jobs for the unemployed and on-the-job promotions for the undereducated or underemployed who work as paraprofessionals. All courses were and are competency based. Flexibility in course selection is allowed according to course content and individual aptitude and interest. Cooperative work experience or field placement forms part of the training.

The target population recruited for the project has included undereducated people, unemployed men and women, and displaced homemakers in the over-30 and over-40 age brackets who need specific training or job-entry skills after many years as housewives. Approximately 25 percent of the paraprofessional students at Madonna College belong to minority groups.

A third component of the Madonna College community service program was the development of the project for the deaf and hearing-impaired in southeastern Michigan. The unique needs of this group of handicapped older adults deserve appropriate consideration.

The profoundly deaf and hearing-impaired are a minority group who, for the most part, cannot communicate their needs orally. Many use a combination of oral and manual communication. For the profoundly deaf, sign language is often the most comfortable means of communication. Deaf speech is sometimes difficult to understand, a fact the deaf realize. They can never become "bilingual" as the speaking world understands that term. By providing practical-living classes—such as health and physical exercise, community resources, basic first aid, leadership, teletypewriting, and nutrition—Madonna College has directly responded to the community service needs of this elderly handicapped group. A principal objective of the project is to provide educational opportunities for leaders in deaf communities. A needs survey was conducted by the college in 1976 to determine what types of educational opportunities are available for the deaf older adult in southeastern Michigan. Educational opportunities for the deaf older adult are practically nonexistent. A second survey incorporating the needs of the deaf adult over 25 years of age is being conducted this year. Results of the 1976 survey indicate that the needs of the deaf older adult are similar to those of their hearing counterparts; that is, transportation, economics, health, housing are all major problems.

Workshops for professionals, paraprofessionals, and volunteers who work for or with the deaf and hearing-impaired are conducted at the college to sensitize service providers to the special problems of this handicapped minority group. Large enrollments in these workshops on deaf awareness indicate the increased interest in and concern for nonhearing persons and their special needs. Through this project, higher education is playing a major role in meeting the needs of the deaf older adult. With a simultaneous curriculum and program development in gerontology, Madonna College has indeed been a meeting ground and a catalyst for interdisciplinary research, education, training, and community service activities.

The Career Training in Aging project, which began in 1976, encompasses a broader perspective on aging. Self-instructional modules on aging are being developed and introduced into all the various disciplines involved. During the past four years, a bachelor of arts program was developed. Students may also elect to pursue an associate degree in gerontology or a certificate of achievement in gerontology. Fifty semester hours in gerontology are offered throughout each academic year. Program development has formed a large part of curriculum development.

Our students, faculty, and staff are of all races, religions, ages, and social backgrounds. We have handicapped persons, including 45 deaf students, in baccalaureate programs throughout the college. Four hundred of our hearing students, administrators, and teachers can communicate in sign language. We are in the fourth year of modifying existing facilities to create a totally barrier-free campus, and our first residential wheelchair-users are being accommodated. We know it takes initiative, creativity, and, most important, total commitment from all members of the college community to respond to the needs of our time and of the next generation.

Gerontology as a Second-Order Change Process for Higher Education
William A. Rogers

In 1971, the Carnegie Commission on Higher Education observed that higher education was concentrated mainly within the first two decades of life.

Apparently, those responsible for higher education were going on in a business-as-usual manner even though technology was changing drastically and life expectancy was lengthening.

The Carnegie Commission stated its concept of "less time, more options" in terms of a need for three years of undergraduate education (because of improved secondary education) and for more opportunity for those who wish to study part-time or return to education during various stages in life, especially women and older adults.

The Carnegie Commission suggested that society would gain if work and study were mixed throughout a lifetime, thus reducing the sense of sharply compartmentalized roles of isolated students. The sense of isolation would be reduced if more students were also workers, and if more workers could also be students; if the ages mixed on the job and in the classroom in a more normally structured type of community; if all members of the community value both study and work and had a better chance to understand the flow of life from youth to age. Society would be more integrated across the line that now separates students and workers, youth and age.

Higher education is rarely the leader in our society. Sometimes, it is a reluctant follower of the obvious. The GI bill, Sputnik, the White House Conference on Aging, and the Carnegie Commission are all examples of the external pressures that slowly move higher education toward the crest of the new wave.

As the supply of 18-year-olds has decreased, administrators and faculty have grown more interested in the older students. The institutional bandwagon effect is obvious, and many times it is motivated by pure economics rather than any genuine, specific interest in older students. Be that as it may, the Carnegie Commission statement on social gain contains three notions that are indigenous to the development of strong and effective curriculum, teaching-learning strategies, research, and public services for the new clientele: first, *break down the compartmentalization* seen in departmental and college behavior; next, *break down isolation* of students and age groups; and third, *mix youth and age* in work and study.

In institutional development, first-order change can be defined as an action that alters outcomes but does not alter the way the outcomes are derived. A second-order change, on the other hand, influences not only the outcome but the process. Five approaches characterize social change. The first three are usually lower order—capital infusion, leadership and group dynamics, and service coordination. The remaining two—pressure groups and natural groups—offer the potential for more profound, higher-order change.

In retrospect, it appears that the development of the gerontology programs at The University of Akron followed the natural-group model. We unwittingly identified the second-order, natural helping networks within faculty and community agencies.

The Institute for Life-Span Development and Gerontology at The University of Akron was organized three years ago by a group of eight faculty and administrators, who foresaw the need to marry Akron's rich experience in continuing education with gerontology. We observed, however, that attracting widespread faculty support made it imperative to build on neutral ground. The institute became a way of bringing together faculty from eight departments in four colleges who were, in some cases, duplicating or working in closely related fields but in isolation. (There are now 50 faculty actively engaged in the institute.) The president of The University of Akron supported the institute concept, perhaps because he saw a way to break down academic compartmentalization in an effort to better serve older clientele in new and realistic ways.

The institute established a bio-socio-psycho-health model that draws support from psychology, home economics and family ecology, speech pathology and audiology, nursing, education, counseling, early childhood, public services technology, developmental studies, and community and nutrition medicine. All of these disciplines focused on establishing and operating The University of Akron/Akron Metropolitan Housing Authority Edgewood Community Services Center Project, located off campus in the inner part of the city of Akron. The Edgewood Project has become a teaching, training, and research model for community service. The key, we decided, was that all previous campus institutes allegedly dedicated to interdisciplinary programs had only given lip service to the concept, but Edgewood has become an interdisciplinary activity that actually works. Interdisciplinary activities have been, for the most part, excellent committee conversation.

The interdisciplinary activity of eight departments in four colleges works because Edgewood actually adds resources to each of them. In no way does it threaten the basic student enrollment pattern of the campus.

Success in external funding of the Edgewood Project has made it easy for the president to support our efforts and for the faculty to enjoy the benefits of additional resources. The programs at Edgewood range from the Title VII Nutrition Site for older adults to the developmental child day-care center, including programs for adolescents. This array projects a life-span model for all of our colleagues to observe and understand. It is interesting to note that several of the departments that actively support inservice and preservice training programs at Edgewood had previously avoided conversation with each other over the years. The institute has also helped the university administration become aware of its responsibility for preretirement and postretirement planning for its faculty and staff.

In summary, gerontology, through a multidisciplinary life-span model, can function as an effective agent of change in academic institutions.

References to Gerontology as a Second-Order Change Process for Higher Education

Atchley, R. C. *The social forces in later life: An introduction to social gerontology.* Belmont, Calif.: Wadsworth, 1972.

Baltes, P. B., & Schaie, K. W. *Life-span developmental psychology: Personality and socialization.* New York: Academic Press. 1973.

Carnegie Commission on Higher Education. *Less time; more options.* New York: McGraw-Hill, 1971.

McClusky, H. Y. *Education: Background.* Washington, D.C.: White House Conference on Aging, 1971.

Pressey, S. L., & Kuhlen, R. G. *Psychological development through the life-span.* New York: Harper & Row, 1957. (Originally published, 1939.)

Developing Interdepartmental Relationships

Jody K. Olsen
University of Maryland

It is quite evident to those active in educational gerontology that effective interdepartmental relations are essential to a good program. The first consideration is that most institutions of higher education are in a period of "resource reassessment," a time when the institution comes to terms with increasingly limited resources and the resultant deployment pattern changes. Under these conditions, it is very difficult to develop a new self-contained program. Only the most fortunate educational facilities would be able to support such a program. Instead, those programs that can build on already existing courses, faculty, active research, field programs, and training opportunities have the best chances for longevity. Most of the resources for program building exist in departments or colleges, which are usually scattered throughout a campus or university system.

The next consideration is that the very nature of gerontology as a body of knowledge dictates an interdisciplinary approach. The intricate interplay among the processes of aging, coupled with the analyses of the service delivery system and its relationship to these aging processes, implies subject matter drawn from a multiplicity of departments, schools, and colleges. This might imply that, to develop an effective gerontology program, one should be as skilled in building the resources as in interpreting the basic body of knowledge within the field. The importance of good interdepartmental relations should not be minimized.

Planning Processes

Before those in educational gerontology embark on a conscious effort toward interdepartmental resource exchange, it is important to plan the process. With planning, an exchange that will have an advantage to gerontology can be established. According to Jacobs (1971), "social exchange" is the exchange of benefits to achieve a given goal. Each person or group has its own goal system, and the achievement of these goals should be done with the minimum of resource loss. Not only are those who are interested in developing a quality gerontology program concerned about goal achievement with the minimum of resource loss, but departments, schools, and even the university or college itself also have similar motivations dictating their actions. In the case of gerontology, however, the risk of losing resources in the process of goal achievement is less than it is with other units because in gerontology there are usually few resources to lose. In institutions with developing gerontology programs, the exchange is more likely one of collecting resources and offering the opportunity to participate in a growing field and the recognition that comes with that participation. Thus, the planning process within the gerontology unit involves organizing situations that will maximize the exchange process for obtaining resources of significance to the program.

In the planning process, both long- and short-term goals for building a gerontology program must be established. Whether or not these goals are established by immediate staff or as a result of key departmental involvement, they must be clearly understood by those building the program. Sometimes it is politically expedient not to reveal the goals to everyone to be contacted, but one must be sure that the goals are clearly defined to those establishing the relationships so that the necessary strategies can be shaped.

Next, an honest assessment of the resources available with which to bargain in building the program must be made. These resources can include, for example, access to a faculty line, a small grant that brings secretarial support, access to information on research guidelines before they are officially announced, potential students looking for a departmental home from which to develop their gerontology interests, training monies, a special friendship with the provost, or three strong gerontology courses already approved by curriculum committees. With more resources already available, it is easier to generate additional resources through an exchange with departments and administrative personnel, but even limited ones can be used and reused.

An assessment of needed resources for goal achievement must also be made. After the resources are listed, it is important to identify where they can come from. Receiving a large grant to hire faculty and build student stipends could be a solution, but growing competition makes this solution less and less likely. More important, long-term program survival is enhanced by university commitment in the form of internal support. If extra resources are not readily available within the college or university structure, resources already in existence can be tapped. The resources can include departmental course offerings, departmental faculty who have demonstrated an interest in research, community contacts established by departments for their influence with key administrative leaders, academic programs, graduate assistants, student assistantships, or space. Once these are identified and located, it is relatively easy to systematically contact the people and departments necessary to help build the program. Once the initial planning process, that is, the identification of what is expected to be accomplished through the exchange, is completed, the exchange process can begin.

The Departmental Exchange Process

The first step in the exchange process is to become well informed about the department, college, or administrative office before making the official contact. Departmental responsibilities, authority, interested faculty, student population, quality of leadership, attitude of the unit to other programs on campus, history of cooperation, and mechanisms for visibility are only a few examples of the kind of information needed in addition to that relating to why the unit would be a useful contributor to a gerontology program. For example, a department may be offering a gerontology course that should be included in the list of recommended courses for a gerontology certificate program. A contact with the department is needed to officially establish the link between the course and the certificate program. If information has been gathered ahead of time indicating that the department is struggling with decreasing enrollment and will lose departmental resources unless this is halted, this information can be used to establish an affirmative relationship for the purposes of the certificate program. On the other hand, if information shows that the department has a history of noncooperation, knowing why could affect the structure of the first meeting and could prevent gerontology from becoming another casualty of the noncooperation.

Generally, it is very complimentary to the department being pursued for the representative from the gerontology program to know strong features about the department and then compliment appropriately. In contrast, points are lost in a meeting if the gerontology representative asks for cooperation in establishing a master's certificate program only to find that that department doesn't have a master's program or is changing its focus. Similarly, making a request of an administrative office over which the office doesn't have jurisdiction hurts further contacts.

Learning the details about other programs ahead of time gives those making contact the opportunity to develop creative ideas for cooperation. When the representative has knowledge of both the departmental operation and the gerontology program, new ways of combining the two can be gently dropped into the conversation as appropriate, giving opportunity for more creative avenues if the standard ideas do not have appeal.

The second step is to ask advice of key faculty, as appropriate. Many faculty members have had experiences that can save time and disappointment later. In addition, the process of asking advice brings new people into the planning process and compliments them at the same time. They will be more likely to see the program as of interest to them if they know that some of their ideas helped shape it. It is important, however, when asking advice about curriculum and program development that it be asked of persons who can give strong answers and that the advice be taken. If advice is given and then implemented and the person giving it is thanked, he or she could become a longtime supporter. If the advice cannot be taken, it is important to get back to the person to talk about other alternatives. This will build the same long-term support.

Third, when talking to departments or colleges about resource sharing, allow the department head or dean some control over how the resources would be shared. For example, if in the department there are two courses that can be listed as part of a certificate program and the head does not want to list both, let him or her select the most important one. If the gerontology program has money to send one faculty member from a department to a conference and two or three are eligible, let the department head decide if possible. By so doing, the head can build his or her own position within the department or rectify some internal political issue. The head will be pleased with this opportunity and will be more likely to reciprocate with resources later.

There is an extension to this same point. If, for example, a faculty member receives a grant in conjunction with the gerontology program, let the department head be involved in making the announcement. Department and administrative officials will support programs that help them advance their own positions. Being able to announce, negotiate, or help make decisions related to successful gerontology programs contributes to a sense of accomplishment in one's own position and will perpetuate gerontology support.

The fourth step is to try to be noncompetitive with departments and colleges. Because gerontology is multidisciplinary, it is more comprehensive when drawn from a broad discipline base. Publicly recognizing (1) the disciplines involved, (2) the faculty involved with their departmental affiliation clearly listed, (3) the courses offered with their departmental affiliation clearly stated, and (4) the administrative units providing funding or related resources gives the message to departments that cooperation with the gerontology program could bring recognition, visibility, and resources. Joint sponsorship of research projects, training programs, conferences, colloquiums, and lecture series builds the feeling of cooperation rather than competition. In most cases, this cooperation will be reciprocated when a particular department sponsors an activity involving someone in the gerontology program.

The fifth step is to support programs and activities sponsored by cooperating departments even though they might not be related to gerontology. Serve on committees when asked, if time permits, and attend functions that are important to or sponsored by the departments. For example, if the department is sponsoring its own lecture program, attend some of the programs and help advertise them when appropriate. Timely letters of support or congratulations show a department that the interest in the department goes beyond its taking the right gerontology course. These symbols of goodwill say that there is a genuine interest in and support for the department in all its activities.

Sixth, as decisions concerning the gerontology program are being made, those departments or administrative units that might be affected should become part of the decision process. If, for example, a certain psychology course will no longer be required in the future for the certificate program, the sponsoring department should be part of that decision or, at least, be made aware of the change as soon as possible and told why the change is being made. Many times, initial contact is made with units on campus and relationships are established; then later, the program structure is changed, and no follow-up contact is made until after the decisions have been made. With regular contact, other groups are, at least, kept up-to-date on potential changes so that they can give correct information about the gerontology program to faculty and students. It is particularly important to share requirements for a certificate or degree program as they develop or change since most students in these programs are also involved with other departments and in contact with other advisors. Receiving information late only makes the department or the advisor look ill informed.

Although committees can be time-consuming, they are essential to good cooperation. Through an effective committee structure, faculty, department heads, and administrative officials can be involved in gerontology program decisions as they are being made, and because these people are made a part of the decisions, they can become advocates for the implementation of the decisions. In order to make a committee effective, we must state the committee functions clearly, and specify the parameters of the committee decisions. For example, a committee on research could have as its members faculty from a variety of disciplines who are known to have an interest in research in aging and who have some influence over colleagues in their respective departments. The committee could have as its goals the development of four new research projects during the year, the development of a faculty incentive program in research, and facilitation of research guideline dissemination. This committee has the potential to bring strong departmental people together to strengthen research in gerontology, and if it has a clear purpose, those involved from the departments can measure what they are getting from their experiences. They can become advocates for the programs shaped by the committee.

The seventh step in the exchange process is to organize informal opportunities for people outside the gerontology program to come together. Receptions, brown-bag lunches, and discussion groups all help those people scattered throughout the campus to get to know each other, making it easier for them to work together on a formal basis later.

Finally, be aware of the limits of influence gerontology programs have over some department or college units. The gerontology program representative can ask for particular faculty members to teach certain courses, but these decisions are usually best left to the departments offering the course. Although there may be a proliferation of courses on the sociology of aging, beyond making that information available, the gerontology program representative can do little without risking the alienation of other units. Student preferences will usually take care of some course duplication over time. Good relationships with departments and colleges will bring opportunities to discuss the course, the research use of faculty time, and the joint programming; nevertheless, individual administrative unit has the ultimate authority on how the resources within that unit are deployed.

Most important, fostering good interdepartmental relationships takes time. There is no shortcut to taking time to meet people, learning about the other programs, and supporting other programs in addition to building an effective internal structure within the gerontology program itself. Time is a scarce commodity; it is also an important commodity. Because of the limitations on time, planning is essential. Through the planning process, priorities are set; time can then be spent where it is the most useful. Once the important links are established, those at the end of the chain can reach out for further links. The stronger the basic links, the more time-equivalents can be spread among many people.

Because of the amount of time and resource sharing necessary to make a program work, those interested in gerontology must have a strong commitment to both the program and the institution in which it is housed. With this dual commitment, the necessary efforts will be made.

References

Jacobs, T. O. *Leadership and exchange in formal organizations.* Alexandria, Va.: Human Resources Research Organization (HUM RRO), 1971, p. 352.

Professional Schools and Interdisciplinary Aging Programs: Problems and Prospects

Donald E. Gelfand
University of Maryland-Baltimore

In recent years, funding agencies at federal and local levels have demanded that an interdisciplinary orientation be evidenced in both training and service delivery programs for elderly populations. Administrators, however, have not often shared the enthusiasm of practitioners or university faculty for interdisciplinary programs. To administrators and some faculty, interdisciplinary programs present threatening as well as rewarding elements. At the worst, they are perceived as drawing students away from intraschool courses, cutting total enrollments, and raising the spectre of underutilized faculty and budget slashes. Likewise, interdisciplinary programs may appear to threaten a loss of control over the rigidly defined programs and curricula that characterize professional education. Finally, in a society where professionals are attempting to maximize employment opportunities by extending the scope of their practice, interdisciplinary programs threaten to further blur the relative expertise of particular professionals.

This paper addresses the opportunities and problems of this new thrust of interdisciplinary aging programs in professional education. Although professional schools appear to be outwardly similar to academic departments in structure and faculty hierarchy, the training of their students for defined professional service roles affects their educational goals, programs, and curriculum development process.

It is difficult to define the parameters of this curriculum for professional education. Whereas relevant topics in aging for sociology students may seem evident, subject boundaries in courses for nurses, social workers, or physicians may be less clear. Complicating these decisions are multidisciplinary service models in aging, which require professionals to understand the basic approach of other professionals. An example would be so-called geriatric evaluation services, which combine the skills of physicians, nurses, and social workers. These fields and pharmacy, allied health professions, law, and dentistry also need to provide students with a background in social policies and programs in aging, an area undergoing rapid change and difficult to encompass in curriculum units.

If the above issues complicate the development of interdisciplinary programs in aging among professional schools, the ambivalence or even hostility of some students toward these interdisciplinary approaches places increased burdens on them. Social work students, for example, are not always convinced about the advantages of a background in biology or the need to understand the relationship between drug reactions and psychotic episodes in preparation for their work in aging. Similarly, many medical students remain unconvinced that living patterns are important to treating organic conditions in an elderly patient.

Bearing this background in mind, let us use the recent efforts at the University of Maryland-Baltimore to develop interdisciplinary programs in aging as a backdrop for discussing issues that apply to professional schools in general.

University Structure and Aging Programs

With its multicampus units, the University of Maryland has a structure similar to that of many large state universities. Maryland may be unique, however, in that its professional schools (dentistry, law, medicine, nursing, pharmacy, social work) are located on one campus in Baltimore. Nonetheless, the goals of the individual schools, despite the apparent advantages of their proximity to one another, have often seemed unrelated. Until 1977, there was not even any commonality to the academic calendars of the respective schools. In fact, whereas all the other schools functioned on a semester basis, the school of dentistry had developed its curriculum on a quarter model. These differences placed obstacles in the way of interdisciplinary programs that required major amounts of energy to overcome. An additional obstacle has been the different classification of graduate and undergraduate students at the respective schools. Social work students earn masters and doctorates, but medical and pharmacy students are primarily enrolled in programs defined as undergraduate in nature. These classification systems are common to professional schools. Developing interdisciplinary courses for students at all of the professional schools must, therefore, overcome a variety of technical problems.

Obviously, the development of interdisciplinary cooperation among professional schools requires a determination to deal with traditional program structures, which are organized without consideration for the problems they might present to new interdisciplinary cooperation. To provide some guidance for interdisciplinary efforts at the professional school level, this article will focus on issues that have been found crucial in the efforts at Maryland to overcome professional and structural obstacles. These include lack of an integrative organizational unit, increased demands on faculty time, status differentials, lack of correspondence in student training schedules, lack of interprofessional relationships of faculty, and mixed functions of professional schools.

Lack of Integrative Organization Although interdisciplinary education programs have been widely discussed and attempted for a number of years, these efforts in the field of aging have often been confined to liberal arts programs. At many universities, the inception of university-wide centers on aging helped focus attention on the programs of individual departments. Lacking identification with any one department, the centers have coordinated research grants and developed academic programs using innovative field experiences for undergraduate students in a variety of service settings.

At a professional-school campus where interprofessional relationships have been limited, the development of similar integrative units to serve as a communications network is even more important. Without these integrative units, individual schools may work along parallel lines without knowing what the others are doing. Each school may thus try to develop new training programs that include common elements or duplicate courses. An integrative unit, whether it is a separate committee or a committee operating from the framework of a center on aging, can help provide resources that further an interdisciplinary focus in general training or individual courses. An integrative unit may also be able to assist schools in sharing resources where an individual school cannot commit faculty time to new programs in aging.

Increased Demands on Faculty Time The activities of interdisciplinary groups are often conducted on the basis of faculty contributions of time, since funds are unavailable to release faculty from other responsibilities for interdisciplinary planning efforts. As activities become more demanding, time limitations on the faculty involved begin to be felt. At Maryland, a training grant attempted to remedy this situation. The bulk of the funds was earmarked for the individual schools to release the time of a faculty member each school designated as its official representative to an interdisciplinary aging committee.

The allocation of funds in this manner helps to legitimize the interdisciplinary thrust. It indicates to administrators of professional schools the seriousness of the commitment to activities within each school related to the development of education in aging as well as to interdisciplinary efforts.

Status Differentials Status differentials among professional-school faculty and staff are often greater than those within academic departments. Nonfaculty personnel hired for pivotal administrative positions in interdisciplinary aging programs within professional schools may encounter difficulties arising from their status as "outsiders." Aside from the problems involved in handling a position requiring constant attention to a multitude of incipient projects, a nonfaculty member may not be accepted as a colleague in an academic setting highly stratified by rank and degree as well as by salary. In many professional school settings, medical-school faculty receive the highest status, with other disciplines lagging behind.

A faculty member may enjoy legitimacy as a spokesman not accorded nonfaculty personnel. This legitimacy can be vital in negotiating programs with administrators. More crucial, perhaps, will be the faculty member's credentials as a peacemaker who can resolve conflicts over resource allocations to the individual schools, especially if suspicions about the degree of correspondence between the needs of individual schools and the thrust of the new interdisciplinary aging programs continue.

Lack of Correspondence in Student Training Schedules At Maryland, Administration on Aging training funds allowed an interdisciplinary group to move ahead on a number of activities. Importantly, it provided for a continuation of the campuswide lecture series, which brings professionals in the field of aging to the university. This function is vital at professional schools because students and service professionals still resist working with the elderly. Distinguished dentists, lawyers, nurses, physicians, pharmacists, and social workers presenting papers at campuswide seminars provide positive role models for students.

The lecture function is also important because of the detailed process involved in curriculum development within professional schools. As already noted, the numbering system of the schools and classification of students as undergraduates and graduates can prove an obstacle and raise questions about the level at which interdisciplinary courses should be developed.

Professional schools also require students to undertake field placements or rotations in many common settings such as nursing homes or senior centers. Because the time students from different professions spend in these settings varies in both duration and intensity, the problems they encounter working with elderly clients may cut across the individual professions. Although the problems of varying time commitments have created scheduling difficulties, students from law, social work, medicine, and nursing can be brought together at a multidisciplinary setting to discuss common training and treatment issues. These kinds of efforts have important implications for the development of an interdisciplinary sense in future professionals who will be entrusted with service responsibilities with elderly clients.

The involvement of students in aging can also be advanced through the type of community lecture series that has been run successfully by the Maryland interdisciplinary committee. These lectures at a variety of community sites have dealt with legal, social, and medical issues and are pitched at a level valuable for many of the present generation of elderly. Delivering these talks or conducting informal workshops following a short formal presentation trains students in important presentation methods. The students are also brought into personal contact with a diversity of elderly, which is not always possible in their field placements.

Lack of Interprofessional Relationships of Faculty The responsiveness of individual faculty to a combined thrust in the area of aging has been surprising.

Obviously, sentiment about the need for an interdisciplinary focus is shared not only at the federal level but by many faculty working in the field. Moving from an interdisciplinary focus to an interdisciplinary project is a major step that is not made easily. Individual faculty continue to be responsible to their respective professional schools, and rewards stem from achievements within their particular discipline rather than from interdisciplinary efforts. Interdisciplinary groups need to take this consideration into account. Designing an interdisciplinary project that benefits the individual school and faculty member as well as the interdisciplinary aging effort will help to increase the commitment of faculty to the project and add to the enthusiasm of school administrators.

Mixed Functions of Professional Schools In contrast to an academic department, the professional school has a complex and often only vaguely defined nature. The academic department usually sees its mission as training students and providing opportunities for scholars to research and publish. The professional school has as its stated mission training students for practice roles and also, at many points, involving the school in providing services. Although the service mandate is often ambiguous, it is related to the practice-teaching nature of the faculty of professional schools and the linkage these schools have with such facilities as hospitals.

It is thus not considered unusual that the university's professional schools should apply for grants to develop clinical multidisciplinary services for at-risk population groups. When grants such as these are funded, it is not automatically assumed that the same individuals responsible for teaching courses in an area will be involved in designing or implementing these services. This split results from differences in practice experience, expertise, or reputation. Faculty involved in teaching courses in aging may be less well known as practitioners, and may not be called upon to become involved in service delivery modules. The university professional-school administrators may attach more importance to the control of service delivery systems than to curriculum content. This is especially true because of the potential income they see in new service-delivery systems.

The disjuncture between teaching and practice faculty can produce two distinct groups: an interdisciplinary committee concerned with education and a second committee concerned with the development of a service delivery system for the aged. Membership on these two committees may be distinct, and the functioning of two groups working in the same field of endeavor may promote "turf" debates that can distract from common goals. These disagreements must be resolved if interdisciplinary efforts in aging are to succeed.

Conclusion

With the pressures placed by government agencies on professional universities for interdisciplinary approaches to aging, responses with potential for long-lasting effects have been made. In some cases, these responses represent external pressures more than shifts in ideological commitment among university personnel. Whatever the motivation, clearly there are important factors that will affect the eventual outcome of these interdisciplinary efforts among professional schools.

As the above discussion indicates, some of these factors are common to both academic departments and professional schools. Others are unique to the professional school. One of the most important elements underlying all the suggestions in this article is the high degree of hierarchical control common to many professional schools. At one extreme, these schools tend to be part of a campus where each professional school functions independently under the benign leadership of a chancellor. In this environment, interprofessional contact may occur only at top administrative levels. At the opposite extreme, of course, are universities where power is shared among the schools, goals are formulated on a campuswide basis, and interschool faculty relationships are widespread at all levels.

In tightly controlled professional schools, decision making flows directly from the dean's office, with heads of individual departments having less flexibility than in academic departments. Policy and programs take their mandate from the dean's office and are channeled through such intermediaries as associate and assistant deans. These administrators occupy positions of greater power than do department heads. Whereas an aging program in psychology may be the brainchild of an individual faculty member and the head, a similar program in preventive medicine may undergo considerably more scrutiny from the dean of the medical school and require his or her support for its success.

Understanding the structure of the individual campus and the decision-making process within each professional school is vital to deciding how to approach interdisciplinary activities among professional schools. A successful analysis of administrative structure can make use of the involvement of senior faculty members who have long-term experience in administrative roles within the individual schools. An analysis of this nature should provide guidance on the best method of obtaining administrative support, the degree of administrative involvement desirable, and the pivotal organizational entities within each professional school.

The second element underlying much of the discussion is the need for interdisciplinary committees or groups to defuse suspicions that the interdisciplinary program competes with the goals of the individual schools. Despite reassurances about the compatibility of intraschool and interschool aging programs, deans and other administrative officials will still be wary of interdisciplinary efforts that begin to use faculty resources, introduce new courses as alternatives to existing intraschool courses, and obtain grants not routed through normal channels. Again, an understanding of the interrelationships of the schools should provide an important background for the interdisciplinary effort. An effort should also be made to note the financial underpinnings of each school's budget. Professional schools that depend on tuition may respond to interdisciplinary programs that make them more attractive to students.

Other schools with a strong base of research grants may feel less concern about enrollment issues.

Interdisciplinary programs in aging are working at three levels: classroom education, clinical training, and service delivery programs. The role of interdisciplinary efforts at all of these levels needs to be clarified at each university before interdisciplinary programs can become full-fledged entities. Under the pressures of grant deadlines, these clarifications are often ignored, causing confusion and a decline in administrative support.

The interdisciplinary model is complex, but it still holds great promise for aging programs in the professional schools. It is advisable, however, that we move into this approach carefully, aware of the obstacles that may be inherent in the structure of the individual professional school. With such caution and careful analysis, it is realistic to expect that accomplishments will come slowly but steadily as the rewards of interdisciplinary efforts become more defined and the threats lessen.

Utilizing Organizational Strengths and Community Resources to Create a University-wide Gerontology Program: An Example

Nona Boren
The George Washington University

The University-wide Gerontology Program at The George Washington University, which began in 1976 and is funded by the Administration on Aging, evolved from previous interdepartmental and interdisciplinary activities within the university, certain fortuitous events, and the planned application of community organization principles. In describing the history, organizational structure, and development of this relatively new program, this paper emphasizes how a community organization process was set in motion and how it contributed to the vigorous growth of the program. The achievements since the award of the first grant have demonstrated the effectiveness of the conscious application of community organization concepts, principles, and practices in developing a new program.

Before 1976 there was no advocate for aging within the university. Although an early survey, conducted in 1976 shortly after we were funded, indicated considerable interest in age-related activities as well as a surprising amount of hidden talent, there was no plan to develop an integrated program, and little was being done in this field in teaching, research, or service. The Institute of Law, which had a record of achievement in the field of aging, was the university's one exception to this general neglect. Other than courses and training programs within the law school, we were able to identify but one course on aging in the 12 colleges, schools, and divisions in the university and only a handful of courses with some aging content. At that time the medical school did not have even one required geriatrics/gerontology course, although problems were touched on during the preclinical years and were included in the clinical experiences of third- and fourth-year students. Electives in geriatric care were offered for senior medical students; however, since no one promoted student interest and involvement, students usually did not sign up for this experience.

Administration on Aging support for the gerontology program provided the university with a principal investigator and a full-time program director to act as advocates for mobilizing the energy and resources of numerous individuals within its interprofessional and multidisciplinary structure and within the community. Major achievements, to date, include: the development of four new courses on aging in four departments; opportunities for several undergraduate and graduate field-placement experiences for credit; the inclusion of aging content in the required curriculum of the medical school; and major conferences and forums on aging, which have done much to stimulate interest both within the institution and the community. In addition, the evolution of three major programs, to be implemented soon, has resulted from the energetic involvement and collaboration of university faculty and community leaders: a geriatric unit within the department of health care sciences with a full-time geriatrician responsible for curriculum development and patient care, a 36-hour graduate program in gerontology in the graduate school of arts and sciences, and a community services center and outreach program to provide a variety of supportive services to the elderly in the District of Columbia. Thus, deliberately applied community organization principles have set in motion a process of cooperation, collaboration, and integration, representing major program achievements.

Concepts, Principles, and Strategies of Community Organization Practice

The community organization process to which I refer is frequently understood to be restricted to the field of social welfare or to the accomplishment of tasks that bring about change in a geographic area. However, it should be emphasized that the principles and process of community organization can also apply to specific areas of interest, such as aging, and to specific functions, such as teaching, research, training, or service. Two interrelated concepts underlie the principles and strategies of community organization practice that are of particular interest to planning interdisciplinary programs in aging.

First is the concept of program goal. The program goal must meet the general consensus of all program participants; it must also be stated in broad enough terms to allow flexibility and freedom of choice regarding the development of specific tasks by individual participants. This allows for the application of an important community organization principle that emphasizes the importance of participant involvement in the planning process.

A second related concept involves the process of community organization practice; that is, the way in which goals and objectives are achieved. A major objective of this process is integration, by which I mean the exercise of cooperative and collaborative practices to increase the capacity to achieve program goals.

Related strategies, principles, and practices that the planner or advocate for change can use to influence the direction of the program include: identifying a problem or a need to change; identifying leadership, both within the institution and within the community, and developing motivation or will to change; applying strategies necessary to meet objectives, such as finding internal and external resources to support program goals; combining planned action with sufficient flexibility to seize unexpected opportunities for growth and expansion; developing constructive power strategies for dealing with conflict; finding ways for individuals to be involved in determining the nature and method of their own contribution without sacrificing integration; accepting that conflict is inherent in collaborative work: and accepting that organizations and individuals move at their own pace.

The developmental and programmatic aspects of The George Washington University program illustrate these concepts, strategies, principles, and practices.

History of the Program

The history of the program incorporated the following specific principles of community organization practice: identifying the problem, developing a plan of action, identifying leadership, and developing the motivation or will to change. It also answers in part the question of how the program originated in the school of medicine and health sciences.

The present program evolved from an earlier Administration on Aging project, which was designed as a career-transition program for older persons interested in a second career in the health care field. This two-year program of working with older persons in career transition and the interaction with different departments in the university, with the community, with persons in the field of aging, and with such organizations as the Gerontological Society, the Association for Gerontology in Higher Education, and the Institute of Medicine unwittingly developed a community base for what was to follow. Simultaneously, the consciousness of those involved was raised. We became acutely aware of education gaps in gerontology and geriatrics in our university in general and in the medical school in particular. We became aware of institutional strengths to fill these gaps. We became aware that medical schools would soon be called on to take a leadership role in addressing gaps in education, training, research, and service.

We were also aware that although we had many resources, we had within our organization few full-time individuals in the field of aging who had reached the stature of faculty at the established institutes or centers on aging at other universities. This raised a major concern: How could we address the issue of providing for high-quality education and training and for the conduct of research in a field where we, as an institution, were comparatively inexperienced?

Two factors made us bold enough to move forward. The first was a growing recognition that we had more resources in our university than were apparent on the surface. The second was a knowledge, based on part experience, that we were indeed fortunate to be in the Washington, D.C., area, where we could draw on the resources of a significant number of individuals who are experts in the field of aging.

We therefore moved to develop these resources and to plan a program that would influence the training of students of medicine, social work, and allied health; residents in primary care, internal medicine, and psychiatry; and students in recreation therapy, sociology, psychology, health care administration, and law. The goal was broad enough to gain consensus from those individuals initially involved in planning the grant proposal, but it also allowed freedom of choice for each participant to take responsibility for developing a task of intrinsic value to themselves.

Program Development

Several activities planned under the initial grant award provide examples of using community organization principles to promote acceptance and recognition of the program within both the university and the community. Shortly after we were funded, forums, continuing-education programs, and conferences were initiated to introduce the program to the faculty, administration, and community and to provide continuing-education credit. These activities continued throughout the first year and contributed to the expansion of the organizational structure of the program. We now have a structure involving five schools and 15 departments. Each of these schools and departments has representatives on one or more of five gerontology program committees: the steering committee and four additional subcommittees on professional services, research, field placements, and continuing education. People were chosen to serve on these committees on the basis of the following criteria: interest, motivation, willingness to take responsibility for developing specific tasks, and power to effect change. These committees involve approximately 40 faculty from the cooperating schools and departments, as well as experts in the field of aging drawn from the community.

Fragmentation and loss of control by the program administration could easily occur without the conscious application of strategies that assure integration of program goals. I will mention only two. One has been provided by the function of the steering committee: Through the monthly meetings of this group all program tasks are reported and a process of integration promoted. An additional strategy for assuring integration of program goals, for managing conflict effectively, and for securing the university's commitment to continuing the program was an early decision to have the program located in the office of the dean for academic affairs of the medical school. This administrative decision makes possible regular and supportive connection to the deans of the cooperating schools, to the vice-president for medical affairs, and to the president of the university. The charismatic administrative clout provided by the dean has been invaluable in negotiating areas of differences and conflict, in promoting acceptance of program goals, and in securing the university's commitment to continuing the program.

The expansion of the program outside the university has been one of the most significant aspects of program development. It illustrates the advantage of promoting recognition of the program within the community. As the gerontology program was developing, the Episcopal Diocese of Washington was planning and seeking funding for a Housing and Urban development #202 project in order to build Saint Mary's Court, a 136-unit congregate housing facility to be located one block from the medical school and adjacent to Saint Mary's Church. Members of the diocese heard about our program and came to us with a request to provide health services within the Court. From the need to plan programs for the semi-independent elderly population in the court has emerged a community service center and an outreach program to provide supportive services for the elderly that will serve the residents of both the court and the wider community. We are seeking funding for a mobile care unit to extend many of these services to other sites throughout the District of Columbia. Sites to be served by the mobile unit would include public housing for the elderly, existing senior centers, and church groups; emphasis will be placed on the development of new services that will complement existing social and health services in the community. Every effort will be made to apply the concepts of community organization practice that promote integration of services.

We have already indicated the need to identify sources of interest, motivation, and power to effect change and meet program goals. A frequently overlooked source of power and energy within institutions of higher education is the students themselves. Many of the activities planned for the Saint Mary's Court and for our expanded community services program stem from student interest and motivation and would not be possible without them. We have planned for the traditional utilization of students, supervised by professionals, to staff many of the programs and services for the center including health care, personal care, health education, counseling, information and referral services, and recreational, rehabilitation, and physical-fitness activities. However, an innovative aspect of student involvement has developed from their inclusion on various committees and from their determination to undertake leadership roles. Students are eager to find avenues for meaningful involvement and for actively contributing to the program.

Conflicts may occur between students and faculty as a result of specific attitudes regarding authority. Student impatience with institutional pace and organizational interaction can threaten program goals. Faculty, by contrast, are frequently guilty of attitudes that are not conducive to student involvement and to using this valuable source of energy. When conflicts arise from such legitimate concerns as a desire to protect boundaries, positive results can be achieved if appropriate strategies such as confrontation are initiated early.

Students at the university have been responsible for taking the initiative to create a health education program for the elderly. They have been involved in developing a new elective designed to train and employ students to collect data through home interviews for program planning and ongoing research. In addition, students and faculty are planning a major intergenerational program to demonstrate that students can fill major service gaps in the community.

Summary

The George Washington experience over the last two years in planning and in developing the University-wide Gerontology Program has highlighted several forces and counterforces that are inevitable whenever several individuals, schools, and departments within a university and institutions outside the university attempt to work together to create new programs. It has also made evident the applicability and effectiveness of concepts, principles, and strategies derived from community organization practice.

The community organization process derives from a capacity, developed and nurtured over time, to promote integration. Identification of interest, leadership, and power within both the university and the community is essential. An attitude of flexibility should prevail to allow for recognizing and seizing unplanned opportunities to effect change. Advocates for change must recognize that institutions have a built-in pace, which must be respected. This concept is much easier to accept if one recognizes that incremental changes, which may appear relatively insignificant, have a synergistic effect when combined with other activities. Program planners must also respect self-determination and academic freedom, allowing faculty to engage in activities of intrinsic value to themselves. Finally, while conflict is an inevitable outgrowth of forces operating vertically within an institution (e.g., the university) and horizontally between institutions, it is not always dysfunctional.

Our program, like any other interdisciplinary effort, has had its share of conflicts growing out of the need of individual departments, schools, and institutions to preserve boundaries and protect turf. There is, however, no doubt that the planned application of the principles of community organization practice, combined with the reality of the Saint Mary's Court and the potential it represents for training, research, and service, has played an enormous role in the vigor of the program. For, through the combination of seizing fortuitous opportunities and consciously applying principles of practice to assure integration, diverse programs within the schools and departments of the university as well as agencies in the community have realized that there is much to be gained by cooperating and little to lose.

The Association for Gerontology in Higher Education as Consultant: A Pilot Project

William C. Hays
Wichita State University
and
Tom Hickey
University of Michigan

This two-part paper describes a pilot project in which the Association for Gerontology in Higher Education (AGHE) provided a team of consultants for one of its developing institutional members, Wichita State University. Analyses of the problems and benefits of this particular consultation experience are given from the viewpoint of both the gerontology program faculty and staff at Wichita State and the team of AGHE consultants, and alternative models and techniques for AGHE involvement in providing aid for its member institutions through consulting activities are suggested.

The Perspective of Wichita State University
William C. Hays

In the fall of 1976, Wichita State University identified a need for external consultants to evaluate the directions that its rapidly developing gerontology program was taking. Limited funding to support consulting activities was available from Administration on Aging Title IV-A training and planning grants. As a member of AGHE, the university decided to ask the association to suggest individuals who would be appropriate consultants for its program. When Tom Hickey, then president of the association, was approached about whom AGHE would recommend as consultants, he stated that the association was studying the role AGHE might play in providing a program consultation service to member institutions. After discussions among Tom Hickey, Bill

Hays (program director at Wichita State), and members of the AGHE Executive Committee, it was agreed that the association would provide consultants to Wichita State University as a pilot project to evaluate the role of AGHE in providing such a service to its members.

Because the program at Wichita State had developed so rapidly, the consulting problem was almost unique. Although a few Wichita State faculty members had long been involved in the area of aging, the existing multidisciplinary bachelor's degree program had expanded recently over a short period of time. Before the fall semester of 1975, only one aging course was offered at Wichita State; by spring semester of 1977, the Wichita State gerontology program offered an undergraduate degree involving 12 new courses. Furthermore, the program had received Kansas Board of Regents approval as a gerontology center and had developed a proposal for a master's degree program (since approved). The gerontology program had grown perhaps too rapidly; it needed someone from outside the university to provide an objective and neutral evaluation.

Because of the scope and rapid development of the Wichita State gerontology program, the first task was to define the areas of consultation. After additional discussion, the following four topic areas for consultation were agreed upon: academic programs, specifically the baccalaureate and masters program; integration of health sciences and health professionals into the program; university and community relationships, specifically continuing education; and issues related to administrative structure and organization. Because of the range of consulting areas to be covered, it was decided that a team of consultants would be used rather than a single individual and that the general framework would be a friendly site visit consisting of four phases. The consulting team was drawn from member institutions of AGHE. The team members, institutions, and primary areas of responsibility were: Tom Hickey, University of Michigan School of Public Health, responsible for administrative issues and university-community relationships; Mildred M. Seltzer, Miami University Scripps Foundation Gerontology Center, responsible for academic-degree programs; and Maxine L. Patrick, University of Washington Department of Physiological Nursing, responsible for health sciences and professions.

The four-phase model for the consultation provided for initial information sharing and briefing, an on-site visit, a written report, and an on-campus follow-up and debriefing.

Phase I: preliminary information. This phase involved the distribution of information. Each member of the consulting team received curriculum materials, proposals, brochures, faculty inventories, catalogues, and other written materials describing the university and the gerontology program. Excluding such items as college catalogues, between 350 and 400 pages of written materials were sent to each team member. Phase I also included a response request from the consulting team specifying the agenda for the phase-II visit and some suggested study questions and issues for the program faculty at Wichita State University.

Phase II: on-campus visit. The site visit occupied a three-day period in

May 1977. It included a preliminary meeting of the consulting team to discuss the written materials and plan the campus visit; a briefing session between the consulting team and the Wichita State gerontology program director to discuss the written materials and fill in any missing information needed by the team; a morning workshop session for faculty, staff, and students at which team members made informal presentations in their areas of specialization and discussed the multidimensional roles of institutions of higher education as they relate to aging; meetings of consulting-team members with individuals and small groups for consultation in particular areas; and extensive team consultation with individual deans and gerontology program staff.

Phase III: written report. The consulting team prepared a 26-page report on the site visit. This report made no attempt to "sugar coat." It identified existing and potential weaknesses in each of the four program areas and suggested directions and solutions that might be pursued in each. The report was submitted to the gerontology program director, who in turn distributed it to key program faculty and staff and to university administrators for discussion and comment.

Phase IV: debriefing. After allowing time for analysis of the written report, Hickey, as team leader, returned to Wichita State to meet with university administrators and gerontology program faculty and staff in order to answer specific questions and provide a follow-up to the written report and site visit.

This procedure summarizes what was, in fact, a long and complex project. Almost a year passed from the original contact between Wichita State and Hickey to the final debriefing. There was a long period of exchange of letters, telephone calls, and discussion before a decision was reached on the appropriate model for the consultation, and many similar open-ended discussions occurred at each phase of the consultation. The following pages present the institution's impressions about this consulting experience and its views about the role of AGHE in providing consultation for member institutions. The report of their impressions will be followed by the reaction of the consulting team leader.

The Institution's Impressions Overall, Wichita State was quite favorably impressed with the AGHE consultation. The consulting team was knowledgeable; its suggestions were specific and candid. The recommendations had both immediate and long-range benefits, and Wichita State was quoted a bargain price for what the association delivered. The friendly site-visit format had the advantages of an accreditation or prefunding grant visit without any of the disadvantages. Since AGHE was providing consultation and not evaluating for possible endorsement or accreditation of our program, we were undoubtedly more open about our program without fear of the consequences. Nevertheless, because of the expertise and experience of the consulting team and the prestige of the association, both the gerontology program personnel and, very important, the top-level university administration took the site visit seriously.

Whereas the detailed recommendations provided by the consultants are unique to Wichita State University both in terms of specifics of program strengths and weaknesses and in terms of suggested alternatives and solutions, the areas covered in the consultation are of more general applicability. Some of these areas are listed in outline form below as a series of questions that may help other institutions identify potential problem areas. This listing also indicates the scope of the AGHE team consultation in these four areas.

1. **Goals and objectives of the gerontology program.** Are the long-range goals and objectives, and the particular academic perspective, well conceptualized? Are the objectives prioritized? To what extent is the program guided by external forces such as grants and "turf" issues? Are continuing education and inservice training related to the academic program? Have procedures for program review been established?

2. **Gerontology center administration and structure.** Does the academic program director have centralized and exact information on courses and curriculum? To whom should the gerontology center director report? What style of center administration is most appropriate to this university (e.g., collegial approach and assigned responsibilities)? How much is the university committed to the program? What is the scope of center activities? Is the relationship between the academic, research, and community components of the gerontology center well defined?

3. **Faculty.** Is there a planned program for faculty development to counterbalance the program's rapid growth? What is the quality of faculty in terms of previous training and ongoing research efforts? How and to what extent are crucial colleges or schools such as health-related professions involved in the program? How many faculty are needed to meet program objectives? Is every faculty member informed about what the others are doing in both institutional and research activities?

4. **Curriculum.** Are student internships clearly defined in structure and purpose? What are the admission requirements for students? How should courses be sequenced? How are biology of aging courses differentiated from health and physiology courses? Are there adequate library resources to support both academic and research programs?

On a broader level, this consultation provided the university important services of an indirect and nonintentional nature, as should be the case in any good consulting experience. One of the most important benefits came from planning the consultation. In deciding the areas of consultation and whom the consultants should see, we were forced to evaluate what issues were most crucial in our program development and which individuals were essential to the success of the program. Even the process of deciding what written information to send to the consultants helped us to focus our program more clearly. In attempting to provide accurate and complete information to the consulting team, we had to clarify issues, to state our goals, objectives, and policy, and better define our own understanding of the problems in administrative structure and function.

Another of the benefits of the consultation was the open-ended process of information sharing. Informal conversation with the consultation team members about what was going on at their campuses and what techniques had proved beneficial in their programs, although often nondirect and diffuse, was very helpful. Perhaps one of the most important functions performed by the consultants, particularly in the debriefing sessions, was that the consultation forced decision making and clarified commitments. For example, in the final debriefing meeting, answers given by the program director, three deans, and the vice-president for academic affairs to questions from the consultation team leader clarified precisely the thoughts of the university officials. These, in effect, became public-policy commitments. Another important result of any consultation is the often-noted "visiting fireman" phenomenon. The consultants could point out the same problem areas to the central administration that had been previously pointed out by gerontology program faculty, but because the consultants were experts from outside the university and had no vested interest, their opinions carried much greater weight.

The major problems in any consulting experience, including this one, are those of dealing with and defining the internal and external political and pragmatic situations. These problems occur at two levels. The first is to describe adequately and accurately to the consultants the complex relationships that exist externally between the university and such agencies as other institutions of higher education in a state system, the state board of regents, the state agency on aging, and local agencies serving older people, and internally between the various university components—colleges, departments, individual faculty members, and administrators. If the consultants are to provide good advice, they must have this information, but it is difficult to provide it clearly and systematically.

The second level of the problem is the relationship between the ideal model for programs and the reality of the situations in which programs are located. Although in the ideal model one should not be led in program development by outside funding agencies, there is a pragmatic need for outside funding to develop programs. Another ideal model is slow, careful program planning; but the reality is a state-board policy under which the first program developed within the state system often precludes the development of later programs, which are seen as duplication of effort. The AGHE team was cognizant of the pragmatic realities and restraints, and it realized that some of its recommendations would not be followed even though it would be "better" for the program if they were. The friendly and open format the consulting team chose allowed issues such as these to be brought into the open.

Suggestions on the Role of AGHE in Consultation It would be ideal if AGHE could provide to all developing programs the extensive service it provided for Wichita State University, but this is impractical. The almost $3,000 the university provided the association did not come close to meeting the real costs of the time and efforts of the consulting team, particularly those of Hickey. If similar consultation services were provided to only ten institutions per year, it might require the full-time services of a three-person consulting team and a secretary. Obviously, the association does not have the human resources to carry out such a project even if the member institutions could bear the financial burden. There are, however, three possible consulting services the association might provide.

The first of these is a clearinghouse function. The association could maintain a list of possible consultants who would be willing and able to provide consulting services to member institutions for a minimal fee. The association could particularly see that this service is made available to new member institutions and those with new, developing programs. Furthermore, the objectives of the consultation could be more sharply focused than they were at Wichita State. Such areas as continuing education and inservice training for agencies serving the elderly or strategies and techniques for faculty development are broad enough and important enough by themselves to justify consultation. A sharply focused approach to consultation would make it easier for the association to identify resources and would force the institutions seeking consultation to prioritize their goals.

A second suggestion is that the association compile a list of existing resources related to gerontology program development and that it sponsor separate publications or projects dealing with program development in the field of aging. Examples of such existing resources might include such items as the booklet *Developing Educational Programs in the Field of Aging* by Atchley and Seltzer, the resources from the Analysis and Selection of Training Resources in Aging (ASTRA) project at Duke University, and handbooks and training manuals such as those prepared by the Syracuse University and Pennsylvania State University Gerontology Centers, to cite only a few. The AGHE publication *Gerontology in Higher Education: Perspectives and Issues* and the results of the AGHE's Foundations for Establishing Educational Program Standards in Gerontology project are also examples of written materials and projects that the association can provide as an indirect form of consultation. Perhaps the association, in cooperation with such programs as ASTRA, could also develop a packet of resource materials, including bibliographic references that could limit the need for on-site consultations.

A third consultation service the association might provide is specialized workshops, perhaps offered on a regional basis or in conjunction with other organizations. These would have to be carefully organized so that they do not greatly overlap topics covered at the annual AGHE meetings. Such workshops could draw together member institutions with similar concerns in what would be a collaborative consultation. This seems to be the costliest and most complex of the three alternatives suggested.

It does seem important that the association provide some consultation service, particularly to new member institutions. Although I realize the association cannot provide all members with the extensive services that were so beneficial to Wichita State University, I do think that providing consultation is important and the association should proceed with efforts to develop such services.

Reaction of the Association for Gerontology in Higher Education
Tom Hickey

On behalf of the Association for Gerontology in Higher Education, Mildred M. Seltzer, and Maxine L. Patrick, I appreciate the opportunity to review and react to Hays's summary paper on the consultation. It is a clear and accurate statement of the thoughtful and conscientious leadership he has provided for the Wichita State University gerontology program.

It is important to say at the outset that this was a pilot project that would be too costly for the association to replicate for other AGHE member institutions. Moreover, there was undoubtedly a certain amount of charisma in this project, given the extensive communication between the university and the association and the close working relationships the three consultants had before the project itself. This does not suggest that many of the components of the model would not be useful for other programs and institutions. In many ways, the preparation and publication of this summary analysis is in itself a useful communication to other programs.

The consultants' perspectives on the important things that happened at Wichita State University as a result of this project fall into four main areas.

1. **The process of assessment.** The multistep assessment was perhaps the most beneficial aspect of our activities. It served to bring together over a relatively short period of time the university's many and diverse elements necessary for the operation of an effective gerontology program—one that by definition must cut across various academic and administrative units. By this process the faculty and administration focused simultaneously on the larger picture and on its prerequisite component parts.

2. **Planning.** Although the stated objective of this project was assessment and evaluation of the Wichita State University gerontology program, the major activity of all participants was planning. This served two very important purposes. First of all, the program director and faculty were required to carefully plan and specify in advance their individual and programmatic objectives. In effect, they were expected to assign the consultants tasks that would reflect present and future directions at Wichita State. For a program that had developed almost too quickly, this was an important step. It served to clarify and even modify some directions and activities at a time when the overall pace of gerontological activity at the university was such that it almost prevented this important priority. The secondary benefit of the planning was to maximize the role of the consulting team by giving it a well-defined agenda. This was a key factor in assuring that our role was relevant to the university. Had this not taken place, the activities of the consultants would undoubtedly have been more limited in duration and effectiveness, and like some "visiting firemen," we might have succeeded at putting out a few brush fires without laying a solid base for fire prevention.

3. **Establishing priorities.** A great deal of useful time and discussion was

spent on the program priorities that were specified by the faculty and administration. In addition, the consultation project served both to rearrange these priorities and to clarify the steps necessary for implementing them. In several instances, we found that the university personnel had simply not thought through the sequence of objectives, nor their interrelatedness, how long each step should take, and what the campus prerequisites were for some activities. For example, approval for a new master's degree program was important internally for many reasons, not the least of which was the local political context. The task of the consultants was to delineate the necessary faculty development that must precede the implementation of a good graduate program.

Similarly, the consultation team served to restore "the horse before the cart." Responses to funding initiatives or dominant interests of individual faculty must be put into the perspective of the mission and objectives of both the university and the gerontology program. In this regard, the consultation team seemed to serve an important role in reminding the gerontology faculty of its particular urban mission in Wichita.

4. **Implementation.** What happens after the consultants leave? If a report is expected (as in this case), one can choose to read it, use it, ignore it, and/or shelve it. An important component of this project was the debriefing phase, which precluded the last two options. We had to be even more specific about our suggestions—to modify, as well as to defend, where necessary. The Wichita State administration and faculty were in a similar position of telling us what they would now do as a result of the entire process. The debriefing was clearly an essential element in the overall effectiveness of the entire project.

Conclusion Each of Hays's three suggestions to the Association for Gerontology in Higher Education represents in some way an approach that AGHE might take to assist member institutions, especially newly developing programs, to further the growth of gerontology on their campuses. I am pleased to report that these suggestions have been recommended to the executive committee of the association, and I anticipate some development on this during 1978–79. Although the consultation activities themselves may take different forms in the coming years, the substantive directions that have emerged from the AGHE-Wichita State project will serve as an important model.

PART FOUR
THE HUMANITIES AND AGING

The richness and diversity of the processes of aging are expressed in the variety of human endeavors. Like the biological, social, and applied sciences, the humanities offer special consideration of the life of the person. Knowledge of human development and of the human condition comes to us from history, literature, philosophy, and religion. These disciplines instruct and expand our sensitivities.

The viability of gerontology in higher education depends more on the awareness of the diversity of our knowledge than on building self-contained, gerontological curricula.

Introduction: The Humanities and Aging

Aaron Lipman
University of Miami

The various sciences deal primarily with data as interpreted within a special type of conceptual framework. This conceptual framework produces a selective identification of aspects of empirical reality for purposes of description, classification, analysis, and explanation. In the subdivision of educational disciplines, the humanities are distinguishable in methodology, conceptual framework, perspective, and content from the biological, physical, and to a less decisive degree, from the social sciences. C. P. Snow (1964) views those in the humanities as literary intellectuals distinguishable from scientists. He believes that literary intellectuals and scientists are members of two unique cultures, which are increasingly being split into polar groups having no common culture and unable to communicate with each other. Scientists generally know little of the humanities and the humanities generally know little of science.

The reasons for the existence of the dialectical positioning and of the barrier between these two cultures are complex. Some are rooted in the inner dynamics of the different kinds of mental processes and activities required and pursued by the scientists as compared with the literary intellectuals. Some are rooted in the historical development of their disciplines, the presence or absence of value judgments, as well as the different symbols with which they deal.

The literary intellectuals, or nonscientists, have a stereotyped impression about the scientists. The literary intellectual sees the scientist as nonholistic or segmented, as unaware and insensitive to the human condition.

On the other hand, the scientists believe that the literary intellectuals are totally lacking in foresight and are, in a sense, antiscientific, antiquantitative, and thus anti-intellectual.

C. P. Snow believes that the polarization of the two cultures leads us to misinterpret our past and to misjudge the present. The dualism of these cultures could be reconciled through increased communication and interaction between them. Under the rubric of literary intellectuals, one would include such substantive areas listed in this section—religion, philosophy, history, ethics, and literature. Their primary focus is on the peculiarly human and humane aspects of knowledge that give meaning to science and distinguish humans from other beings and the rest of nature. These disciplines signify values, wisdom, inclinations, feelings, and other qualities and characteristics proper and peculiar to humankind. A guiding principle is the primacy of the dignity of the human being that gives meaning to existence. Humanistic knowledge is often viewed as expressive—an end in itself—rather than instrumental—a means to an end.

Partially as a consequence of this instrumentality, the physical, biological, and social scientists have been able to sell the techniques and information of their disciplines to business and government, and thus have entered nonacademic positions more frequently than have those in the humanities. With the economic and enrollment crunch limiting the number of positions in the universities, it has become a challenge to utilize the surplus of humanists with doctoral degrees.

The National Endowment for the Humanities, for example, has recently funded a grant for the business school program at New York University to train and educate people in the humanities in business techniques that might be salable in the business world.

A far better use of the humanist would be to assist in the integration of the humanities into the field of gerontology, for aging is a holistic process. Aging will be comprehended only when its multiple facets—social, physical, biological, medical, and cultural—are synthesized into a fully humanistic totality.

The field of gerontology would benefit from the orientation of the humanist. The humanities are a necessary component of our understanding of the human condition. In science, dealing as we do with both the physical and social areas of aging, all of us have been increasingly confronted with questions that transcend scientific determinations and require assistance from the vantage point peculiar to the humanities. Should human life be prolonged artificially? How important is the quality of the aged life-style? Should the individual or the state decide when a person may die? How are old people treated in historical eras in our own and other cultures? What has been the contribution of the elderly authors? How have older people been portrayed in literature? All of these are questions that are of interest to the gerontologist and geriatrician; for answers we must look to the philosophers, religionists, historians, and literary analysts.

The following papers demonstrate how the integration and utilization of the humanities with the discipline of gerontology can contribute in a sensitive, creative, intellectual, and practical manner and can help reduce the impoverishment created by this cultural divide.

References

Snow, C. P. *The two cultures: And a second look.* London: Cambridge University Press, 1964.

Biblical Mythology and Aging

Gerald A. Larue
University of Southern California

The Bible is probably the single most powerful socio-psycho-religious literary force operating in Western society today. It remains the world's best seller; it is found in many American homes and in the rooms of hotels and motels throughout the nation. Its precepts are administered to millions of people every day and every hour through personal devotions, Bible-study classes and prayer groups, by chaplains, ministers, priests, and rabbis in sermons, in churches, and on radio and television. Popular religious books and pamphlets interpret the Bible and apply its teachings to human life and living.

Religious teachings in the home and in preschool church or synagogue classes initiate conditioning that may continue throughout the life of an individual. Even those who reject Judaism or Christianity as a way of life, or as a guide, are not free from religious influences. Indirect pressures abound in a society that gives token adherence to Judeo-Christian ethics. For example, large newspapers and local community newspapers report extensively on synagogue and church activities; business organizations commercialize religious festivals. It is almost impossible for modern Americans to be untouched by Biblical teachings, which impact in both direct and indirect ways.

Not everyone uses the same Bible. Jews have as their source of guidance what Christians call "The Old Testament"; Christians add "The New Testament"; and Roman Catholic and Eastern Orthodox Christians include portions of what Jews and Protestants call "The Apocrypha." No matter which Bible one uses, the contents, which consist of selected literature from Hebrew-Jewish-Christian communities, were gathered, composed, compiled, and edited between the tenth century B.C. and the second century A.D., or between the time of the reign of Solomon and the establishment of Christianity as a separate religion. In other words, the primary source material is between 2,000 and 3,000 years old and reflects mind sets and life styles from another-time-and-place world.

Biblical literature can be labeled generally mythic. Myth, a term derived from the Greek *muthos*, originally meant "the word spoken," "the tale told." In classical usage, it designates literature in which divine beings (gods or goddesses, or a single god or goddess) play primary roles, in terms of interaction not only on a superhuman level but in the world of humans, also. Like other mythic literature, the Bible establishes limits, sets standards, defines roles, and explicates relationships (Larue, 1975).

Biblical literature, promulgated by the cult as divinely revealed or inspired or divinely authoritative, contributes both directly and indirectly to the formulation of concepts about the nature of the universe, an individual's place in the world, the meaning of existence, patterns for living individually and societally, and attitudes toward birth, aging, and death. As the central interpreter of the myth, the cult, by its very organization as an institution, is conservative and, at the same time, immensely powerful. The influence exerted by cult and myth may be positive, life-affirming, and nourishing, or it may be negative, life-denying, and toxic. Where cult and myth combine to enable individuals to achieve inner psychic balance or harmony or peace, or a sense of self-actualization as well as adjustment to societal situations, the cult and myth may be said to be exercising nourishing influences. Where the cult and myth serve to create inner tensions, feelings of guilt or despondency, where they develop social estrangement, disharmony, and social disease, they may be said to be toxic.

In discussing myth and mythic, we go far beyond the early Greek meaning of the term as something spoken and recognize the classical association of *muthos* with *dramaena*, which involves the interpretation, the dramatization, and the expansion of the myth. Hence, it is not only through the written Bible that mythic influences become conditioning factors in individual life and in society, but also through rites, through festal observances that are both private and public, extending from baptism, bar mitzvah, marriage, and funerals to Hanukkah, Christmas, Easter, and Passover. Moreover, the place world is spotted with cultic symbols that recall, remind, or point to the mythic traditions.

In relating Biblical mythology to aging, I think of aging both as a process—the process of aging that begins at birth—and, with reference to the aged, as a condition—those who have grown old. The term *aging* is, therefore, fluid.

The Work Ethic and Retirement

The earliest cosmological myth in the Bible begins in Chapter 2 of Genesis, verse 4, and ends with Chapter 3, verse 24. This myth was recorded as temple literature during the reign of Solomon in the tenth century B.C. It tells how humans rose above the animal state by eating of the tree of knowledge of good and evil and how, because they had expressed individuality and had not blindly obeyed divine rules, they lost their positions as gardeners for the Hebrew god, Yahweh. They were expelled from Eden lest they eat also of the tree of life and acquire immortality and thereby become divine. They were cursed by the god to labor to survive. The function of the male is defined agriculturally; he is to till the soil, battling against a hostile nature that attempts to produce weeds rather than life-sustaining foods. The female bears children in pain and is to be subservient to her husband. The myth establishes roles and destinies. For woman not to bear children is to fail to fulfill divinely ordained destiny (one need only check through Biblical literature and much religious literature written since the Bible to see how this edict has functioned in human life). For man, not to work is to be a failure, to function in ways that are other than those ordained by the god "in the beginning."

In one of my classes, a 20-year-old woman expressed her convictions that if people don't work they should be allowed to perish. She, a very "religious" person, has accepted the Biblical work ethic—for others and for herself.

To work is to be in process of fulfilling destiny and to be meaningful in the divine scheme of things. Not to work is not to be fulfilling destiny and to be meaningless. The guilt potentials are great, and guilt can be anything but nourishing or life-enhancing.

Biblical Mythology and Life Span

Biblical mythology establishes the human life span as a divine "given." As one psalmist put it: Our life span is 70 years, or, if heaven decrees, 80 (Ps. 90:10). The length of life is determined by "heaven." Good persons, according to most Biblical thought, died old. Longevity was a gift of God. Heroes of the faith, such as Moses, Abraham, and the patriarchs, lived to be over 100. But heroes are models and assume a removed-from-real-life dimension in terms of their faith and their personal, intimate contact with the deity. (Post-Eden and pre-flood figures lived hundreds of years, but because their characters are never developed, they play no hero roles. It is generally assumed that the excessive life-span motif was a literary device to cover long periods of time about which nothing was known and to separate cosmological beginnings from historical time. See Gen. 5.) In actuality, the death rate appears to have been high in ancient times. Those who enjoyed old age were the hardiest and the fortunate and were assumed to be blessed.

The mythic cliché that the good died old was, of course, not always the experience of the community. Some deemed to be good died young; some considered to be wicked died old. These contradictory experiences raised the issue of theodicy—the justice of God. The myth proclaimed the goodness of God and postulated divine rewards and punishments on the basis of adherence to divinely revealed regulations and mores. Where was God when the wicked thrived and lived to a ripe old age and the good died young?

Answers to theodicy varied in different historical periods. At one time it was taught that the sins of the father could burden the children for generations (Exod. 20:5). If a wicked father lived to a ripe old age, his children or grandchildren could suffer for his evil and might be short-lived. Another answer argued that each person suffered from personal sins, but obviously that did not work out in reality (Ezek. 18). Still another implied that humans could not know what went on in the mind of God. When ill fortune befell the faithful, all one could do was keep the faith in the hope that the god would act in accordance with mythic assumptions (Job). As belief in afterlife developed, rewards for goodness and punishment for evil were projected into an afterworld. (See Daniel, Chapter 12, in the Old Testament. The New Testament reflects the mythic assumption of life after death throughout.) But no matter in what historical period particularistic mythic assumptions developed, longevity and health were among the rewards for goodness.

These mythic assumptions placed burdens of guilt on believers and yielded tremendous power to the state and the cult as arbiters and interpreters of mythic presuppositions. What happened to the individual psyche was of little concern and seldom surfaced except in writings such as Job.

Two toxic results can be related to mythic assumptions about life span. The first is the current attitude that once people are past 35 or 40 they are on the "down slope" or "over the hump." One of my colleagues, who sees himself as a scientist, maintains that if a scientist hasn't made it by age 30, there is little hope that any important scientific findings will come from that person. During the late 1960s, some youths believed that after the age of 25 individuals had nothing to communicate to younger persons. I recall from 1968 the trauma with which one of the protestors approached 25. Five years later, he was even more disheartened about reaching 30. A neighbor woman is convinced she is past her prime at 43. Our youth-oriented society has swallowed the life-span myth, has determined middle points, and has associated with various age groups relatively fixed patterns of conduct and activity. Assumptions concerning the attitudes, tastes, and behavior patterns of different age groupings have been capitalized upon by advertisers. Colorful pronouncements on billboards, television, radio, and in magazines and newspapers reinforce the stereotypes, and even induce persons in specific age groups to accept these determinants of what is normal, proper, suitable, or acceptable in everything from food and clothing to activities.

Another toxic effect of the life-span myth relates to beliefs in rewards and punishments in the afterworld. Personal responsibility for what happens after death tends to produce feelings of guilt, fear, and doubt in the minds of some. There may be those who long for death and the joys of heaven: but in my limited experience, people who express such longings are caught in impossible human situations—heaven becomes an escape to that which can only be better. They are confident that their misery in this present time guarantees joy in the next world. Often those concerned with rewards and punishments in the world after death become occupied increasingly with cult-approved activities that guarantee blessings. In my own family, my Roman Catholic father's concern with what his fate after death might be occupied him increasingly as he aged, prompting my brother to comment that he "worked like hell to stay out of purgatory."

Biblical Mythology and Respect for Elders

What was, perhaps, a most nourishing societal mythic emphasis within the Bible, so far as the aged are concerned, has become a fading mythic pattern within our culture. Much Biblical thinking de-emphasizes individuality and stresses the corporate nature of the group. Individuals achieved identity by membership within a larger whole—a concept of psychic unity that has been labeled "corporate personality" (Larue, 1970). In such a societal structure, what happened to one happened to all; what happened to the group affected each member. The group, therefore, was conceived of as having a personality of its own, and the individual was recognzied and evaluated as a member of the group. Injury to or killing of one was loss of the strength and the life of the group and called for retaliation. Nor did the group exist only in present time, but its identity stretched backward to progenitors and forward into the future. What ancestors did affected the well-being of the unit. The sins of the fathers could be punished in the descendants to the third and fourth generation. What an individual or group suffered now could be punishment for the actions of a previous generation (Deut. 5:9).

The close-knit nature of the group in ancient society placed responsibilities for mutual protection and care on members. Widows, orphans, the aged were to be cared for. The closer the relationship, the greater the responsibility.

Biblical legislation assumed mythic overtones because the laws were believed to be god-given. The Torah demanded of individuals: "Honor your father and mother." A promise or threat accompanied the statement: "that your days may be lengthened and it may go well with you in the land Yahweh, your god, gives you" (Deut. 5:16).

In the royal wisdom schools eatablished in the Solomonic and subsequent courts (as they were in royal precincts in other nations), instructors were wise old men. Their teachings reflected not only mythic authority of divinely revealed insights and rules but also knowledge based on practical experience and reflection. The instructors became as parents to their pupils: "My son, heed your father's instruction and don't reject your mother's teaching" (Prov. 1:8); "If a person curses his father and mother, his lamp will be put out in utter darkness" (Prov. 20:20); "Listen to your father who begot you, and do not despise your mother when she is old" (Prov. 23:22).

Joshua ben Sirah, who had a wisdom school in Jerusalem during the second century B.C., counseled his pupils as follows:

Listen to me your father, children;
and act accordingly, that you may be kept in safety.
For the Lord honored the father above the children,
and he confirmed the right of the mother over her sons.
Whoever honors his father atones for sins,
and whoever glorifies his mother is like one who lays up treasure.
Whoever honors his father will be gladdened by his own children,
and when he prays he will be heard.
Whoever glorifies his father will have long life,

and whoever obeys the Lord will refresh his mother;
he will serve his parents as his masters.
Honor your father by word and deed,
that a blessing from him may come upon you.
For a father's blessing strengthens the houses of the children,
but a mother's curse uproots their foundations.
Do not glorify yourself by dishonoring your father,
for your father's dishonor is no glory to you.
For a man's glory comes from honoring his father,
and it is a disgrace for children not to respect their mother.
O son, help your father in his old age,
and do not grieve him as long as he lives;
even if he is lacking in understanding, show forbearance;
in all your strength do not despise him.
For kindness to a father will not be forgotten,
and against your sins it will be credited to you:
in the day of your affliction it will be remembered in your favor;
as frost in fair weather, your sins will melt away.
Whoever forsakes his father is like a blasphemer,
and whoever angers his mother is cursed by the Lord.

In local villages, issues affecting the community were judged by elders, who met in the gate area. These older men were repositories of experience, wisdom, law, principle, and norms for the group. They were living storehouses of group history. They were honored and respected. For much of the Hebrew period, parents had absolute control over the life and death of their children, and local elders assumed this same responsibility for persons in issues affecting the well-being of the community. Old men were persons of importance and power.

Except in some Muslim communities where old customs prevail, these ancient Semitic patterns, despite their presence in the Bible, have faded from our way of life. In some areas of the contemporary Middle East, where modern Western values have not penetrated too deeply, parents and grandparents are accorded love, respect, honor, authority, and protection much as they were in the ancient Near East.

In our Western world, the extended family is no longer the norm, and the role of older persons has changed. Elders are no longer viewed as repositories of wisdom; they cannot compete with libraries, photo records, news reports, history courses, and so forth. Rapid technological changes and new knowledge have turned our thinking away from the wisdom of experience to innovation, change, productivity and profit. Margaret Mead (1970) has pointed out that the 80-year-olds have "traversed the greatest and most rapid change the world has ever known . . . have crossed more boundaries more successfully and learned to live with more funny kinds of things and more strange people they never dreamed of meeting than have the young." Despite the demonstrated flexibility of older persons, they have been overtaken by a work ethic that denies identity when they cease to be involved in production, when they cease to be wage earners, or when their retirement funds are inadequate for full, free living and they become powerless. Many are segregated in communities of the aged or in "rest homes" that become final resting places. Poverty, loneliness, numb existence, confinement within institutional premises, bland foods, sedation, and lack of interest or lack of encouragement in maintaining physical health ossify inmates physically, mentally, and spiritually until merciful death relieves them of their meaningless, dependent, unwanted existence. These old persons, having lost any semblance of human dignity, recognize themselves as burdens and know that they are tolerated because they are alive in a society that forbids killing. They do the only thing they can do—exist.

The old myth does not function any longer in any significant way. We are no longer where we once were. We have abandoned concepts of corporate personality, of respect for elders and the wisdom they have accumulated. We do not honor them for having lived and for having contributed to human life and growth. We have surrendered our responsibility for them to the city, county, state, nation.

One positive ripple in the sea of negatives, one small response revealing respect for the aged, has occurred in the search for identity among some youth. For them, identity has assumed a meaning larger than "Who am I at this moment?" and includes "What are my antecedents?" "Who are my parents and grandparents?" The result has been a probe into backgrounds. Long, tape-recorded conversations with parents, grandparents, and older relatives have mined repositories of family history, family thinking, attitudes, and life styles that give uniqueness to the group and the individual. Old family documents have been unearthed, love letters and photographs rescued from nearly forgotten hiding places. The results, in instances where I have been involved, have been growth in love, respect, and understanding between generations and the enhancement of the role of the elders, who became accepted and respected for their unique experiences and for the ways in which they had moved from the world of their youth into the world of present youth—and kept their balance (Larue, 1976).

But this is only a small ripple.

Potentials for a New Mythic Emphasis and a New Ethic for Aging

In calling for a new mythic emphasis and a new ethical stress, I assume that the cult and the Biblical myth will be with us for a long time. I assume also that the influence of the cult and the myth will continue to permeate society and affect life patterns directly and indirectly. The suggestions I make can have meaning for noncult members, for those who reject Biblical mythology—they need only be removed from their mythic or Biblical setting. I assume also that just as in the past, the organized cult has discovered in the Bible mythic support for whatever causes it has embraced (both for and against war, for and against slavery, for or against asceticism or social action or whatever), so now the cult may need to discover Biblical prooftexts to lend mythic support to the ethic I propose.

I believe we must move away from emphasis on the work ethic to the development of a life ethic. For some people at retirement age, it may be too late to begin. The education must begin now with little children, with youth groups, with young and middle and older persons—it must span varying age groups. The training must be in self-actualization, in potentials for self-fulfilling adventures, in discovering meaning not only in work, employment, and tasks, but in the rich possibilities of life. Dreams, visions, hopes need not be projected to the future, to retirement; their realization begins now. The key is simply that life is more important than work and that life is more than existence.

For many older people life is dull and boring because life for these people has always been dull and boring. Apart from employment, they developed few interests, experienced few adventures, embarked on no voyages of discovery. I counsel continually with youths and adults whose existence is a continuum of dull, wasted moments. It is no surprise to me that there are so many frustrated retired old people since there are so many frustrated young people.

Simply because Biblical cosmological myths reinforced by Biblical societal myths project the image of humans destined to survive by working, there is no need to limit life to work alone. A Biblical writer, whose advice is generally ignored, counseled: "I commend enjoyment, for man has no good thing under the sun but to eat and drink and enjoy himself, for this will go with him through his toil through the days of life which God gives him under the sun" (Eccles. 8:15). He says further: "Light is sweet, and it is pleasant for the eyes to behold the sun. For if a man lives many years, let him rejoice in them all; but let him remember that the days of darkness will be many. . . . Rejoice, O young man, in your youth, let your heart cheer you in the days of your youth; walk in the ways of your heart and the sight of your eyes" (Eccles. 11:7–9).

Admittedly these texts are lifted out of a total context of a writing which, like the black humor of today, finds existence meaningless. Nevertheless, the quotation reflects the writer's option to the work ethic and to the simplistic play ethic and invites involvement in what one wants to do, in what brings satisfaction and joy and meaning—now. This implies a rejection of the hypothesis that there are social oughts that must be obeyed even if they force one into someone else's preconceived ideal mold.

The life ethic calls for accepting individuals as wholes, as entities in themselves, and for diminishing emphasis on age, class, and status groupings. Personhood is more significant than year of birth, income, or social rank.

We exist in a category-happy society. We succumb to labels and social stereotypes projected by those who find it simpler to treat persons as members of groups expected to perform in certain fixed ways rather than as individuals who have had varying life experiences that have made them uniquely different from every other living person. Jesus, in the so-called Sermon on the Mount, emphasizes individual uniqueness (Matt. 6:25–30). The same emphasis can be found in modern science, which enables us to realize that each individual is the end product of the four-and-a-half billion years of evolution of our solar system, and that with our individual DNA plus our unique life experiences we can never be duplicated or replaced.

The life ethic calls for greater emphasis on human potentials and less on human limitations. In other words, the list of "Thou shalts" and "Thou shalt nots" can be replaced by an emphasis on "You may, providing you do not injure or infringe on the rights of others." It calls for more emphasis on the varied ways of experiencing life and less emphasis on sin and guilt for violation of concepts that may have been useful in a Palestinian or Mediterranean setting some 2,000 to 3,000 years ago. It suggests that less heed be paid to rules that inhibit and produce guilt and that more importance be given to possibilities for self-awareness and self-realization.

The new ethic encourages investigation of aging as a process that begins at birth, and of death as an event that can occur at any moment. This emphasis is one that I find particularly important in classes in death and dying and in counseling with those facing their own or another's death. One basic question is, "How do I live the time between now and the time of my death, which can come at any moment?" Another is, "How do I treat those about me in the time between this moment and their death?" Responses to these questions can have a great deal to contribute in determining philosophy of life and patterns of living. Life can be interpreted as a cup to be drained rather than as a measure to be filled.

The new ethic calls for emphasis on the explosive potentials of each moment as we move from space to space, recognizing that each change in state or position or role is alive with creative possibilities. The trend is not simply to move away from goal orientation, but to underscore possibility orientation.

Finally, we should look again at the standard retirement age and the waste of human potential. Perhaps this suggestion also involves a consideration of the redistribution of wealth. To live with dignity invites involvement in creative exploration, in exploitation of one's own potentials. This may sound like a return to the work ethic, but some of us are engaged in expanding the frontiers of life and living, and this is exciting, energizing, life-sustaining. For those who wish to retire, there should be ample resources to permit individuals to live with dignity as befitting persons who Biblical myth proclaims were formed in the image and likeness of the deity.

The life ethic is idealistic. But there is a tide flowing at this moment affecting the attitudes of young and old and of some psychologists, humanists, and religionists. It seems to me that gerontologists and humanists can cooperate in establishing new attitudinal watermarks.

References

Larue, G. A. *Ancient myth and modern man.* Englewood Cliffs, N.J.: Prentice-Hall, 1975.

Larue, G. A. *Old testament life and literature*. Boston: Allyn and Bacon, 1970.

Larue, G. A. "Religion and the aged." In I. M. Burnside (Ed.), *Nursing and the aged*. New York: McGraw-Hill, 1976, 573–583.

Mead, M. The cultural shaping of the ethical situation. In Kenneth Vaux (Ed.), *Who shall live?* Philadelphia: Fortress Press, 1970.

Philosophy and Aging

Cyril P. Svoboda
University of Maryland

Prejudices against old age are many and long standing. Though attempts have been made in literature, education, or government to combat these prejudices, they have met with little success. It is this author's contention that ageism continues to exist because countermeasures have been overly practical, without sufficient theoretical base. Neither education, feeding, housing, nor caring for the elderly can occur devoid of theory. One's theory about old age will determine, for example, not only if and why we supply aid but also what aid is given and how we deliver it. Practices flow from theory or the lack thereof.

Our current interest in gerontology and in the problems of the elderly is not unique. Throughout history, people have been concerned with senescence. What has differed is the approach taken by individuals. In the earliest stages of our civilization, humankind employed myth and ritual to give explanation to the puzzles of life. The Greco-Roman philosophers emphasized reasoning. Plato (*Republic*, Book X) stressed the superiority of the philosopher's rational argument as a means of solving life's problems. Still later, answers to questions were sought through the empirical approach: the scientist's experiment. The latter methodology prevails today in the study of old age, in suggesting "what it all means." Thus, little attention is paid to the philosophical approach, which preceded and, to some degree, forms the underpinning for today's science.

Since human beings have searched for truth for more than 20 centuries by primarily employing reason, we could expect this particular approach to have great impact in forming our civilization's concepts and associated attitudes concerning the major issues of life. For this reason, we should look at what philosophy has to say about old age.

This paper argues that the source of meaning and attitude concerning old age in our civilization is found in the writings of the philosophers. Representatives of the ancient, medieval, modern, and contemporary eras are surveyed and their ideas presented in four main categories: concept of old age, the character of the elderly, the capabilities of the elderly, and the social role of the elderly.

As one reads through the philosophers to locate their specific remarks concerning old age, one realizes that they used various terms: *old age, the aged, the elderly, age*, and *old man/woman.* It is impossible to know why so many different terms were used. Perhaps the proliferation of terms reflects that old age was not seen as an important enough problem to merit effort in concept formation. Yet a search of ten recently published books on aging forced this author to conclude that contemporary gerontologists speak with similar imprecision.

Both philosophers and gerontologists have difficulty in defining old age, in setting parameters for old age (When does it begin? or How is it characterized?), and in determining which behavioral changes in the elderly are age related and which are illness related. This author suggests that failure to distinguish old age from disease is one of the causes of our negative feelings for old age. If the two terms are not kept separate and distinct, the fear and repulsion that most feel for disease could be felt for old age.

Ancient Philosophers

Concept of Old Age Plato[1] argued that between youth and age each individual undergoes "a perpetual process of loss and reparation" until such time, in old age, as the "body begins to fail." Evidently, according to Plato, the aged human body is not able to repair the constant losses and eventually becomes "an old, worn-out mortality." Aristotle[1] maintained that heat is the necessary condition for a vigorous human body and that old age is a time when the body begins to lose its heat. As its heat is dissipated, he believed, the body begins to dry out, the skin of the eye becomes thicker (thus vision is impaired), and hair grows coarser.

Plato[2] noted that old age is a time when the body is "overcome and decays," concluding that old age is the curse of every animal. In his theory, Plato believed that the material body traps and encumbers the spiritual soul. He seemed to despair that in old age the soul is even further burdened by the deteriorating body. For Aristotle[2] it was natural for the body to reach its prime around age 35 and to "advance" until about age 50. At this very point when the soul finally reaches its perfection, he noted that the body begins to decline. A more idealistic picture of old age was given by Seneca[1]: it is "natural" and "good," a time in which there is "no falling away."

Nevertheless, the attitudes associated with old age in the ancient mind were generally negative. Cicero[1] staunchly maintained that the opinions commonly held about old age are nothing more than "prejudices," but even he had to admit that most people "hate" it. The elderly, Plato[3] suggested, should make use of wine "to lighten the sourness of old age." Aristotle[3] mused that "happiness in old age is the coming of old age slowly and painlessly" and that joy depends on the "excellence of one's body and good luck." Painful is the old age, he was certain, that comes to a person too early or too tardily; it is to be avoided if at all possible.

Character of the Elderly Plato[2] used gentle terms to describe the psychological condition of the elderly. He said that old age brings "an immense peace and liberation"; the elderly undergo a "greater modification of character," which "increases the honor and respect due to them." The elderly find great "pleasure and charm in conversation" and turn their backs on the activities of the young. Aristotle[3] countered the idea of the tempering effect of age. He asserted that the self-controlled character of the aged is merely an illusion: "the fact is that their passions have slackened and they are slaves to the love of gain." According to him, only in the prime of life are the "excesses or defects" of both the young and the aged "replaced by moderation and fitness."

A whole chapter of Aristotle's *Rhetoric* is devoted to a description of the character of the elderly. The picture he painted could hardly be more scathing or negative. He advised the novice orator to adapt his speech to the character of the audience; if the audience is elderly, the orator should be mindful that they are apt to be "cynical," "distrustful and therefore suspicious of evil," "small-minded," "not generous," and "cowardly . . . always anticipating danger." Since Aristotle believed that the elderly are constantly on guard, he concluded that "they are too fond of themselves," "more utilitarian and less noble," certainly "not shy but shameless rather," that they lack "confidence in the future," and therefore they "live by memory rather than by hope." The elderly, he decided, are loquacious and "given to sudden but feeble fits of anger"; they may feel pity, but only "out of weakness," not out of kindness. Since they, as Aristotle wrote, "guide their lives by reasoning more than by moral feeling," the elderly feeling pity actually are selfishly imagining that what has happened to someone else could easily happen to them.

Lucretius[1] echoed many of the same sentiments: "The whole nature of the soul is dissolved, like smoke; just as the body is liable to violent diseases and severe pain, so is the mind to sharp cares and grief and fear." Cicero[1] called old age "an intolerable state," but Seneca[1] waxed idyllic, proclaiming that the elderly no longer feel the need for pleasure; since their souls have "no great commerce with their bodies," they "burgeon" during this time of life. This runs counter to Aristotle's[2] contention that age is a process "blunting the mind." Because of this dulling effect, sensations must be strong to make an impression on the elderly and beauty must be deep "to free man from the deformities of old age." Lucretius[1] agreed that with age the body is "shattered" and "the frame has drooped with its forces dulled." Nevertheless, Aristotle[2] maintained that the "wise" old person "can bear all vicissitudes with greatness of soul." Plato[4] felt that the elderly are to be envied for the way they face life's final vicissitude: the death of old age "is the easiest of deaths . . . accompanied with pleasure rather than with pain."

Capabilities of the Elderly The early philosophers neatly dichotomized subjects that they studied. The world was seen to be composed of a world of ideas and a world of matter; individual objects comprised coprinciples of matter and form; humankind was a combination of body and mind. In old age the powers of mind and body were both affected. Plato[2] felt that the elderly lose the ability to enjoy physical pleasure. He complained that because of old age, a person grows weak and "can hardly get to the city." His advice was that when the elderly begin to fail, they should be allowed to "range at will and engage in no serious labor." Even the guardians, his philosopher-kings, reach a time when they should be freed of their duties, so that they can "raise the eye of the soul to the universal light which lightens all things and behold the absolute good."

Aristotle[3] attributed an "inherent slowness" to old age, which was due to the loss of the body's vital heat. Given that loss, the elderly males procreate female rather than male children: the homunculus contained in the sperm of an old man does not possess sufficient body heat to develop into anything better than a female! The reason for their failing sexual potency is to be found, he believed[5], in the fact that the elderly "do not sufficiently concoct their food." The loss of powers in old age extends[6] even to the arts: "The old, who have lost their powers, cannot very well sing the high-strung modes, and nature herself seems to suggest that their songs should be of the more relaxed kind."

Cognitive powers are also affected by old age. Plato[5] complained that the elderly do not easily "tolerate distractions" and cannot remember as they once could. He wrote[6] that the elderly are "too old to learn" and that they "can no longer improve." Aristotle[7] explained that, in comparison to children, adults are obviously superior in learning and in forming judgments because they are "less restless" and not so much in motion. But the elderly find themselves too much at rest; they are thought by Aristotle,[3] "too slow." Their defective memories and other mental processes are caused by their decaying bodies. Separating mind and body, Aristotle[4] argued that deficiencies are to be found in the mind's vehicle, not in the mind itself, "as occurs in drunkenness or disease." Just as when the effects of alcohol or illness are gone, the mind is found to be fully functioning, so, he thought, would it be for the elderly. If the blunting effects of old age could pass, an old person would be found to have a mind with undiminished powers, since "mind itself is impassible." Lucretius[1] held a different position: "The mastering might of time causes the intellect to halt, the tongue to dote, and the mind to give way, all faculties fail and are found wanting at the same time . . . worn out with age."

Social Role of the Elderly Plato[2] felt that the elderly should be given a position free of the burden of "serious labor." Thus freed, they were expected to be happy and concerned only with "seeking knowledge," "contradicting for the sake of amusement," and "assuring happiness in another life." Aristotle[8] argued that just as freedom from pain is more desirable in old age because it is of greater consequence at that time, so, too, prudence is more to be expected in the elderly because it is then of greater consequence: "No man chooses the young to guide him, because he does not expect them to be prudent." Thus, the elderly are expected to be prudent because they are to be the guides of the young. Indeed, the young are seen by Aristotle[2] to seek objects of passion (action), whereas the elderly "seek knowledge." "Nature herself," he wrote,[6] "has provided the distinction . . . between old and young . . . (in that) she fitted the one to govern and the other to be governed."

Medieval Philosophers

Concept of Old Age Roger Bacon[1] regarded old age as a disease, the effects of which could be mitigated with proper hygienic care. Little else was said of the process of aging during the Middle Ages, perhaps because few individuals survived to any age that could be called "elderly." Montaigne[1] steered clear of the argument whether the body or the mind brings about "the decrepit age of man." He assured his readers that he has seen enough individuals who "got a weakness in their brains before either in their legs or stomach."

Character of the Elderly Machiavelli[1] felt that certain emotions were out of character in the elderly. For instance, he advised that gallantry toward women should be left to the young for "love is revolting in the old." Aquinas[1] reflected Aristotle's ideas concerning the elderly: they are lacking in hope, because of the experiences they have endured. The bitterness found in so many of the aged was, he believed, due to the "many evils that have befallen them." Machiavelli[2] reasoned that luck, like a woman, favored youth rather than age, because the young are less cautious, more violent, and more audacious than the aged.

Capabilities of the Elderly In *The Coming of Age*, de Beauvoir[1] asserted that the Middle Ages, because of its emulation of the vigorous human body, despised the bodily condition of the elderly. Erasmus[1] praised those few aged individuals he knew who were not "wrinkled," "white-haired," "spectacled," and "sallow." Twice Aquinas[1] cites Aristotle as his authority for asserting that "the powers of the sensitive soul are neither weakened nor corrupted when the body becomes weak" in old age. Thus, only bodily powers deteriorate with age; mental powers remain unchanged in themselves, though heavily encumbered by the condition of the body in which they reside.

Social Role of the Elderly There is nothing to report under this topic. None of the philosophers surveyed spoke about the social rights, duties, or position of the elderly. Certainly little was said; perhaps little needed to be said because the elderly were too few to merit concern.

Modern Philosophers

Concept of Old Age Rousseau[1] felt that old age is the "illness which can least be alleviated by human aid." From his viewpoint, old age is a time of infirmity when a person is faced with formidable foes, "illness of every kind." For Hegel[1] the old age of the spirit must be contrasted with that of material nature: the former is a time of perfect maturity and strength, while the latter is characterized by weakness. In his view, matter is a mere exteriorization, a frozen instant, of the constantly perfecting spirit. Any moment of the spirit's development contains its whole past, through which it was brought to this point and which points toward a more perfect future. Seen this way, the old age of spirit could be a time when the highest peak of perfection was reached, a time very different from that of one's material old age. Rousseau[2] referred to old age as the decline of an "innocent, yet innocent life." John Stuart Mill[1] saw aging as a time of ravaging, when the "freshness of youth and curiosity" withers. Rousseau[2] spoke of the soul sinking, being "clogged and darkened by the body," and of "the spirit of life . . . little by little going out." Hegel[1] likened old age to a "watch winding down," a time when "customary life comes to an end."

Character of the Elderly Hume[1] stated that aging brings about a "gradual change of our sentiments and inclinations," which gives rise to the general "maxims which prevail in the different ages of human life." Rousseau[2] analyzed the "sentiments and inclinations" of old age as "a mixture of sad and gentle feelings." In his eyes, the aged individual possessed a "heart still full of eager sensibilities" and a "spirit still adorned with flowers."

In speaking of the temperament of the elderly, Schopenhauer[1] felt that the "old lack the appetite for activity."

Schopenhauer[1] was especially concerned with the psychological condition of the elderly. He maintained a generally negative view of human effort and purpose, calling it all useless vanity. For him, old age is a time when the elderly lose the illusions of youth that "gave life its charm and spurred on our activity." Free of these illusions, the "burden of life is lightened" in old age. Yet this does not result in the elderly turning their gaze to some "universal light," as suggested by Plato. Instead, the world of the elderly "becomes dreary and faded," and they find themselves "condemned to boredom."

When modern philosophers considered the behavior of the elderly as a reflection of their condition, they gave quite different reports. Whereas Hegel[1] felt that "aging made men more tolerant" and understanding, Rousseau[2] noted that the aged "cling to life and leave it with less good will, a poorer grace" than do the young. Schopenhauer[1] granted that the elderly only partially agree with his view of life. They "more or less" become convinced of the emptiness of everything in life; "yet most people turn into automata. For them, old age is no more than the *caput mortuum* of life."

Capabilities of the Elderly Rousseau[1] reported briefly on the physical capabilities of the elderly. They had "less need for food," though this was probably the result of being "less able to provide it." In addition, he observed that the elderly "were less active and perspired little." He concluded that with advanced age "a lukewarm weariness drains the faculties of their strength."

Schopenhauer[1] seems to have argued more from a consideration of what ought to happen in old age than of what does happen to the elderly. He asserts that as we grow old the discovery of the vanity of all vanities gives us an "intellectual calmness," which is the sine qua non for happiness. Hegel[1] spoke of a general "ripeness of judgment" in the elderly brought about by "the grave experience of life," which leads them "to perceive the substantial, solid worth of the object in question." In *The Coming of Age*, de Beauvoir presented Darwin as an old man realizing that his memory has become quite selective: Ideas that ran counter to his beliefs vanished from recollection much more easily than those that agreed with his ideas.

Rousseau[2] was concerned not so much with the powers of intellection as with the faculty of imagination. As a person grows older, Rousseau believed, the "imagination is less vivid," that it "no longer glows." There results a gradual termination of creativity: the imagination of the elderly "no longer has the strength to launch itself" on creative ventures. Even an old person's dreams were "less intoxicating."

Social Role of the Elderly Schopenhauer[1] believes that the ideal man of advanced age becomes convinced of the worthlessness of the world around him. With this conviction, his personal worth becomes "of more value to him." Locke[1] was concerned more with the social rights and privileges of the aged. He felt that "age . . . may give men a just precedency," without ever putting a "scepter into the father's hand." Locke argues that although the aged have no sovereign power of commanding, they do have a claim on "that honor and respect, support and defense, and whatsoever gratitude can oblige a son to." Quite apart from filial relationships, he concluded that "a man may owe honor and respect to an ancient or wise man."

Adam Smith[1] felt that old age gives an individual a certain "superiority": "An old man, provided his age is not so far advanced as to give suspicion of dotage, is everywhere more respected than a young man of equal rank, fortune, and abilities." He gives examples of how age is the "sole foundation of rank and precedency" both among preliterate societies and "the most opulent and civilized nations," concluding: "Age is a plain and palpable quality which admits of no dispute."

Contemporary Philosophers

Concept of Old Age With relatively little development in the meaning of and attitudes toward old age, contemporary philosophers seem to echo familiar sentiments. William James[1] described how the elderly gradually slip into such automatic routine that eventually their "years grow hollow and collapse." Proust[1] suggested that the elderly are merely living what they were, that the behavior patterns of youth are carried forward to old age. Camus[1] concurred.

For him, the past prepares one for the future. However, Sartre[1] seemed to disagree with such unidirectional thrust. He mentioned that age does not lead to ever greater perfection and certainly not to any summit. Instead, throughout life we learn and forget, become enriched and impoverished. He asserted[2] that old age belongs in a category of "unrealizable" projects, an attempt to have a full, inward experience of something that is beyond or outside of one's life. For him[1] the old are defined more by *exis* than by *praxis*, by being rather than by doing. If we achieve "objectification" (and thus realization) by our actions and if, when elderly, we are limited to being rather than doing, then old age is, indeed, an unrealizable project.

Character of the Elderly Freud[1] only obliquely mentioned old age, while commenting on a colleague's statement that "traces of a primitive *oral* phase of development survive in the sexual life of later years." Sartre[1] felt that the elderly bear the burden of the reification of the past, what he called the "practico-inert." From this point of view, the elderly have recognized that the present can have no meaning, for theirs is a "solidarity with the past."

Proust[1] felt that old age marks a drastic change in the character of the aged. Whereas the aged were formerly concerned with activity and with others, he and Gide[1] believed that they now become constantly distracted by their deteriorating "bodily condition." To Gide, the body, which had been a trusted vehicle to be taken for granted, had lately become "a hindrance." Old age seems to him to consist of "a plethora of little indispositions," which makes these last years of life "a wretched time." Adjectives used by Gide to describe old age drive home the depressive wretchedness of the state: It is last, slow, past, repetitious—it is the end. Ineffectual, the elderly have "a desire to create," but find themselves "unable." They reach for wisdom, but find some ersatz substitute derived by "weariness or loss of warmth," and this is "despised." The spirit "falls into boredom when it has no goal": the spirit of the elderly becomes a "prey to leisure."

Characteristically, Sartre[2] maintained that the elderly suffer "an identification crisis" in that the feedback they receive from the world tells them what they have not yet experienced: that they are old. Gide[1] reported that as he grows old he becomes aware of "a narrowing of interests, powers, and will" and that he must keep reminding himself of his advanced age. Indeed, he confessed to having "to make a great effort" to convince himself that he is of the very age that, as a youth, seemed to be so ancient. Sartre[2] posited that "the elderly come to feel that they are old by means of others, not by their own realization, and they often refuse to accept the label."

Capabilities of the Elderly Gide[2] reported in his own old age that he had not yet experienced any weakness of intellectual powers, but that he expected he eventually would! All he could do is wonder: What then? James[1] stated that in old age time (days, months, and years) seem to pass more quickly: "The same space of time seems shorter as we grow older," and with advancing age "the days and weeks smooth themselves out in recollection to countless units." With obvious implications for motivation, he observed that in old age we choose those stimuli "connected with one or more so-called permanent interests" and restrict our attention only to these.

The memories of the elderly were observed by James to be "so transient that in the course of a few minutes of conversation the same question is asked and its answer forgotten half a dozen times." The acquisition and loss of memories seems to be based on the formation and decomposition of "brain-paths." In old age, "the old paths fade as fast as the new one forms until finally forgetting prevails over acquisition, or rather there is no acquisition." He explained that the memories formed in youth have a "superior tenacity" over those formed in old age, so that "the dotard will retrace the facts of his earlier years after he has lost all those of later date." Gide[2] explained the withdrawal often seen in the elderly: they are afraid of repeating themselves, for they have nothing new to say.

Social Role of the Elderly de Beauvoir[2] complained that there is a taboo associated with old age; people do not want to be reminded of it. And if they must be reminded, they demand that the author be "optimistic." Gide[3] pictured "a fine old age" as a series of "perpetual victories and recoveries" but admitted that this was an ideal state. He explained the dearth of information about old age: The elderly themselves do not write about it, and the young, who do write, are uninterested in the elderly. Indeed, he concluded dourly that "an elderly man no longer interests anyone at all."

Conclusions

If one looks for some pattern of development in the concept of old age in these thinkers, one may be destined for disappointment. Little progression seems to have been made in our understanding of the final segment of the lifespan. Contemporary thinkers appear not to think or feel anything significantly different from ancient philosophers. The ideas about old age have not become more precise; the attitudes about old age are not much less negative. When philosophers talk of the ideal state of old age, they tend to paint a positive picture; when they describe the actual state of old age, the picture is generally more negative.

The social role of the elderly in ancient times seems to have been one of honor, not power. As society moved to mercantilism and industrialization, the social role of the elderly was stripped of all vestige of power. The elderly were not important in the later societies requiring strength, speed, and endurance. Energies, even philosophic energies, are most often directed at those objects that are most highly valued. The small number of positive references to old age in the last two historical periods might well reflect our society's value of old age.

When this author has shared the results of the present investigation with students and colleagues, he has received objections that such a recounting of negative comments does not help the situation. This strikes at the core of the issue. The purpose of this discussion is precisely to challenge us to demonstrate that we think differently about the elderly today. Our concepts and attitudes are not kept in isolation from our practical activities. What we think about old age will color our actions toward the elderly. Our theories will set practices in motion.

Notes

Aquinas: (1) *Summa Theologica*
Aristotle: (1) *Generation of Animals*, (2) *Ethics*, (3) *Rhetoric*, (4) *Soul*, (5) *Generation of Animals*, (6) *Politics*, (7) *Physics*, (8) *Topics*
Bacon: (1) *History of Life and Death*
Camus: (1) *L'Envers et L'Endroit*
Cicero: (1) *De Senectute*
de Beauvoir: (1) *The Coming of Age*, (2) *La Force des Choses*
Erasmus: (1) *Colloquies*
Freud: (1) *General Introduction to Psychoanalysis*
Gide: (1) *Journal*, (2) *Ainsi soit-il*, (3) *Les Faux—Monnayeurs*
Hegel: (1) *Philosophy of History*
Hume: (1) *Human Understanding*
James: (1) *Principles of Psychology*
Locke: (1) *Civil Government*
Lucretius: (1) *Nature of Things*
Machiavelli: (1) *Clizia*, (2) *The Prince*
Mill, J. S.: (1) *On Liberty*
Montaigne: (1) *Essays*
Plato: (1) *Symposium*, (2) *Republic*, (3) *Laws*, (4) *Timaius*, (5) *Laches*, (6) *Theaetetus*
Proust: (1) cf. de Beauvoir's *The Coming of Age*
Rousseau: (1) *Inequality*, (2) *Reveries*
Sartre: (1) *Critique de la Raison Dialectique*, (2) *L'Etre et le Neant*
Schopenhauer: (1) *Aphorisms on Wisdom in Life*
Seneca: (1) *Letters*
Smith, Adam: (1) *Wealth of Nations*

References

de Beauvoir, S. *The coming of age.* New York: G. P. Putnam's, 1972.
Hutchins, R. M. (Ed.). *Great books of the western world.* Chicago: Encyclopedia Britannica, 1952.

Ethics and Gerontology

Gari Lesnoff-Caravaglia
Sangamon State University

The guiding and ordering of life belong to wisdom—a wisdom that has traditionally been the province of philosophy. There are, however, many indications that the basic enterprise of philosophy has lost its relevance to human existence. Unfortunately, philosophy has disintegrated precisely when sound and realistic cultural goals are urgently needed, when people are questioning the basic nature of society and their personal roles within it. In response to such needs, philosophy is mute or chooses to remain silent.

Societal groups, regardless of their endeavor, are made up of a number of individuals who, although free and independent, are drawn together in a spirit of cooperation. If they are to cooperate willingly and effectively, their group must be guided by mutually accepted standards for direction in life. They must possess an ethical view of their particular world. Further, their standards or value system must be sound and justifiable, coherent and appealing, as well as in tune with the nuances of human existence—like sex, age, and personal predisposition.

The absence of such ethical direction becomes particularly apparent when people attempt to deal with the needs and problems of older individuals. As Svoboda agrees in the preceding paper, there is now no philosophy of aging. Instead, a collection of myths and beliefs basically unchanged for generations is responsible for the development of current attitudes and convictions about older people and about the human process known as aging.

The interplay of myth and belief upon societal attitudes has made it difficult for people to realize that much of what they know or believe to be true about the processes of aging, and consequently about old people, is very likely erroneous or slanted to serve some utilitarian purpose, which may act more against than for the best interests of older individuals.

Much has been said and written about disadvantaged people in our society. Programs to meet their needs and interests develop and fade as effortlessly as the snow receding from the sun. Older people in our society have begun to be singled out for seasonal efforts, which are doomed to fail unless disciplines such as philosophy and, specifically, ethics move toward expanding their doctrines and positions to incorporate those who live beyond middle age. Philosophers are particularly guilty of viewing the human race as having been made of fully rational individuals who are, in every sense, in their prime. Society and philosophers alike suffer from what I refer to as the Jack Benny syndrome—no one ages beyond 39.

The primary concern of ethics is to order human existence in terms of duty and obligation. The ethical dimensions of human existence—that is, the principles of conduct that govern individuals or societal groups—that impinge most radically upon the lives of older people are considered to fall within the classification of possibility. It is possibility, of which freedom and choice are integral parts, that characterizes human existence. An ethical examination of the nature of possibility in the context of the experiences of older people demonstrates strikingly the restricted nature of life in later years.

Throughout life an individual is faced with a variety of possibilities. In each situation, however, choices are limited. In some instances choices may be quite numerous; in others there may be only one. Situations exist in which the choice may lie only between unfavorable alternatives. In no instance, however, are the possibilities offered to an individual identical or of equal value. Such individuality of choice gives urgency to the moment of experiencing. In other words, each human experience, characterized as it is by possibility, is unique.

Central to the notion of possibility is the idea of duality—a possibility can be or it cannot be. This duality, of course, is reflected in human existence itself, which can or cannot be. In the case of possibility, the decision of whether a possibility will indeed exist is made by personal choice. As individuals move through life, they must continually choose. The awareness of choice and the personal responsibility for that choice make each person an individual.

In weighing one choice against another, people experience anxiety or dread, for there are no guarantees that a particular choice is the right one. The element of risk is forever present. There is the constant need to weigh and contrast the probable outcomes of choices before making a final decision.

Once a choice has been made, it can be regarded as right or authentic if it becomes a decision that the person would repeat. That is, the person, having made the choice, confirms its authenticity by acknowledging that he or she would make the same choice again. Repeatable choices are those that form the fabric of our lives; these are cumulative decisions, ones that build upon one another. This function of choice is perhaps best illustrated in the choosing process experienced in selecting a career. In effect, the norm of the choice lies within the choice itself.

When a choice can no longer be regarded as repeatable and does not provide additional opportunities for choice, then the person must recognize the impasse and make a totally new choice. This calls for an ability to assess possibilities and to see oneself as capable of choosing. It must be borne in mind, however, that not to choose is, in itself, a choice. Severe limitations upon the exercise of choice can result in injustice or in a lack of self-fulfillment.

The limits of possibility are real. They may be due to age, sex, physical condition, educational attainment, cultural conditions, and so on. These limits, however, can be pushed to their extremes; we can exhaust the limits of the possible. Again, this perspective requires that the person see himself or herself as the sole creator of his or her existence.

It is a unique human capacity to foresee possibilities. Of course, possibilities have a future orientation, as all possibilities lie within the future. In this way life can be regarded as a human endeavor through which we project ourselves, ahead of ourselves, in terms of possibilities. The very personal aspect of possibilities is underscored by our sense of possession. The possibilities I perceive to be my own are linked to my perception of myself—my identity—and are closely linked to my personal process of becoming. For this reason the ethicist can hold to no single description of human nature; there are only individual interpretations of self.

Superimposing the category of possibility on the contemporary experience of aging leads to some interesting interpretations. To begin with, societal attitudes toward aging and the aged severely limit the possibilities for older persons. Some possibilities are rendered nonexistent. Possibilities are limited in such vital areas as educational opportunity, employment, health care, housing, aesthetic appreciation, and life style.

This restricted view of one's life project seriously blocks the processes of self-development, and, in the broader philosophical sense, it curtails the process of becoming. Since part of the perception of self is based upon future self-projections, older persons, who are unable to participate in life through a free choice of possibilities, are effectively alienated from a society that permits the same freedom to other age groups. This is at the heart of discrimination against the elderly.

If the attitude toward life changes as one ages, the reason may be the dwindling array of possibilities presented to an individual, not any change toward life and its possibilities inherent in aging itself. This very restriction of life space and self-expression significantly alters older persons' perceptions of life and their personal freedom within it.

Successes and failures of life, unexpectedness of experience, dreams, and their attendant emotions are what provide life with meaning. Being cut off from life, even in terms of such possible experiencing, is the real loss that comes with age. This closing off of experience creates a sharp discontinuity between self-concept and the ability to maintain a future orientation.

Once persons are expected to alter their life styles, they are supposed to create a life cut loose from any of the reference points that have previously given life its moorings, such as work, a routine, expectations in terms of role, and self-determined position in society.

For example, upon retirement, one is faced with the problem of redefining life—the meaning of one's very existence. As often as not, such definition is difficult, largely because of the limitations imposed on the financial, social, and health capabilities of the older individual. These limitations come from without, and they sharply curtail the ability to act on one's possibilities or to seriously entertain them. Individuals are forced to look primarily to themselves for both emotional and intellectual satisfaction. If a person has not been prepared for such eventualities earlier in life, identity shock may occur. Suddenly, and quite effectively, the identity that presumably was one's own has evaporated.

The contrast to death is telling. In death, the biological body remains, but the person (mind/spirit) is absent. In old age, both body and spirit remain but are devoid of meaning. The struggle against meaninglessness must be understood on the same level as the struggle against annihilation.

There is always the option of living "for others"—the others being either the community or the family. What such arguments fail to take into account is that the individual's previous life has been "being with others," with his or her own existence as the primary consideration. To expect older persons to forgo concern with primary existence and to live at one remove, as it were, concerned only with the welfare of others, is a form of martyrdom that we could scarcely regard as a personal possibility. In fact, such a depersonalized existence clearly indicates the emptiness of the individual's life—in other words, a living death. Ethically, there is a world of difference between a person who endures, wishes, experiences, and a person who takes what is given, realizes it, and shapes his or her own existence.

Furthermore, the value system that has been part of one's inheritance does not appreciably alter as one grows older. A person's value system, internalized at an early age, emphasizes productivity, acquisition of wealth and power, youthfulness, health, and competitiveness. Older persons can only chafe under the knowledge that they represent none of these values. The low image that older people often have of themselves is based precisely on this inability to score favorably on such a value scale.

Is There Any Sense and Any Vital Meaning in Old Age?

We need to develop a new system of values that is meaningful to older people now. But this need is exceedingly difficult to satisfy, for the elderly often have been conditioned to regard themselves from the perspective of past association, goals, and roles. The choice appears to be either to develop a minority-group culture based on differences in values or to seek new alternatives for the aging within the framework of existing values.

In order to insure that aging is not a poor imitation of life or the mirroring of past achievements, goals at advanced age must be developed on the same bases as prior self-projections. The ability to continue one's concept of self, built upon such self-projections, permits continuity within existence and maintains the framework of time with present, past, and future as constant points. Without a positive outlook upon the self and possibilities, people will inevitably fall into despair, no longer choosing existence but drifting into lives of quiet desperation. Depression in the aged is existential anxiety taken to the limit.

The more older individuals withdraw from existence—from actively participating in their own existing—the greater is their guilt, and the greater their frustration and hostility. The negative stereotyping of old age has led older individuals to look on themselves as bereft of possibilities. Rather than projecting into the future, the older person is left with only the opportunities to reminisce and to rework past possibilities futilely.

Cut off from the heart of existence, is it surprising that older persons are often apathetic, unhappy, depressed, suicidal, or hostile? Those who do not fall into this class are those for whom possibility continues to operate.

The element of possibility is crucial to life, to living. Only individuals can assess their own possibilities. When older people are not permitted to make decisions—no matter how small—they frequently lose interest in life. They may become ill and die. Many of the morbid behaviors observed in institutional settings may well be protests against rules and regulations over which the individual has no control. The opportunity to regulate one's own life, by saying no, is limited for many older persons.

A single anecdote illustrates this point. Burnside describes an 83-year-old man who refused to eat. Meals were brought to him, set by his bedside without comment; wine, eggnog, and snacks were occasionally set on his table quietly. He stayed in bed for two to three weeks and then began gradually to eat. Within a period of three months, he gained 29 pounds, became more active, got out of bed, and improved in physical appearance. The staff caring for him was uncertain about what had happened. According to Burnside, allowing the patient to decide for himself may have been the turning point in his living or dying. He could decide when to eat, what to eat, how much, and could also decide when he was ready to get up. This clearly indicates the importance of the decision-making process for the aged, even in the case of those who have been institutionalized for long periods of time.

The importance of seeing oneself as a self-directed human being regardless of age, physical condition, mental condition, or state of dependency, is vital to survival. If people are convinced that they are beyond hope, not worth the trouble, pain, or interest, they may give up as human beings and die. But if they are treated sensitively and considerately as individuals, with every opportunity accorded them for controlling their own lives, they will continue to regard themselves positively. That there are still choices to be made, choices that rest upon oneself, makes the difference between meaningful existence and meaninglessness. There must always be something that the individual can control, regardless of age or state of health.

It is important for people to learn that they are, in a very real sense, holders of their own freedom. To be a human being is, by definition, to exercise the possibilities of choice. Unschooled to freedom in this sense, many older persons too soon abrogate their freedom and begin to die long before the onset of biological death.

Anxiety enters when one is engaged in the process of choice. The more one attempts to come to grips with life and its personal meaning, the greater the dread or anxiety. The anxiety is due in part to the fact that one must give meaning to life; if it is meaningless, the fault is one's own. To take on such a responsibility for one's own existence takes a great deal of courage—a person must go beyond himself in order to become himself. That is why "to be" is described as a process of becoming. An individual is never complete. If there is such completion, it is unobserved. The final human act lies in the taking over, not the acceptance, of one's own dying.

We are very much aware of societal expectations through middle age. We can choose to abide by them, to ignore them, or to modify them. It is only when we approach old age that we realize how alone a human being really is. When an individual reaches old age and is no longer in a position to satisfy some of society's expectations, society loses interest. Then the individual realizes that existence was lonely all along. There is the sneaking suspicion that one may have been a pawn. It is this cold, sharp realization that comes to many people at the onset of retirement or when they first experience the physical infirmities associated with old age. They sense that as long as society had a use for them—a role to play—they were important enough to elicit societal expectation.

To be cast adrift into the world at an advanced age is a trauma of unprecedented proportions in terms of human experience. The basis of life has been inauthentic. In old age comes the discovery of authenticity and its component—despair. The anguish of existence is felt at a time when the individual has few reserves to fulfill the possibilities he or she would like to envision.

Authenticity in old age is painful. Some may say they enjoy old age because now they can say what they think, possibly do what they like. They are not bound by convention. But what is there to do? How prepared are people to take their lives into their own keeping? Few have experienced authentic living. The false gods of employment, procreation, recreation, and the like, no longer smile on the old, the indigent, and the halt.

Personal commitment to self and to one's possibilities is rare at any point in personal history, but such commitment is called for if one is to give life integrity and meaning in old age. To regard oneself as in flux—in the process of becoming—eliminates some of the fear of aging, and allows one to see life as a process rather than as a static set of stages of development or life phases. Life is thus seen as a span of experience built upon possibilities that can or cannot be, but that are individually determined. Unless life continues to have this duality, existence is unhuman.

References

Burnside, I. M. "Depression and Suicide in the Aged." In Burnside, I. M. (Ed.), *Nursing and the aged*. New York: McGraw-Hill, 1976, 165–181.

The Humanities and Aging: A Historian's Perspective

W. Andrew Achenbaum
Canisius College

Aging as a New Area of Historical Research

These are the worst of times and the best of times for historians. Job opportunities in teaching for junior scholars have drastically decreased since the 1960s. Pessimists predict that an already grim situation will get worse. Even the most optimistic attitudes toward employment outlook are guarded. The growing fragmentation of the discipline itself, moreover, has undermined professional morale. As historians increasingly identify themselves as experts in relatively narrow areas of specialization, they too often find themselves unwilling or unable to keep abreast of developments in other parts of the field. Yet these disturbing circumstances are counterbalanced by more sanguine trends. Although some academic critics and popular pundits have been bemoaning "the death of history," the recent bicentennial festivities and the "Roots" phenomenon have inspired a greater public appreciation for our collective and individual antecedents and have afforded scholars a wonderful opportunity to demonstrate the relevance of historical research to understanding contemporary society.

Indeed, much of the most exciting research in history today attempts to elucidate the hopes and fears of hitherto anonymous people and to investigate the daily experiences of ordinary men and women in past times. Anxious to study history from the bottom up, researchers have made a concerted effort during the last decade to describe and explain the varieties and contrarieties in life situations at earlier moments in historical time. For example, scholars of U.S. history have been analyzing how much the occupational status, household structure, value systems, concerns, and ultimate destinies of various groups in pre-industrial and industrializing American society diverged from the typical patterns of the time. New England Colonial women, antebellum Southern Blacks, Wisconsin pioneers, Pittsburgh steel workers, late-nineteenth-century college professors, Italian immigrants in Buffalo, Great Plains Indians, and Japanese-Americans in Los Angeles during World War II, among others, have all been the subjects of intensive research by American historians trained in the latest techniques of the social sciences and humanities.

Whereas scholars have long been aware of the importance of race, ethnicity, gender, occupation, and location in the shaping of people's circumstances in past times, they have as yet paid scant attention to the importance of age. Philippe Aries opened a new frontier of historical research with the publication of *Centuries of Childhood*, which argued that childhood was not considered a distinct stage of life until the end of the Middle Ages (Ariès, 1962). Researchers have also determined that the concept of adolescence is the product of cultural and structural forces that reshaped Western civilization in the nineteenth century (Demos and Demos, 1969; Gillis, 1974; Kett, 1977). Still others have shown the value of a life-cycle approach in explicating crucial transitions in adulthood in past times (Elder, 1974; Hareven, 1976; Modell, Furstenberg, and Hershberg, 1976). In this context, it is not surprising that historians have started to investigate the history of old age. Two book-length essays have been published thus far, and several major research projects, monographs, articles, and dissertations are in progress or in press.

It is already clear that historians have much to contribute to gerontology, even though aging as a field of inquiry has barely emerged from Clio's womb. The crucial link between the humanities and aging, from a historian's perspective, is the need for a temporal perspective in old-age research and course development. Historical milieu and societal context, as I hope to suggest, greatly affect the images and realities of being old at any given point in time. By reconstructing the past record, by illuminating current challenges and opportunities, and by forecasting trends, historians can underscore the fundamental importance of studying aging over time.

Reconstructing the Past Record

Because of predilection and training, historians prefer to study the evolution of cultural trends and societal patterns over longer periods of time than most other investigators. To be sure, since the earth is at least four billion years old, any time segment that a scholar chooses is really a very modest slice of the whole pie. Nevertheless, since historians generally examine events and developments that occurred during a decade, an era, a century, and sometimes even a millennium, they are in a position to differentiate between the timeless and time-bound features of the particular problem under investigation. This orientation becomes especially useful in efforts to distinguish between the eternal and the transitory meanings and experiences of old age.

The historical record reveals that three characteristics of being old are age-old. First, old age, unlike childhood and adolescence, has been perceived as a specific stage of life since ancient times. The Biblical "three-score and ten" definition of adult life expectancy has proved remarkably durable. The chronological boundaries of the last stage, moreover, have typically been defined in roughly the same way. Owing to an incessantly fluid but ultimately resilient combination of biological factors, cultural assumptions, and personal quirks, 65, give or take 15 years either way, has long been considered the benchmark of old age (Philibert, 1968; de Beauvoir, 1972).

Mainly because old age has persistently embraced such a large segment of the life span, a second generalization about old age has been invariably true: Throughout the centuries, the aged have been a diverse group. Marked longitudinal and cross-sectional differences in the elderly in physical health, intellectual capacity, interests and activities, economic resources, marital status, and social integration have always existed though they have not always been recognized (Laslett, 1976; Thomas, 1977; Smith, Friedberger, and Dahlin, 1978).

The heterogeneity of the older population, in fact, partly explains a third universal of old age: the attitudes and feelings about growing and being old expressed by men and women of all ages, races, places, and stations in life have been a mixture of negative, positive, ambivalent, ambiguous, and conflicting sentiments. Thus, it is highly unlikely that Americans in the 1970s have discovered any assets or liabilities of old age that previous commentators had not already detected (Kastenbaum and Ross, 1975; Achenbaum and Kusnerz, 1978).

Yet, despite all its perennial qualities, old age definitely has a dynamic history. The prevailing images of old age and the actual conditions of the elderly have changed over time (Van Tassel and Cetina, 1978). Since the American Revolution, for example, commentators usually have referred to the eternal advantages and disadvantages of old age in describing the overall worth and status of the aged. But their evaluations of the presumed roles and the social position of older Americans have also reflected the interplay of the diverse and ever-changing cultural and structural forces transforming their society at a given moment. Hence, the aged were ascribed a comparatively favorable place in America when people thought they fulfilled essential social functions, such as serving as guides to healthful longevity, guardians of virtue, veterans of productivity, and keys to the ultimate meaning of life. When these tasks seemed less vital to the well-being of the republic or when others (such as physicians, psychologists, corporate managers, or younger people) seemed better equipped to assume roles once assigned to the elderly, Americans increasingly questioned the utility of heeding the advice of the aged, following their example, or even including them in activities. Perceptions of the old also shifted insofar as observers accentuated the negative features of senescence or believed that old age itself constituted a significant social problem (Achenbaum, 1978).

It should also be noted that significant changes in ideas about the functions and values of old age were not directly related to profound alterations in the absolute or relative numbers of elderly, their occupational or household status, or even the nature and incidence of old age dependency. Modernization—a concept social scientists frequently employ to analyze the impact of industrialization, urbanization, bureaucratization, and secularization on personality, culture, and society—clearly affected the meanings and experiences of the elderly in the past, but definitely not at the same time nor in the same way nor for the same reasons that it affected other age groups. It would be historically inaccurate, in fact, to assert that modernization either suddenly, inexorably, or irreversibly caused the position of aged people to deteriorate in Western societies (Fischer, 1977; Stearns, 1977). The actual relationship between old age and modernization is far more complex; the distinctive features vary from place to place and even within countries.

In the United States, for instance, a striking discontinuity between the rhetoric and the reality of old age arose during the last third of the nineteenth century. Americans steadily undermined the antebellum notion that the old could and should perform important functions in society and concluded instead that elderly men and women had become obsolescent because of the new ideas and conditions taking hold in society (Achenbaum, 1974). Federal and state census reports indicate, however, that there really was very little change in the nineteenth century in the actual demographic and socioeconomic status of the elderly. It appears, therefore, that prevailing definitions of the needs and opportunities of the aged have developed, over time, a dynamic of their own. They did not necessarily change as or because the situations of older Americans altered. Hence, in the past, images of old age did not invariably fit the "real" circumstances of the elderly, at least insofar as a historian can objectively reconstruct that reality through quantitative and qualitative analysis.

Illuminating Present-Day Challenges and Opportunities

The discovery that there once was a difference between the perceptions held by Americans of the aged's situation and the empirically verifiable circumstances of the elderly helps us to understand our present difficulties in challenging and extirpating misconceptions about what it means to be old. Gerontologists are particularly sensitive to the prevalence of virulent stereotypes about the conditions of the aged in contemporary American society. Some of the deleterious ideas about old age, researchers have determined, arise from ageist assumptions embedded in our value system and social structure. Others are deliberately or inadvertently fostered by media reports that emphasize the tragic features of growing old today and slight the positive aspects. Still other stereotypes, however, have been historically conditioned. They consist of notions about aging that once enjoyed considerable scientific and popular support, but that now have become anachronistic in light of new evidence and changing circumstances.

Tracing shifts in American attitudes toward aged sexuality during the past century aptly illustrates this point. In *Plain Facts for Old and Young*, the best-selling guide to sexual matters in its day, John Harvey Kellogg (1881) recommended abstention in old age and documented his case with medical evidence couched in moral tones. Those who defied the dictates of nature risked serious consequences: "When the passions have been indulged and their diminishing vigor stimulated, a horrid disease, *satyriasis*, not infrequently seizes upon the imprudent individual, and drives him to the perpetration of the most loathsome crimes and excesses." Doctors reasoned that women were less vulnerable to this malady because they generally recognized that menopause signaled the end of sexual interest and activity; thus, physicians directed most of their literature to men. Such ideas gained increasing credibility over time. In *The Psychology of Sex*, Havelock Ellis (1933) argued that sexual activity in old age was often accompanied by egotism, callousness, exhibitionism, and homosexuality; elderly men who engaged in intercourse sometimes suffered heart attacks, cerebral hemorrhages, and a hastening of their demise. The Kinsey report, it is worth noting, attributed the decrease in sexual responsiveness and activity with advancing age to physiological decline and psychological fatigue. Sex research conducted since the 1950s, however, has overturned much of the scientific basis for the proverbial myth of the dirty old man. The best currently available evidence indicates that sexual interest in later years is perfectly normal, and sexual activity at all ages is healthy and natural for both sexes. But, tragically, many Americans prefer to sneer along with television comics than to read the findings of Masters and Johnson. As a result, outmoded ideas about aged sexuality continue to predominate. One solution to this predicament, of course, is to communicate the latest findings about sex after 60 as broadly as possible. In fact, the case for eliminating old-fashioned sexual attitudes would be made all the more plausible if advocates provided a temporal perspective. In that way, Americans could better appreciate the historical basis for many assumptions about aging that current research challenges.

The general public is not the only group whose perspectives on aging have been biased by the persistence of ideas that previously made sense, but that subsequently have grown outmoded. Professional gerontologists and policy makers also have sometimes been unwitting victims of their adherence to principles and methods that may no longer be useful in addressing the current needs and opportunities of the elderly. Is it not possible, for instance, that our definition of old age as a social problem is less appropriate now than it was 50 years ago, when scientists, demographers, and economists first began discussing the medical and financial predicaments of the elderly in terms of their implications for the health and vitality of the nation? To be sure, perceiving old age as a national problem served several useful functions. It helped to focus attention on social trends and intellectual currents that were undeniably rising in importance, and it led to constructive action that assisted many older persons in need. Nevertheless, in perpetuating the image of old age as a social problem, we might be aggravating the situation because we view the aged— the targets of our concern—as passive, helpless objects, incapable of caring for themselves and unable to recommend feasible alternatives to ineffective or obsolete programs.

Indeed, from a historical perspective, it is apparent that many of the advantages and predicaments of the elderly in contemporary American society are novel. We have an unprecedented opportunity to improve the quality of life in later years. The growth of a vast institutional framework in public and private sectors since the passage of the Social Security Act in 1935 has done much to improve the overall well-being of citizens over 65 and to increase our knowledge of the current assets and liabilities of the older population. The emergence of a "gray lobby" (Pratt, 1976) provides a means for older men and women themselves to energize their individual and collective resources in identifying priorities and in securing needed legislation. Yet there are many obstacles in our path, some of them unforeseen or underestimated even a decade ago. Despite all of our efforts, for instance, the extent of poverty among older Americans exceeds the national average, and its incidence among minority groups and women is truly alarming. Furthermore, changes in the population structure, labor market, and energy supplies make many astute observers question whether we can afford to ensure the aged a greater share of this nation's resources, much less whether we are able to honor our present commitments.

Forecasting Trends

Although it is crucial to realize that the current situation of the elderly in America is unprecedented in many respects, and although it is necessary to recognize that the needs and resources of the aged will continue to change, to attempt to predict what old age will be like in 2001 is not quixotic. To be sure, it is humanly impossible to forecast with absolute certainty the next steps and major developments in the evolving history of old age in the United States. But an understanding of the events and forces that have culminated in the present circumstances of older Americans offers both a fresh perspective and a vital baseline worth using as we seek to prepare for the future. Creating old-age policies requires far more than remedying existing deficiencies and satisfying present goals. Policies must make sense in the light of well-established precedents, current programs, and philosophies, as well as anticipated trends. The temporal aspects of all policy deliberations and decisions that affect the aged now, or will do so in the future, merit just as much scrutiny as demographic, fiscal, ideological, and political considerations (Achenbaum and Stearns, 1978).

Historians can help legislators, policy makers, and experts in other disciplines evaluate the short-term efficacy and long-term impact of various old age programs in the most comprehensive framework possible. The distinction between matters that do not require major action by policy makers and developments that policy makers dare not ignore must be more sharply drawn, as the debate over the future of Social Security painfully illustrates. It is indisputable that the composition of the American population in general and the dependency ratio of the old upon the young in particular will change profoundly as the children of the postwar baby boom mature and attain the age of 65. In light of this demographic trend, if the present institutions of mandatory and early retirement continue to operate as they do today, and if the phenomenon has been successfully integrated over time into people's expectations about old age, then there can be no doubt that financing Social Security on a pay-as-you-go basis will become an increasingly costly enterprise. Yet what if the practice of quitting work at a prescribed age becomes increasingly anachronistic as the conditions and attitudes that caused it to arise and justified its continuance decrease in relative importance? How would such a structural and ideological change affect cost estimates for the first quarter of the twenty-first century? This historian's crystal ball is as cloudy as everyone else's, but the question is of foremost significance and it cannot be answered by actuaries alone.

As the Depression experience dramatically reminds us, unexpected crises forced our predecessors to reconsider options and reforms that earlier had been rejected as un-American or impractical. We must, therefore, remain flexible and ready to accept the necessity of having to enact radical measures if unexpected crises or compelling new evidence warrants a significant departure from the status quo. We also must become increasingly sensitive to how much our personal and collective values affect both the way we articulate society's responsibilities toward its aged citizens and the way we believe they ought to be defined in the future (Neugarten and Havighurst, 1977). Above all, we must vigilantly scrutinize the assumptions and methods we employ left they become outmoded as the increasing interplay among cultural values and structural forces creates a new context for the meanings and experiences of old age in the years and decades to come.

Conclusion

I have set forth an ambitious task for historians. They cannot confine their interest in gerontology to analyzing and interpreting past events, ideas, and conditions. Historians must increasingly join humanists, social and behavioral scientists, government officials, and others in the field who are concerned about present realities and future possibilities. I do not claim that the task will be easy. The relationships among old age, human values, and social policies are difficult to investigate at any point in history; efforts to trace changes and continuities over time are even more problematic. But a broad-gauged examination of old age in as wide a sociohistorical context as possible is urgently needed.

References

Achenbaum, W. A. The obsolescence of old age in America, 1865–1914. *Journal of Social History*, 1974, 8, 48–62.

Achenbaum, W. A. *Old age in the new land: The American experience since 1790*. Baltimore: Johns Hopkins University Press, 1978.

Achenbaum, W. A., & Kusnerz, P. A. *Images of old age.* Ann Arbor: Institute of Gerontology, 1978.

Achenbaum, W. A., & Stearns, P. N. Old age and modernization. *The Gerontologist,* 1978, *18,* 307–312.

Ariès, P. *Centuries of childhood.* New York: Vintage Books, 1962.

de Beauvoir, S. *The coming of age.* New York: G. P. Putnam's, 1972.

Demos, J., & Demos, V. Adolescence in historical perspective. *Journal of Marriage and the Family,* 1969, *31,* 632–638.

Elder, G. *Children of the great depression.* Chicago: University of Chicago Press, 1974.

Ellis, H. *The psychology of sex.* New York: R. Long & R. R. Smith, 1933.

Fischer, D. H. *Growing old in America.* New York: Oxford University Press, 1977.

Gillis, J. *Youth and history.* New York: Academic Press, 1974.

Hareven, T. Modernization and family history. *Journal of Women in Culture and Society,* 1976, *2,* 190–206.

Kastenbaum, R., & Ross, B. Historical perspectives on care. In J. G. Howells (Ed.), *Modern perspectives in the psychiatry of old age.* New York: Brunner/Mazel, 1975.

Kellogg, J. H. *Plain facts for old and young.* Burlington, Iowa: Segner & Condit, 1881.

Kett, J. *Rites of passage.* New York: Basic Books, 1977.

Laslett, P. Societal development and aging. In R. Binstock & E. Shanas (Eds.), *Handbook of aging and the social sciences.* New York: Van Nostrand Reinhold, 1976.

Modell, J., Furstenberg, F., & Hershberg, T. Social change and the life course in historical perspective. *Journal of Family History,* 1976, *1,* 7–32.

Neugarten, B. L., & Havighurst, R. J. (Eds.). *Social policy, social ethics and the aging society.* Washington, D.C.: U.S. Government Printing Office, 1977.

Philibert, M. *L'échelle des âges.* Paris: Editions du Seuil, 1968.

Pratt, H. J. *The gray lobby.* Chicago: University of Chicago Press, 1976.

Smith, D. S., Friedberger, M., & Dahlin, M. *The construction of households by older blacks in the south in 1880 and 1900.* Unpublished manuscript, 1978. (Available from The Family and Community History Center, The Newberry Library, Chicago, IL 60610.)

Stearns, P. N. *Old age in European society.* New York: Holmes & Meier, 1977.

Thomas, K. *Age and authority in early modern England: proceedings of the British Academy.* London: The Academy, 1977.

Van Tassel, D., & Cetina, J. *Aging over time.* In preparation. 1978.

Literature, Mentality, and Aging

Edward F. Ansello
University of Maryland

Literature is both mirror and matrix of cultural theory. Literature serves the functions of both reflecting and changing cultural values. Perhaps distinct from other media, it maintains this duality. Some literature has changed the way people think. *Mein Kampf*, superbly polemic, altered political and social history. The Bible has certainly changed the interactions of much of human-kind. More often than not, however, literature reflects what has been and what is, rather than creates what is to be. Even catalytic works like *Mein Kampf* and the Bible are quintessentially products of their times.

Literature, reflecting cultural character, acts as a socializing agent. Its importance in value-transmission with one specific audience has been recognized by the Council on Interracial Books for Children (1976). The Council states:

> Let us start with the fact that children's books are not merely a matter of text (which may be lively, entertaining and stirring, or not) plus pictures (which may be well done or not). Children's books are not merely exciting, imaginative and full of good characters or the opposite. . . . No writer is just a reporter, and artists put more on paper than their eyes see.

> Most of us who work with children's books know this. We realize that such books do carry a message—a moral, a value or set of values—and that they mold minds. But how often do we stop to consider the source of those values? Do they come from the personal beliefs of the writer? Do they come from the publisher's mind? If so, then we must ask in the persistent way of children themselves: Where do their values come from?

We propose . . . that those values are not simply individual, not creatures of a series of vacuums, but that they rise from the total society. In any given society, children's books generally reflect the needs of those who dominate that society. A major need is to maintain and fortify the structure of relations between dominators and dominated. The prevailing values are supportive of the existing structure; they are the dominator's values (p. 1).

Of course, these same observations apply to literature addressed to audiences of any age. The reason is that the basic unit of all literature is words and there is no meaning in words of print themselves. That is, there is no inherent denotation in a word. A printed word is merely a symbolic trigger of consensual associations. To illustrate this point simply open to a page in a book on astrophysics and see what sense it makes. To most of us it would be meaningless. But we could hardly say that the book is nonsensical. All we could honestly say is that we have no stored associations that the symbols on the page stimulate.

The process of reading is one of learning the "proper" associations between a printed symbol and a stored experience. If by consensus, we all decided that c-o-w could stand for a winged machine that transports passengers, henceforth c-o-w would trigger this image. Those who researched the area of disadvantaged youth and IQ in the late 1960s were quick to point out the associative-experiential basis of reading and learning.

Literature, then, having its basis in consensual associations, can be seen to reflect the prevailing theories of *aging* of the time.

In his review of the Great Books, Charles (1977) says that if literature does indeed reflect its times, then there was surely no golden age of aging. There appears to have been no time when unequivocally positive things were said about growing older. In his concluding remarks Charles notes:

While the foregoing obviously is not an exhaustive study of the literature of the Western world, it should be apparent that there are remarkably few old people appearing in literature at all. In part, this neglect probably reflects the relative sparsity of old people in the real world; not too many people survived early life and lived to grow up. For example, parish records in London during Shakespeare's time show that of every 100 children born in 1583—a plague year—70 survived to the first birthday, 48 to the fifth, and only 30 to the fifteenth! (Toches, 1970). But still, there have always been some people surviving to an age as old as today's oldest. In some periods, the threatening and physically demanding nature of society may have reduced older persons' involvement, and thus their role in literature. But these physical explanations of neglect do not seem adequate.

In such appearances as they have been allowed in literature, old characters' status has not generally been very high. There exists a popular notion that old people fared a great deal better in the past than is true today, that they were loved, cared for, respected and the like. This may be so, but literature from Old Testament times to the present does not confirm this.

While there is variety and range of treatment of elders in the literature of most periods, in general there is neglect, and for most of history a high inci-

The Humanities and Aging

dence of scorn, ridicule and disparagement. Rather than suffering from low-
ered status in contemporary society, the literature reviewed in this study
would suggest that modern times—the nineteenth and twentieth centuries—
have been better for them than was true of past centuries, or at least no worse
(pp. 249–250).

We can infer from literature, then, that the theory of aging, for centuries
of Western civilization up to the present time, has been one of loss and deterioration. Consider how often, in print and in conversation, people excuse
their behavior with the explanation, "Well, I guess I'm getting older." If one
forgets someone's name, or is late for an appointment, or really does not want
to do something, or commits a silly error, one might excuse it as the effect of
aging. Or one's colleagues might say, "Looks like you're getting too old for the
job," and a laugh, good natured or otherwise, may follow. We all join in this
collusion because it is acceptable to blame aging for loss.

There is an association, then, between age and loss. Neugarten (1968)
has researched the concept of "on-timeness" and demonstrated how broadly
people agree, across generations, on the time when it is appropriate to do
certain things. We agree that it is on-time for a five- or six-year old to start
school. It is on-time for someone in late adolescence to begin seriously to
consider a career. Until recently we tended to agree that it was "off-time" for
a woman to reach 30 without marrying.

Examining on-timeness as a function of age—that is, looking at it
developmentally—one finds that with an older "target" on-timeness becomes
an increasingly negative phenomenon. Behaviors ascribed become increasingly constrictive. As one gets older, it is on-time to let loose one's friends, to
quit one's job, to venture socially less often, and so on. The concept of on-
timeness has been reified in Havighurst's (1972) developmental tasks. Of the
tasks assigned to late life, some two-thirds are associated with loss.

A cycle operates, then, among theory, literature, and behavior. Literature reflects theory; theory determines cognitions or expectations; these, in
turn, predispose behaviors or practices. The current practices of associating
age and loss find in literature the roots that, as can be seen, substantiate a
theory of aging relatively unchanged for centuries. The Roman playwright
Plautus observed, "He whom the gods favor dies young." Two thousand
years later, Lord Byron would parallel in *Childe Harold*, "Heaven gives its
favorites early death." Virgil penned, "Age carries all things, even the mind,
away" some 18 centuries before Shakespeare reiterated the sentiment in the
"Seven Ages of Man" soliloquy in *As You Like It*; the seventh age ends "in
second childishness and mere oblivion—sans eyes, sans teeth, sans taste,
sans everything."

Reviewing the contributions of philosophers to our cultural concept of
age, Svoboda (1977) concludes that their postulations, too, reflect a relatively
unchanging equation of age and loss:

There seems to be no progression in the understanding of the final seg-
ment of human lifespan. What contemporary philosophers proclaim about old
age does not significantly differ from what the ancient philosophers asserted.

On this topic Whitehead's remark rings true: All philosophy is merely a foot-note to Plato. An immediate impression of the attitudes associated with old age through history is similar: There has been little change; the attitudes are generally negative. When philosophers talked of the ideal state of senescence, they painted a positive picture. But when they described the actual stage of old age, their strokes grew heavy and their colors dark (p. 232).

The writings of philosophers from four historical periods (ancient, medieval, modern, and contemporary) were analyzed for descriptions and explanations of old age, the psyche of the elderly, the powers of the elderly, and the position of the elderly. Svoboda (1977) concludes that the associations with "age" have remained relatively constant; the meanings of today "have appeared in each previous historical period." And so, echoing concepts stated centuries before, Sartre described the elderly as "strangers from another time."

So culturally pervasive is the association of age and loss that it operates at a higher level than theory. The association transcends theory. It is, more accurately, an element of what Kuhn (1970) calls a mentality, the composite of a culture's belief systems. According to Kuhn, a mentality provides the climate within which "paradigms" can grow and support groups of similar-minded thinkers who advance disciplines, say, scientific inquiry. Promoted by individuals who are products of a mentality, scientific inquiry does not always grow in an upward linear progression. Rather, it starts and spurts in an erratic evolution as one group of thinkers "fall out" with another; scientific "reality" is very much the product of personal human influence. It is from these paradigms that theories are generated. Theories, then, must be compatible with the paradigms that spawned them. The definitions of premises and hypotheses, that is, what is real and what is researchable, are, therefore, relative. Again, these definitions must agree with the parent paradigm. When individuals within paradigms disagree, counterparadigms sometimes develop, which, in turn, create their own theories. In any event, theories generate models or abstractions of theoretical interactions; and models may eventuate in applications to practicality. Applications and models are constantly changing; to a lesser degree, so are theories and paradigms. Least resistant to questioning, least resistant to change is the mentality.

Since the literature on aging is fairly uniform across millennia, we may conclude that this literature reflects mentality. If so, it will not change significantly until the entire knowledge substructure (paradigms, theories, etc.) changes. Consider how difficult, how marked by religious, social, philosophical, and cultural upheaval, was the acceptance of our heliocentric solar system.

With such a potent factor as literature conveying a negative theory of aging—the association of age with loss—it is appropriate to ask if all age changes are internally induced. Is "acting one's age" only, or even mainly, the manifestation of biological decrement? Or are age changes internally and externally induced? The answer seems to be obvious.

The culture cannot reinforce deviance from its norms (its definitions of reality), the norms that have been conveyed through its literature. Its norms say that age and loss are synonymous. So we look for, and indeed we find, loss in intelligence with age because we use a cross-sectional assessment technique, insensitive to cohort differences (Baltes and Labouvie, 1973). We look for and we find increasing conservativism with older samples for the same reason. We have ignored cohort effects and other potential explanations because we have been induced to ignore them.

Even the discrepancies between attitudes toward aging and the experiences of older people themselves are not likely to be easily rectified because the culture cannot tolerate threats to its mentality and to the whole knowledge structure that underlies it. So Ahammer and Baltes (1972), Borges and Dutton (1976), and Harris and Associates (1975) have demonstrated disparity between younger and older respondents' estimations of the autonomy, instrumentality, and quality of life of older people. The Harris survey of over 4,000 individuals in a cross-section of the United States found 67 percent of the public believing that "most people over 65 spend a lot of time watching television," 62 percent agreeing that "most people over 65 spend a lot of time sitting and thinking," 39 percent feeling that those over 65 spend their time sleeping, and 35 percent believing that older people spend their time doing nothing. In each instance only about one-half of the older respondents concurred with the public's estimation. The discrepancy between projected reality and experienced reality is great. Pointedly, some 54 percent of the public believed that if they themselves were over age 65, they would feel "unwanted."

Again, the impact of the mentality, and of the literature reflecting it, is felt in various social interactions within the culture, including the research interactions. One's paradigm, one's circle of professional colleagues, determines expectations of what is; it determines the questions asked, the methods of investigation, and the interpretation of the data. Researchers, being part of the society whose mentality associates age with loss, do not often go beyond the findings to explanations other than the confirmation of expectations in the research design. Consequently, to some degree, developmental stages/tasks "norm" loss. Again, for decades researchers have employed cross-sectional techniques to quantify mental loss with age, failing to scrutinize the research modality because the data fit expectations. For example, Wechsler (1955) formulated an "age credit" in IQ points to compensate for the "normal decline" in ability with age. Only recently have cohort differences been considered.

In part, changes in the entire knowledge structure (Kuhn, 1970) have been retarded, at least in the area of gerontology, by the very changes in population that have substantially increased the numbers of older persons and stimulated the development of the discipline. In the twentieth century, demographic changes have been so rapid and so ill-timed as to preclude a reworking of the knowledge structure and a rewriting of the literature that reflects it. For example, the most rapid demographic changes (i.e., increases in the number of older people) occurred during the 1930s and 1940s. In those years the number of people over age 60 increased approximately 32 percent and 34 percent (U.S. Bureau of the Census, 1976), but the change came at the very time that the country's attention was diverted elsewhere to the Great Depression, a world war on two fronts, and so on. Typically, government, researchers, and social scientists responded to the burgeoning of the older population amidst crises in ways that were ill conceived but consonant with the mentality. It can be argued that in time of crisis "instinctive" responses close to the core of the mentality occur. And so the government manufactured old-age assistance, the Social Security Act, specifying an age of recipiency that statistically only about half of the then 40-year-olds could expect to reach. Social scientists adapted the child-development research methodologies that suggested asymptotes in adolescence in most physical and mental functions, and they adopted a monotonic theoretical and research design predicting nearly linear increments in performances to adulthood and nearly linear decrements thereafter.

Contemporary popular literature can be shown to reflect this same mentality, which is predictive of age and loss. An analysis of literature along two developmental perspectives demonstrates the efficacy of this influence (Ansello, 1977a). We content-examined literature developmentally from the historical standpoint (ancient to contemporary works) and, within contemporary works, from the standpoint of the chronological age of the readership (child to adult readers). The historical-developmental perspective has been alluded to (Charles, 1977; Svoboda, 1977); the chronological-developmental analysis is as telling.

Ansello (1977b) systematically analyzed the content of almost 700 circulating children's books, classified as easy readers (E) or juvenile picture (JP). These levels represent the first literary experiences of children and their initial exposure and socialization to the values of aging in the cultural mentality. The books were analyzed and categorized for the presence of older characters, their sex and race, relationship to the main character, occupational role, behaviors, appearance in illustrations, and their physical and personality descriptions. (*Older* referred to any story member who met at least two of three criteria: being drawn, verbally described, or socially positioned—for example, "retired"—as older. *Character* described any story member who uttered one word or more, thus eliminating crowd scenes from consideration.)

The analyses found that only some 16 percent of the books contained any older character at all. Of course, omission is a message in itself. The literature maintained a skewed proportion of males to females (55 percent to 41 percent); the sex of the remaining 4 percent was indeterminate, as in the case of fictionalized inanimate objects. Minority older characters were significantly underrepresented. Moreover, in less than 4 percent of all the books examined the main character was older. Older characters are most frequently strangers in the story, with indeterminate occupational status, existing on the periphery to drift in and out of the plot.

Each instance of behavior by an older character was fitted into a behavioral category matrix adapted from Saario, Jacklin, and Tittle (1973). The behavioral analysis revealed substantial constriction of performance of older characters, as shown in Table 1.

Table 1   Older Characters' Behaviors

Rank	Type of behavior (with examples)	Total behavior (%)	Male behavior (%)		Female behavior (%)	
1	Statements of information (nonevaluative observations)	21.07	(1)	21.58	(1)	20.05
2	Directive (initiating, directing, demonstrating)	11.79	(2)	12.39	(4)	10.55
3	Routine-repetitive (walking, rocking, turning on light)	11.44	(3)	10.88	(3)	12.53
4	Nurturant (helping, praising, serving)	10.79	(4)	8.03	(2)	16.29
5	Social-recreational (games, greeting or visiting someone)	6.42	(7)	6.24	(5)	6.80
6	Physically exertive (lifting heavy objects, chopping)	6.37	(5)	7.85	(10)	3.40
7	General verbal (listening, asking questions, looking)	5.65	(6)	6.78	(10)	3.40
8	Aggressive (hitting, kicking, verbal abuse)	4.87	(8)	4.99	(6)	4.65
9	Expressions of emotion (crying, laughing, shrieking)	4.75	(9)	4.90	(7)	4.47
10	Constructive-productive (building, sewing, magic acts)	3.98	(10)	4.09	(8)	3.76
11	Passive-supportive (non-active involvement, complying)	2.91	(12)	2.85	(12)	3.04
12	Problem-solving (producing idea, unusual combinations)	2.43	(11)	2.94	(15)	1.43
13	Statement about self (overall)	1.90	(13)	2.40	(16)	0.88
	(positive)	0.90		0.98		0.71
	(negative)	0.53		0.80		0.00
	(neutral)	0.47		0.62		0.17
14	Fantasy activity (silliness, daydreaming)	1.54	(16.5)	0.62	(10)	3.40
15	Self-care (dressing, washing, shaving)	1.36	(14)	1.78	(18)	0.53
16	Conformity (conveying rules, norms, expectations)	1.13	(15)	0.80	(14)	1.79
17	Passive-exertive (unwilling part of other's actions)	0.95	(18)	0.26	(13)	2.32
18	Avoidance (run away, stop trying)	0.65	(16.5)	0.62	(17)	0.71
	Total	100.00		100.00		100.00

Source: E. F. Ansello, "Age and Ageism in Children's First Literature," *Educational Gerontology*, (2)3, p. 267. Reprinted with permission of the Hemisphere Publishing Corporation.

Regarding the dispersion of behaviors, Ansello (1977b) noted:

For both sexes combined, 4 of the 18 categories (statements of information, directive, routine-repetitive, and nurturant) comprise some 55.09 percent of all behaviors. The predominance of these relatively mundane, routine portrayals contrasts sharply with the frequency of more creative, personal, and autonomous behaviors, e.g., constructive-productive, problem-solving, statements about self, and self-care, which total only 9.67 percent of all behaviors. Substantiating the definition of ageism, constricted roles and constrained behaviors are the norm here" (p. 268).

Again reflecting their relatively unimportant status, older characters appear alone in less than 0.5 percent of the 22,000 illustrations inspected, and are given flat, one-dimensional physical and personality descriptions. One adjective, *old,* accounts for about three-fourths of all the physical descriptions of older characters. Adding *little, elder,* and *ancient* accounts for 86 percent of all such descriptions, even though an extensive vocabulary analysis of literature for kindergarten through the third grade revealed at least 136 adjectives in "common" use. Although the descriptions of older characters' personalities vary more, these appear less than one-third as often as physical descriptions. The most frequent personality characteristics are *poor* (17.3 percent) and *sad* (6.8 percent), followed far less frequently by *wise* (4.5 percent) and *dear* (3.8 percent). This suggests ambivalence, at best, toward growing older. Significantly, negative ascriptions far outweigh positive.

In related research, Robin (1977) content-analyzed two samples of children's school readers, 47 published from 1953 to 1968 and 33 published in 1975, for age, sex, race, positions, and descriptions of older characters. She found that, while more than 70 percent of the books examined contained stories with older characters, less than 6 percent of the total characters in each set of texts were old. These were found to be predominantly white, with scant minority representation; they were circumscribed by the single adjective *old,* likely to have no other descriptors applied to them, and to be "supportive" behaviorally. Comparing the earlier and later sets of books, she found "little change over time." She concludes:

> *Children are not being socialized to the society as it is—at least not through elementary school readers. It is probably reflective of our basic ethnocentrism and of the social power of the dominant group that there has been little concern for the world view presented by texts among the writers or editors of texts, or among parents, teachers, and school administrators, or among those who study cultural processes. We do not know the extent to which textbook presentations of population segments (including age groupings) mold or reinforce the formation or maintenance of these attitudes, values, and knowledge. Children read elementary school readers over a period of six years. Perhaps a major concern should be the cumulative impact of these and other materials to which the child is exposed as a contributor to anticipatory socialization. Old age is the single minority status into which all people will move if they live long enough; children do not belong to that minority group but presumably should want to do so in the future. The impact of the misleading and inaccurate pictures of age that we have described may well influence children's future personal desires as well as their treatment of those who are currently members of that group (p. 291).*

Peterson and Eden (1977) assessed the depiction of old age in the best of early adolescent literature, the Newbery Medal winners, from the period 1922 to 1975. The Newbery books include novels, biography, fantasy, and nonfiction. Because of their quality and the attention afforded them by the Medal, these books "have some effect on the attitude teenagers form in the course of seeking to clarify their relationships with individuals and society," according to Peterson and Eden. The books were analyzed to answer questions about: the extent of development of older characters, their positive or negative descriptions, their social relationships, the trends that have occurred over time in positive-negative portrayals, trends in the numbers of older characters and in their complexity.

These researchers found that older characters were present in some way in 51 of the 53 books examined. However, they were judged to be not well developed. "Only 4.6 items of information were available on the average older character, which provided minimal insight into their personalities and behavior. This meant that the older character was seldom judged to have a major role in the story (16 percent) and was generally peripheral to the development of the plot" (p. 319).

The valence of the positive-negative portrayals of older characters was considered inconsistent because the number of positive versus negative descriptions was not statistically significant and the plurality of their appearances was neutral. Social relationships were also distributed; men were more likely to have an occupational identity than women, who were more often placed in a family relationship.

Looked at over time, the books showed that behaviors of older characters tended to become more negative but descriptions of them became more positive. Older characters increased in number around the time of World War II, perhaps because of wartime exigencies, followed by a sharp recent decline. Finally, Peterson and Eden concluded that there was no greater complexity in the roles of recent older characters since occupations, economic status, and activities did not seem to increase.

The authors hold that, although there was no apparent ageism, a more subtle prejudice pervaded the literature. As in children's literature, the lack of development and the constriction of activities tend to make older characters flat, uninteresting, and boring. According to Peterson and Eden (1977):

There are few role models acceptable to those of us who see the process of aging as providing the potential for continuing growth and development. . . . What is needed is a collection of literature that provides the vicarious experience necessary to assist teenagers to move from the stereotype to the attitude stage. It is neither surprising nor inappropriate for adolescent literature to have younger people as the major characters in these stories. Role models and personal interest are extremely important. However, it is also important for well-developed, complex characters of other ages to be included so that additional insights may be acquired. This currently is not occurring.

The adolescent literature tends to support the youth culture with the emphasis on strength, beauty, and physical activity. There seem to be few characters who gain the respect of others through the use of their wisdom, insight, or patience. The strengths that can be gained through the process of aging are not recognized nor rewarded in the stories. There seems to be little reason or value in being old or in having older people present (p. 323).

Schuerman, Eden, and Peterson (1977) investigated the images of aging in current women's periodicals. Choosing nine magazines (*Cosmopolitan, Family Circle, Good Housekeeping, Ladies Home Journal, Mademoiselle, McCall's, Ms., Redbook,* and *Women's Day*) on the basis of their extensive readership and ready availability, the authors reviewed all fiction stories in the 1975 issues. In addition, several representative humorous and childhood-recollection articles were included. In all, the study covered 216 stories from 108 issues.

The researchers tallied by sex the total numbers of characters, of older characters, and of major and minor characters. With stories containing older persons, each description and action of an older person was recorded verbatim. These transcriptions were then analyzed by a panel of 15 gerontologists and judged positive, negative, or neutral. In addition, older characters were assessed for age, health, marital and financial states, family role, occupation (present or previous), retirement status, and housing situation.

Schuerman and colleagues found that 121, or 13.4 percent, of the 902 major characters were older, compared to 222, or 8.5 percent, of the 2,878 minor characters. The researchers found more positive than negative descriptions and actions for older persons, though negative descriptions outnumbered negative actions.

With regard to the various demographic variables, the researchers noted significant discrepancies between older characters in women's periodicals and older persons in the total population. Essentially the literature of the periodical was found to reflect the mentality of that periodical, rather a microcosm of the relationship between literature and mentality spoken of earlier. Examining the readership data (age, education, etc.) provided by each publisher showed that women's current periodical literature projects images of old age congruent with the backgrounds and expectations of the readerships rather than with real life. So there were equal numbers of male and female older characters, and they were married, blessed with good health, and were quite comfortable financially. Many were in professional occupations, and few had chosen to retire. The single exception to this positive projection was in the area of housing where a higher than actual percentage of older characters was institutionalized. Schuerman and colleagues suspect that "the authors' solution to older characters who were no longer able to maintain their independence was to place them in nursing homes where they would not have a direct claim on the time and energy of the young characters" (p. 344).

The researchers' conclusion recalls the previous discussion of Harris and Associates' (1975) quantification of the discrepancy between realities of aging projected and experienced:

In summary, then, the image of aging presented through these stories is both positive and inaccurate. Older characters are present and perform essential roles and functions, but are shown as extensions of the readers themselves, rather than as realistic older people. Old age is described more through cosmetic changes in appearance, i.e., white hair and wrinkles, than through the characteristic changes in survival, marital status, health, financial status, and retirement that actually mark transition to old age (p. 344).

Conclusion

It would appear evident that literature has been both mirror and matrix with regard to the processes of aging. As mirror, it has reflected and perpetuated, perhaps more steadily than other cultural institutions, the association of age and loss. As matrix, it has served to socialize untold generations, conditioning them to expectations of aging dissonant with actual experience at least, and inferior to potential experience at worst. The denial of continued human development throughout the lifespan is evidenced historically in philosophical and literary great books. It is also apparent in contemporary literature, in the uninspiring, vapid, unidimensional routinism of older characters in children's literature, through the age-denying, self-reflective unreality of women's periodicals.

Literature, after all, reflects the almost timeless mentality equating age with deterioration. Perhaps it would be unrealistic to expect literature to portray much else with regard to aging. Literature will probably not provide significantly more positive role models until the mentality evolves and changes. But herein lies the final paradox: as mirror and matrix, literature continues to condition people to avoid aging as a subject and older people as contacts. We are thus estranged; and the opportunity for direct experiences that would challenge personal, social, and literary attitudes—indeed, the very knowledge structure—remains frustrated.

References

Ahammer, I. M., & Baltes, P. B. Objective versus perceived age differences in personality: How do adolescents, adults and older people view themselves and each other? *Journal of Gerontology*, 1972, 27, 46–51.

Ansello, E. F. (Ed.). Old age and literature: A developmental analysis. *Educational Gerontology*, 1977a, 2(3).

Ansello, E. F. Age and ageism in children's first literature. *Educational Gerontology*, 1977b, 2(3), 255–274.

Baltes, P. B., & Labouvie, G. Adult development of intellectual performance: Description, explanation and modification. In C. Eisdorfer & M. M. Lawton (Eds.), *The psychology of adult development and aging.* Washington, D.C.: American Psychological Association, 1973.

Borges, M. A., & Dutton, L. J. Attitudes toward aging: Increasing optimism found with age. *The Gerontologist*, 1976, 16(3), 220–224.

Charles, D. C. Literary old age: A browse through history. *Educational Gerontology*, 1977, 2(3), 237–253.

Council on Interracial Books for Children. *Human (and anti-human) values in children's books.* New York: Author, 1976.

Harris, L., & Associates. *The myth and reality of aging in America.* Washington, D.C.: The National Council on the Aging, 1975.

Havighurst, R. J. *Developmental tasks and education.* New York: David McKay, 1972. (Originally published, 1948, 1952.)

Kuhn, T. S. *The structure of scientific revolutions.* (2nd ed.) Chicago: University of Chicago Press, 1970.

Neugarten, B. L. (Ed.). *Middle age and aging.* Chicago: University of Chicago Press, 1968.

Peterson, D. A., & Eden, D. Z. Teenagers and aging: Adolescent literature as an attitude source. *Educational Gerontology,* 1977, *2*(3), 311–325.

Robin, E. P. Old age in elementary school readers. *Educational Gerontology,* 1977, *2*(3), 275–292.

Saario, T. N., Jacklin, C. N., & Tittle, C. K. Sex role stereotyping in the public schools. *Harvard Educational Review,* 1973, *43*(3), 386–416.

Schuerman, L. E., Eden, D. Z., & Peterson, D. A. Older people in women's periodical fiction. *Educational Gerontology,* 1977, *2*(3), 327–351.

Svoboda, C. P. Senescence in western philosophy. *Educational Gerontology,* 1977, *2*(3), 219–235.

U.S. Bureau of the Census. *Demographic aspects of aging and the older population in the United States.* Current population reports, special studies series P–23, no. 59. Washington, D.C.: U.S. Government Printing Office, May 1976.

Wechsler, D. *Manual for the Wechsler adult intelligence scale.* New York: Psychological Corporation, 1955.

PART FIVE
THE HEALTH PROFESSIONS
AND AGING

The health professions in general, and medicine in particular, are facing the same developmental issues that other areas of gerontology have been addressing: Should concern for aging be integrated into basic disciplines and professions, or should it have a specialized area, such as geriatric medicine? The five papers in this section suggest that both models may exist in the health professions.

The Health Professions and Aging

Tom Hickey
University of Michigan

The title of this paper has about it something paradoxical. Health professions are institutions, whereas aging is a process. Institutions seem to be static structures that have evolved in relation to fairly well defined functions. Processes, however, indicate something dynamic and changing both in nature and in outcome.

Let us assume for the moment that what we should be addressing here generally is the role of the various health professions in the treatment of the aged, and, specifically, that our task is to delineate the educational needs of health professionals who serve older people. What do these future health professionals need to know?

Among other things, they need to know about the settings and (institutionalized) systems where health care is provided for elderly people. They also need to know about the implications and interactions of the aging processes as they affect the diseases or illnesses of their older patients. It is perhaps somewhat less important to know about aged people themselves, since they are changing anyway. For example, people now 65 years of age are much healthier than their parents were a generation ago. Therefore, to adequately address our task of discussing the education of health professionals for gerontology and geriatrics, we need to know about the institutional context of health care and the clinical implications of the aging processes. Thus, we are indeed focusing here on both processes and institutions, and the title may turn out to be somewhat fitting after all.

That we are dealing with educational content suggests to me that we have gone beyond verifying the need for educational programs. Incidentally, in this regard, it is somewhat refreshing to note that many of the newer texts in gerontology do not begin with the general statement: "Ten percent of this country's population is over the age of 65." Similarly, I hope that we are familiar with the demography of health needs among our older population. I am assuming that we all know that this same 10 percent of the population accounts for at least one-fourth of all of the health dollars spent in this country annually. I further assume we know that the older population, especially the very aged, are the principal consumers of drugs and of the time of most health professionals. At least one out of three acute-care beds and nine out of ten long-term care beds are occupied by the elderly. This is the well-documented demand for health care by the aged in our society. The need for health care is undoubtedly greater. In fact, the continuing discrepancy between need and demand results in a significant stress on our planning efforts—both for services and for personnel (cf. Kovar, 1977; *Occupational Outlook Quarterly*, Fall 1976).

Institutions

We must begin by recognizing that the paramount role in future health care for the elderly lies with the medical profession and its medical education. From an institutional perspective, leadership must begin there. It is refreshing to see that much activity has begun in recent years (cf. Dorsey in this volume; see also Libow, 1976, 1977). In addition, the American Geriatrics Society conducted two major study conferences on geriatric education, with findings and recommendations published in the November 1977 issue of the *Journal of the American Geriatrics Society.*

It has been too easy for many of us to criticize the medical profession for its lack of interest in older patients. Until these recent developments, for the most part, we have forged ahead in gerontology and in allied health care areas without the assistance and leadership of the medical profession. In the clinical and health service sector, public health, nursing, and related social services have maintained a sense of priority for the elderly, despite frequent physician resistance and related difficulties in dealing effectively with the geriatric patient. We have been heard to say quite freely that doctors want to "cure" people, not "care" for them; since the chronic diseases of many older people are considered incurable, doctors have been said to ignore them.

However, this issue has posed real problems for medicine. Should there be a new specialty in geriatric medicine? This is a territorial issue of great conceptual and clinical significance to schools of medicine and to medical practice. It is not unlike the argument we have been debating in gerontology for many years: Should we have degree programs in gerontology rather than aging-related curricula and emphases integrated into basic disciplines and professions? In gerontology we now have both, although much more of the latter. In medical education, we will probably have various types as well. I would argue, however, that the field will strengthen through the process of integrating clinical research and education in aging into basic medical curricula—for example, internal medicine, psychiatry, and physiatry. In the past year or so, much praise has been given to the Cornell University Medical College for being the first American university to establish a chair in geriatric medicine. I would hope that we will find equally praiseworthy the successful integration of aging content into all basic disciplines in the curriculum of a medical school. As we are currently discovering at the University of Michigan, this is no easy task. A great deal of planning has yielded only the beginning of collaboration within the five health science schools and an initial small-scale offering of a senior-year elective for medical students.

I trust that we will not see our role here as one of complaining about and criticizing the past. Let us move forward to look at the improvement of curricula in all of the health professions, and develop clinical programs of treatment and services that will meet the important health needs of older people. I do think that leadership from medicine will facilitate this integration more rapidly, increasing the feasibility of other institutional changes in health care for older people. To put this another way, we no longer have time for the somewhat academic disputes about leadership for educational programs in this area. Far more important issues require our immediate attention. The ethical issues and value questions inherent in policy development at the national level are crucial at this time. This is a leadership issue for the health professions, and it is not to be left solely to legislators.

Another institutional issue that cannot be ignored—and one that is slow to change—is the pattern and structure of available care dictated by methods of reimbursement. Ideally, there should be a range of services to match needs along the spectrum from full independence in the home, to the near total dependence of older patients in a skilled-nursing facility. This goal has been realized only partially. Among many problems, the present reimbursement mechanisms do not generally make it easy to accomplish this goal. We have a major "educational" challenge at the level of community awareness and advocacy and also at the level of state legislative and policy activity—not an easy task. It is somewhat simplistic, for example, to think that home health care is the unchallengeable answer. I recently examined this service in my own state, only to find that the cost of a professional nursing visit in the home ranges from $15 to $50 and that of a health aide visit from $5 to $15. Nevertheless, we do need to facilitate (and reimburse) the use of home health services for the elderly.

Speaking of institutions, families and neighborhood are important, underused societal institutions. The "24-hour discharge dilemma" faced by many older people in an acute-care facility is something more than simply a reimbursement problem. It is as much a family issue as it is a Medicare issue. It is also somewhat simplistic to think that we can depopulate our skilled-nursing facilities, thus reducing the continuing trend of adding more and more beds. The proportion of the population moving into the over age 75 classification is increasing dramatically, and one out of every three or four of these people will need institutional care in the future, if only briefly. Thus, there is a need for all kinds of health care services, including the present institutional system. Something like home health care is an additional and necessary option, not an alternative to institutions.

Aging and Chronic Illness

This brief paper does not permit a detailed discussion of normal aging changes and chronic illness (cf. Hickey, 1979). Let me simply say that if we are going to develop sound curricula and train qualified health professionals, we need additional research to better differentiate disease processes from physiological aging and to further elucidate the effects of their interaction for health care. I might add that much of this could occur through modifications and extensions of many ongoing biomedical research programs. Furthermore, despite the high cost of longitudinal data, cross-sectional research with older people is very time-limited in its usefulness to us for the development of educational content, since these data represent a somewhat biologically elite group of survivors, who may not be comparable to others. Furthermore, this type of research begs the question of the interactive phenomenon of aging and chronic illness, which needs to be examined at earlier points in the life cycle.

Students and future health professionals need to know what is clinically and functionally important in older patients and what should be and is treatable. They also need to see this demonstrated in a context that includes old people. Given the dynamics of the aging process and the multiple etiologies of various health problems in old age, we need to be able to diagnose accurately. We further need to be able to monitor ongoing health problems and their rapid changes in this population with greater frequency. In summary, we have diagnostic problems and treatment problems that change much more rapidly with the aged than with other age groups. Quite apart from the incidence and prevalence of disease among older people, their qualitatively different health care needs require a significant upgrading in the knowledge base and clinical treatment skills of all health professionals. Moreover, this same base is necessary for the realistic training of health planners and administrators. Once again our program experiences at the University of Michigan's School of Public Health have demonstrated to us the importance of clinical observation experiences in geriatric care for future health planners and administrators. Nonmedical personnel in the health care setting need to know firsthand of the particular concerns and problems of the elderly population, as well as some of the important personal and environmental dynamics involved in their health care.

I hope that explorations in this area will further our own search for more accurate and useful information (i.e., curricula) for all health professions and for the techniques to develop opportunities for these students and future professionals to practice their skills and test their knowledge base.

References

Hickey, T. *Health and aging.* Monterey, Calif.: Brooks-Cole, 1979.

Kovar, M. G. Health of the elderly and the use of health services. *Public Health Reports*, 1977, 92(1), 9–19.

Libow, L. S. A geriatric medical residency program. *Annals of Internal Medicine*, 1976, 85(5), 641–647.

Libow, L. S. The issues in geriatric medical education and postgraduate train-
ing: Old problems in a new field. *Geriatrics*, February 1977, 99–102.
Occupational Outlook Quarterly, U.S. Department of Labor, Bureau of Labor
Statistics, USGPO, Fall 1976, *20*(3).

Health Gerontology: Select Ethical and Planning Issues

Jerome Kaplan
Mansfield Memorial Homes
and
Ohio State University-Mansfield

Preventing disease and trauma may improve and lengthen life. However, if we accomplish this by involving governmental protection designed for large groups of people, we are likely to compete with individual freedom. Thus, the view that absolute costs for health services should be controlled and that new facilities and beds should be restricted is incompatible with the view that one should have the freedom to select from a number of facilities that offer ever-increasing service in amount and quality.

In the continued effort to attain new knowledge, we need to avoid politicizing research or applying controls that are not scientifically acceptable. In addition, the use of gerontological knowledge should be free of political restraints as well as inappropriate judgment on the interpretation of such knowledge. Neither taking care with research nor using knowledge free of restraints implies that people's views would be disregarded. On the contrary, they suggest an ethical and moral structure supported by appropriate governmental guidelines instead of government serving as the value base that molds ethics and morals. The extent to which researchers and the providers of health, human service, and enrichment programs should be autonomous or should operate within a publicly defined context is still being debated, but the publicly defined context appears to be accepted by our society.

To some people, the knowledge provider is an individualist pursuing his own intellectual interests, a contributor to society. To these people, structures tend to control research and stultify the development of new knowledge. Others see the individualistic researcher as primarily pursuing his own interests regardless of public need. From this perspective, management is needed to make the development of new knowledge responsive to public need and, also, to protect older people as research subjects. Mediation of these viewpoints will decide the productivity of our evolving research system and the direction of the effect such knowledge has on policy, planning, and practice.

The equitable distribution of health, human service, and enrichment programs is one of the great problems facing American society. But how is equitable need to be determined? We must increase assessment activities and refine our assessment instruments so they can be easily used. We must also develop improved methods of assessing the consequences of added knowledge and the resultant use of such knowledge. Finally, we need to use these new approaches toward assessment if we are to proceed with rational policies.

Further, as a concomitant step, the older person should be encouraged to participate in policymaking. The dissemination of information through such means as open meetings and publications is critical to these decisions. In order for the informed older person to make knowledgeable decisions, valid information should be transmitted; hence, the call for studies of the implications of our ever-growing knowledge about aging and for requests to government to disclose sufficient information to the older American public.

Individual Freedom Versus Social Good

The older person should be responsible for his or her own actions and should be free to decide what is best, provided that society has no compelling interest in the outcome. Compelling interest does relate to those elderly who are considered by society to be incapable of making their own decisions. Decision making is also a matter of degree and type. Hence, our perspective of individual freedom and of governmental intervention in private affairs becomes more clear as we consider the consequences.

That concern for social good can overwhelm and erode individual freedom of choice is a real possibility. There are people who wish to be left alone even if they choose to be unhealthy. Individual freedom of choice is still more important than either the attainment of knowledge or the pursuit of health or social well-being. This perspective, however, may not hold true in the future.

Generally, different policies adversely affected minority or disadvantaged groups. Control of advances may restrict access to minority groups; promotion of technologies may open minority groups to abuses. It is at least arguable that this reflects a tendency to use the disadvantaged as symbols in making a point, for we must not forget that biomedical and behavioral research and technology do exist in a larger cultural and social context.

Where individual responsibility is involved, as in the relationship between smoking and heart disease or lung cancer, individual solutions have taken priority. Thus, we provide general education to promote personal choice based on information rather than governmental regulations. In general, although society allows individual responsibility in such cases as the decision to participate in a risky experimental treatment, society is inclined to enforce conformity to social good where an individual's behavior or choice is a detriment to others.

Advances

Many people, when considering desirable advances in behavioral and biomedical research, tend to think of things that have major health effects, for example, a cure for heart disease or cancer. In addition, they think that the means by which these health benefits will be attained are themselves good, or at least do not conflict with other equally important values. However, when advances in knowledge are specified and methods for attaining them are pinpointed, issues of value come to the forefront. Careful analysis can show that benefits may not be as great as once imagined; there may even be the potential for impairment. More important, the means by which these benefits are to be attained may harm the rights of people. Examined at this level of detail, advances may no longer look so attractive. For example, if the prevention or treatment of heart disease or cancer could be accomplished only through the rigid control of individual behavior, it is doubtful that it would be regarded as highly desirable.

Advances that might be expected to occur in the last part of this century have the potential to:

contribute markedly to the solution of the world population growth problem; contribute to the general improvement of individual health care for all members of society; significantly decrease certain health care costs, particularly the costs of custodial care; enhance research and development in epidemiology and preventive medicine; and ameliorate the individually debilitating effects of anxiety and depression and the socially debilitating effects of criminal aggression.

However, they also have the potential to: . . . substantially alter the sex ratio of American society, if not all the world; substantially alter present values regarding life and death . . . euthanasia, privacy, human rights and individual responsibility; substantially alter basic American social patterns of marriage and family life; create entirely new "minority" or disadvantaged groups based on health status; and cause redistribution in the economy through prolonging the average life span. (A Comprehensive Study of Ethical, Legal, and Social Implications of Advances in Biomedical and Behavioral Research and Technology, Note 1.)

Knowledge Application

The effect of culture and its particular morality and conflicts is dramatically presented in a question I developed for a training program. Knowledge about sex in the later years came into conflict with how trainees responsible for a situation viewed sexual expression:

Mrs. M., age 84, invited Mr. L., age 79, to join her in her room and "see if my bed has room for two and we can push the chair against the door." You have overheard the discussion, and your immediate thought is: (a) She's a dirty old woman. (b) He's a dirty old man. (c) They're a dirty old duo. (d) Ha! Who are they kidding? They can't do anything. (e) Hmm! Not a bad idea! (Kaplan, Note 2).

Knowledge about sexual interest in older people and about the differentiation of such interests among older individuals is important to programming within any group environment, whether it is a nursing home or a senior center. Social relationships are important factors in making major policy decisions about how emphasis should be divided between group nutrition programs and home-delivered meals-on-wheels programs.

The same training examination asks about the effect of knowledge about crystallized and fluid intelligence and memory, which directly affects programming:

The activities director of the Heterosexual Senior Center could not decide whether or not to proceed with a word-building activity and sought out your counsel. You, as the administrator, suggest: (a) It's ridiculous. Our seniors have enough problems remembering words they used to know. (b) It's an interesting thought, but why don't you stay with bingo instead because most people have played bingo. (c) It's an interesting thought. Let's add this game to our repertory of activities. (d) Foolishness. You can't teach an old dog new tricks. (e) Why don't you bring in an erector set, instead? (Kaplan, Note 2).

Knowledge Implementation through Planning

The influence of knowledge and its application form the cornerstone of social planning. For example, a recent article by Teaff and colleagues (1978) reports that age-segregated living arrangements in public housing have favorable effects. The authors discovered small but reliable relationships between such arrangements and on-site activity participation, housing satisfaction, and neighborhood motility. Yet another study notes that the majority of the general elderly population does not prefer age-segregated housing (Lawton, 1975). Even so, reservations about close contacts with young people were common to both studies. Policy planning, then, requires appropriate assessment of such knowledge to pursue a facility, services, or a personal-enrichment approach to enhance the living conditions of older people.

The broad purpose of any plan to assist old people is to provide a framework for the future development of resources. To meet this end, the goals set forth in such a plan must express the desired status of older people and the health, human service, and enrichment systems that serve them. Objectives that would lead to the achievement of the goals are also part of the plan.

In order to evaluate progress in meeting goals, we must be sure that both goals and objectives are measurable. One kind of measurement is to classify goals as priority, rate the level of the priority, and then incorporate these priority goals within a plan.

In determining the priority level of a goal and its objectives, we take as a major consideration the expected positive effect on improving health, human service, and enrichment status. To do so, we need sufficient information to express these expected changes quantifiably. Further, the feasibility of achieving goals and objectives is also a primary consideration. The application of gerontological knowledge is an essential key toward any such implementation. Priority goals, therefore, are the ones that express desired changes in an ever-extending range of importance about older people's health care, human service, and personal-enrichment systems. These priority goals are considered highly significant because of their potential to enhance accessibility, continuity, and quality of care and service or personal enrichment; to meet identified individual and social needs; to incorporate cost-effective and cost-containment measurements; and to develop a positive feeling.

Any good plan includes the importance of mental, physical, and psychological screening; the prevention of disease and maintenance of well-being, which would incorporate the dissemination of assessment instruments and training in their use; nutrition education and meals programs; integration of the social and public network systems (the family, educational institutions, community and tax resources—Medicare, Medicaid, Title XX of the Social Security Act, and Older Americans Act, to name a few); the understanding of the various roles of older people; the effects of isolation on older people and the implementation of specially designed mobility programs; the implications of death and dying, which confront the old more than the young; and the understanding of how minority and female status necessitate precise knowledge to allow for individuation within planning.

Priority Goals and Objectives

Examples of priority goals and specific objectives affecting older people are listed below to demonstrate how a plan puts aging knowledge into usable form. These are only illustrative and are not to be considered comprehensive (Kaplan, Note 3).

Purpose I Health promotion and protection
Goals
1. Local health directed services to improve the behavior, health, and security of older people
2. Decrease detrimental environmental actions
Objectives
1. A local coordinated county or multicounty system for older person information and referral services
2. Patient education on accidents, arteriosclerosis, cancer, diabetes, heart disease, hypertension, learning and memory, nutrition, strokes,

and other topics of import to older people by hospitals, rehabilitation, ambulatory-care centers, and long-term care facilities

Purpose II Prevention services
Goals
    1. Promote optimal physical and mental well-being through identifying disease or ill health at the presymptomatic stage
    2. Protection against the development of detected disease
Objectives
    1. Screening programs for cancer, arteriosclerosis, diabetes, heart disease, hypertension, and strokes available and accessible to all older people
    2. Congregate and home-delivered meal programs serving a specified percentage of all older people
    3. Therapeutic programs to prevent suicides by older people

Purpose III Treatment services
Goals
    1. Diagnosis to identify disease
    2. Treatment of specific diseases or their symptoms.
Objectives
    1. Distribute short-term acute beds in an equitable manner at the national ratio of per 1,000 population
    2. Primary care available to older people 24 hours every day
    3. Continuity of care coordination among the various types of care levels offered

Purpose IV Rehabilitation services
Goals
    1. Assist the ill or disabled older person to maximize capacities
Objectives
    1. Coordinate the mental and physical therapies for older people
    2. Provide therapies within congregate centers and apartments for older people

Purpose V Maintenance services
Goals
    1. Assistance in activities of daily living
    2. Provision of services to older people with chronic mental or physical conditions to prevent or minimize deterioration in these conditions
Objectives
    1. Homemaker health services available to all older people
    2. Day-care services available to all older people
    3. Effective transportation to maintain usual mobility and to use available services

Purpose VI Enabling services
Goals
    1. Enrichment programs for older people within educational institutions and congregate older people residences
    2. Accessibility to the opportunities for creative group and interpersonal relations

Objectives

    1. Variable creative educational opportunities by schools and within senior centers, homes for aged, and retirement apartment complexes

    2. Opportunities for older people to participate in college courses

    3. Indoor and outdoor recreational resources and their refinements, including appropriately structured camping

    4. Group outlets for relationships and the enhancement of leadership and volunteer potential

Again, these purposes, goals, and objectives illustrate how a plan for priorities is developed to improve the well-being of older people through the effective use of gerontological knowledge. They are not in priority order nor comprehensive in content.

Minorities

The United States population comes from many backgrounds. An adequate perspective about older people includes knowing the parameters of membership in officially recognized minority groups and knowing how these data refine our overall gerontological knowledge. Not only are these data of worth by themselves, but the interpretation of such information is a crucial factor in putting this knowledge to work, since health, service, and enrichment program development and subsequent use relate to how different groups of older people see needs and how they adapt to aging. We have learned that American ethnic groups view aging differently (Sterne, Phillips, and Rabushka, 1974), just as American racial groups do. Thus, elderly white Americans have a more positive view of aging than elderly black Americans, who, in turn, have a more positive view of aging than elderly Mexican-Americans.

One should, however, keep two important facts in mind. First, there are individual elderly Mexican-Americans who view aging positively, whereas some elderly white Americans perceive a stigma attached to aging. Therefore, there are individual differences to be found within any one group of the elderly and among groupings of older people. Second, it is the totality of sociocultural influences, which include how ethnic and racial groups have developed life styles and evolved the satisfactions obtained from these life styles, that sets the tone of individual perceptions of aging and not one's ethnic nor racial background.

Ethnicity and Race

Most older people prefer to retain their own households while maintaining valued relationships with relatives. Very few families (3 percent) that have an older person as a head of the household also include grandchildren, and only 3.3 percent of all older heads of households have dependent children under the age of 18 residing with them. But, in the case of older people with Spanish surnames, the percentage with dependent children under 18 rises to 10 percent. Obviously, sociocultural factors, whether from tradition or late marriage or economics or adequate housing, or some combination of these and other sociological factors, set this group apart from the elderly population as a whole. Planning and subsequent services, therefore, must make use of this datum about this particular ethnic group.

In understanding ethnicity, it is very important to recognize that ethnicity has provided a group identity predicated on centuries of evolution. The creation of a large block of older people is new to our times. In turn, these older people represent varied backgrounds. Although older persons may respond to a particular happening because of societal expectations of aged behavior or because of available chronological age roles, they are influenced in thought and action by ethnic-root variables, including the moral base of their particular ethnicity. Thus, policymaking, planning, services, and educational programming must take into account how such ethnic knowledge affects and modifies gerontological knowledge.

Although there is remarriage in the older years, six widowers remarry for every one widow who does. This is due to variable factors such as the much greater number of older women. In addition, our culture more readily accepts marriage between an older man and a younger woman than between an older woman and a younger man. Since the marriage rate among the nonwhite older people is higher than among the elderly white or the older person population as a whole, an apparent subcultural factor is at work. Again, this knowledge affects plans and resources and has a direct relationship in planning for specified gerontological entities, such as numbers of nursing home beds, transportation, home services, and numerous other program approaches.

It further appears the elderly nonwhite person is worse off than the older white person in education, finances, health, and longevity, even though older people as a group do not fare well compared to the whole U.S. population.

Older Women Identity and Support Systems

The declining ratio of older men to older women is a modern phenomenon that will probably continue and accelerate. Women tend to outlive men. As this tendency continues, the ratio of elderly women to elderly men may be two to one by the end of this century.

A great many women lose their source of emotional support when their children become adults and move out of their household. Others lose their status and social function when they become widows. Consequently, the development of services and programs that provide opportunities for such emotional support and for the maintenance of status and social function is of great value.

For older women, as well as men, age-related losses can create a predisposition to a change in sexual identity. The rapidly decreasing ratio of older men compared to older women—a 1960 sex ratio of 82.6 males per 100 females compared to 72.1 older males to 100 older females in 1970—suggests these age-related losses will have a much more substantial effect on many more older women than on older men. These losses are aptly described by Butler and Lewis (1973) as social-type loss, such as family, friend, job, social status; physical-type loss, such as health, strength, appearance; and psychological- and cognitive-type losses, such as change in self-esteem, rote memory, creativity, conditionability, senses, speed, and timing. Losses are not absolute for all older people since there are some individuals who may have little diminishment.

Specific adaptability is required of older women. The low remarriage rate of widows and its effect on planning have already been noted. Such adaptability suggests modified services, encouragement toward living-style changes, and—among other approaches—specially designed health care programs.

A Perspective

A great, current plague in the fields of human service and health care has been the reversal to the "do-gooder" role of the late nineteenth and early twentieth centuries, except that this time, the do-gooder is the paid non-professional rather than the volunteer humanitarian. In aging service, we have flitted from the idea of love is enough, to love is not enough and needs supplementation, to professional applicability that seemed to override scientific knowledge, and finally to the current era of love (only incidentally) and knowledge (applied peripherally).

The ultimate test should be, Who can make the most modern gerontological knowledge available in a form acceptable to a person or a family? The lack of gerontologically trained professional clinical workers is very serious and very obvious. Of equal concern is the relative lack of opportunity for such professionals to practice directly with old people and their families. Likewise of much concern is the unresolved role of the trained gerontologist, who is not trained to be a clinician but is trained to be a person highly knowledgeable in aging. But in a direct helping role?

Ethical considerations draw from American and Western value clusters. Gross (1967) identifies 15 such major value-belief clusters: (1) activity and work, (2) achievement and success, (3) moral orientation, (4) humanitarianism, (5) efficiency and practicality, (6) science and secular rationality, (7) material comfort, (8) progress, (9) equality, (10) freedom, (11) democracy, (12) external conformity, (13) nationalism and patriotism, (14) individual personality, and (15) racism and related group superiority.

Almost two-thirds of these value beliefs belittle the elderly, as can be seen by comparing these value clusters for the elderly with the American population as a whole. Gross (1967) states that "running through these complex orientations . . . is an emphasis on the worth of active mastery rather than a passive acceptance of events . . . and a high evaluation of individual personality rather than collective identity and responsibility." If Gross's formulation is accurate, and it is one with which I concur, then the aged are still excluded from high-value considerations.

Morality and values with the aged: Are they in conflict or in consonance? Are they for individual or the social good?

Notes

1. *A comprehensive study of the ethical, legal, and social implications of advances in biomedical and behavioral research and technology. Summary of and final report.* Policy Research Incorporated and the Center of Technology Assessment, New Jersey Institute of Technology, 1977, 30–31.

2. Knowledge utilization test developed by J. Kaplan.

3. Based on a schema originally designed by J. Kaplan for inclusion in *Working with older people* (Vol. 2). Washington, D.C.: Gerontological Society, in press.

References

Butler, R. N. & Lewis, M. I. *Aging and mental health: Positive psychological approaches.* St. Louis: C. V. Mosby, 1973.

Gross, B. M. Individual and group values. *Annual American Academy Political Social Science,* 1967, 371.

Lawton, M. P. *Social and medical services in housing for the aged.* Philadelphia: Philadelphia Geriatric Center, 1975.

Sterne, R. S., Phillips, J. E., & Rabushka, A. *The urban elderly poor: Racial and bureaucratic conflict.* Boston: D. C. Heath, 1974.

Teaff, J. D., Lawton, M. P., Nahemow, L., & Carlson, D. Impact of age integration on the well-being of elderly tenants in public housing. *Journal of Gerontology,* 1978, 33, 126.

On Ethnic Variations in Aging Behavior: Some Problems for Future Research

Wilbur H. Watson
National Center on Black Aged

Historical and Ethnographic Research on Community Organization and Aging Behavior

The histories of race relations and the social and behavioral science literature amply document the association between racial discrimination, residential segregation, and low frequencies of black use of public accommodations including medical service centers in the United States (Pinkney, 1969; Norman, 1969; *Double Jeopardy*, 1964). However, little ethnographic research has focused on how black Americans and other nonwhite ethnic Americans, living in communities that developed under the constraints of race-related social oppression, learned to perceive, assign meaning to, and formulate social means of coping with disabled elderly members, physical illness, and irregularities in the social behavior of community members at large.

We need historical and comparative ethnographic research on community adaptation to elderly members and illness. This kind of inquiry will help deepen our understanding of the forms of community health care and of the alternatives to costly long-term institutional care for the elderly and other impaired people. Further, through systematic historical and comparative ethnographic research, we can begin to take steps toward preventing what Lipman (1978) calls the "error of implicit social, psychological, and valuational homogeneity." This is the fallacy of assuming that once people enter old age, however that may be defined, they become an undifferentiated mass. There is great risk of falling into this error if comparative methods in research are not developed. For example, an investigation may simply fail, albeit unwittingly, to take into account possible ethnic variations in behavior. Lipman writes (1978): "While there are undoubtedly certain correlates to poverty and minority living, there is little question that the native American experience differs from that of the Blacks, which differs from that of the Puerto Rican, which differs from that of the Japanese" (p. 224).

Further, although it is correct that the elderly population in the United States is predominantly female when undifferentiated by ethnicity, Kalish and Moriwaki (1973) have pointed out that Chinese-American elderly are predominantly male: "If Chinese-American, the elderly person is probably a man; the ratio of males to females, all ages combined, in California was 107:100 in 1970; the same ratio among the aged would be higher" (p. 196). This fact is probably explained by late-nineteenth century patterns of Chinese male migrants who came to the United States in search of gainful employment without their families (Lyman, 1971; Kitano, 1974). However, this important observation would probably be obscured or neglected entirely in the absence of comparative ethnographic analysis.

In addition to an accurate factual portrayal of ethnic variations in the United States, comparative ethnographic research will help to document some of the historical and contemporary relations among racism, patterns of discrimination, and health care for black and other nonwhite Americans; identify sociocultural factors in definitions of health and illness; and help reveal various informal intervention systems, such as institutional aspects of folk medicine that have developed to provide health and social-supportive care in spite of discriminatory treatment in public accommodations.

Differential Life Expectancy

It is common knowledge that black Americans and other ethnics of color live, on the average, fewer years than their white ethnic counterparts in the United States. It is also relatively well known that women—Asian, Hispanic, black, and white—have a longer average life expectancy than men, with white women having the greatest life expectancy overall. Yet very little systematic research has aimed at explaining these differences. There has, however, been a variety of small-scale piecemeal studies and many more journal articles devoted to speculating about the differences and either romanticizing about the life styles, diets, and sociocultural environments of centenarians or lamenting the supposedly harsh conditions under which ethnics who manifest significantly shorter life spans must have lived.

In a country, such as the United States—where endless lip service is given to the personhood of all people despite race or religion, where liberal politicians often call attention to the equality of all citizens under the law, where it is proclaimed that all citizens have a right to life, liberty, and the pursuit of happiness—these differential rates in longevity raise a variety of moral and empirical questions. Although this is not the place to belabor the moral implications of differential longevity and the white ethnic biases represented by other factors, such as age 65 as a criterion of eligibility for receiving

Social Security and other benefits, it is appropriate to raise a number of important researchable questions in this area.

It has been well documented that older people suffer disproportionately from chronic rather than acute illnesses (Watson, 1979, Note 6; Neugarten and Havighurst, 1976; Illich, 1976). And, where the life span has been increased, it seems that those increases have been associated more closely with improved controls over disease (Neugarten and Havighurst, 1976) than with a slower rate of aging. It appears on the surface that further improvements in life expectancy overall or for any particular group portend advances in two areas of inquiry. The first is carefully detailed studies to distinguish the incidence of chronic disease and other factors that differentiate ethnic groups with statistically significant differences in life expectancy among them. The second is experimentation with various techniques of disease control or preventive geriatric care such that the incidence of mortality from uncontrolled disease can be somewhat reduced. This call for experimentation harbors no illusions about a relationship between improved medical knowledge, more medical doctors, and subsequent intervention by them. Illich (1976, pp. 32–33) has studied clinical iatrogenesis, that is, the damage that doctors inflict on patients with the intent of "curing" or of exploiting the patient and those other consequences that result from the doctor's attempt to protect himself against the possibility of a suit for malpractice. There is little solid evidence to warrant the conclusion that increased medical intervention in the course of a disease or illness group will decrease the incidence of compound disease or increase longevity. It may very well be that to improve the longevity of black Americans and other ethnic minorities, our efforts will be more likely to be rewarded if we concentrate on socioenvironmental improvements, including life styles, the management of stress, and food consumption. As Illich says (1976, pp. 17, 21): "For more than a century, analysis of disease trends has shown that the environment is the primary determinant of the state of general health of any population. . . . In contrast to environmental improvements and modern nonprofessional health measures, the specifically medical treatment of people is never significantly related to a decline in the compound disease burden or to a rise in life expectancy."

A variety of other studies corroborate Illich's emphasis on the need for careful attention to environmental correlates of health and longevity, including collective and individual attitudes toward illness (Cannon, 1942; Slack, 1974; Watson, 1976), the quality of food, water, and air (Howell and Loeb, 1969; Albanese, 1977), and differentials in sociopolitical equality and social structures that help to maintain stable communities (Leiberman, 1961; Watson and Maxwell, 1977; Watson, 1979, Note 6; Durkheim, 1951). Further research focusing on comparative analyses of disease correlates of differential longevity between ethnic minorities and white ethnic groups will doubtlessly help to establish the role of various diseases and biochemical factors in the explanation of life-span variations. However, other factors besides iatrogenesis do not conveniently fit the medical model of disease but may be no less significant in our attempts to understand differential longevity. Stress from uncontrollable or erratic external environmental changes, psychological conflicts, and psychophysiological tensions can also be detrimental to health and longevity. For example, there is some evidence that people undergoing involuntary change in residence may experience increased levels of psychophysiological stress and have a lower likelihood of surviving that experience than those who either migrate voluntarily or at least participate in the decision to move (Lawton and Yaffe, 1970; Marlowe, 1972, Note 4; Watson, 1979, Note 6). Like differential longevity, coercive migration between places of residence, sometimes called transplantation shock, is an area of inquiry with many unsettled questions. For example, we now have evidence that black elderly may manifest a high degree of external locus of control under conditions of rapid uncontrollable social change (Watson, 1979, Note 6). Further, external locus of control among blacks seems to be associated with an incidence of mortality lower than predicted by some studies of elderly white persons in which the interpretations of data seem to be based on a form of Lipman's error of aged homogeneity: In the latter studies, there seems to be an assumption that elderly persons are relatively homogeneous in social and cultural characteristics (Leiberman, 1961; Pastalan, 1976, Note 5). There are also a number of findings about health, performance, and personality differences between the "young-old" and the "old-old" elderly, which foster other questions about the assumption of aged homogeneity and point to the need for comparative research designed to take into account developmental as well as ethnic and class differences in aging (Neugarten and Havighurst, 1976; Butler, 1976, Note 1). Clearly, differential longevity and variations in patterns of coping with stress in old age remain major areas of inquiry in behavioral studies of aging.

Sustaining the Elderly in Community Settings: The Bearing of Congregate Meal Programs

Research aimed at finding alternatives to institutional long-term care of impaired elderly persons has also received growing attention in recent years (Moss and Halamandaris, 1977; Townsend, 1964; Watson and Maxwell, 1977). Without question, there are humanitarian issues in this area. However, economic motives have been equally influential in turning research in this direction.

The costs of long-term care have skyrocketed in recent years, and the costs of highly skilled nursing care have been prohibitive for many individuals except where Medicaid, Medicare, and other supplemental benefits have been available. Further, maintaining large numbers of poor, chronically ill persons in specialized state-supported institutions has been financially devastating to many state treasuries and families as well.

Class, Ethnicity, and Eating Behavior

One of the many questions in the field of long-term care about which there is still too little concrete information is the extent to which community-based centers for older adults can function effectively to sustain elderly infirm members in their homes in community settings. The relative value of congregate and home-delivered meals to the poor elderly is a major question in this area. For example, there is little definitive information on measurable effects of Title VII nutrition programs on the health and quality of life of the elderly poor and the extent to which these programs are accessible to the minority poor elderly, who presumably need them most.

According to Gemple (1973, Note 2), white elderly are served in the largest numbers through nonprofit meal service programs in the United States. And, judging by the Administration on Aging's 1977 year-end report on Title VII AoA nutrition programs for the elderly (see Table 1), Gemple's observation still holds largely true. One explanation for this state of affairs is a shortage of programs that are financially accessible to the elderly poor and that do not discriminate racially against black American and other nonwhite elderly. For example, it has been shown that when the elderly are both poor and black, they are more likely to be excluded from public services in America than if they were only poor or only black (*Double Jeopardy*, 1964; Lindsay, 1971). Poor health, physical disability, fear of venturing into public places beyond the symbolic security of their neighborhoods, and short supplies of low cost public transportation also help explain the behavior of black elderly in public places and their low consumption of meals through congregate programs.

In spite of the significance of nutritional meals and the potential contributions of other health services in the maintenance of productive and healthy living, there has been a lack of careful research focused on factors related to the participation of the low-income elderly in meal service programs (Howell and Loeb, 1969, p. 15). The need for more research is suggested by the fact that, although there is no doubt that ability to pay is an important factor in determining participation, lack of money is not the sole cause of nonparticipation (Watson and Figgures, 1975).

A recent study by Watson (1977, Note 7) found support for the hypothesis that ethnic-oriented recreational programs are positively associated

Table 1   Minority and Nonminority Participants in Title VII Nutrition Programs[a]
For Fiscal Year, 1977

Minority/Nonminority Groups	Numbers	Percentage (Excluding Caucasians)	Percentage (Combined)
English-speaking Caucasians	2,219,200		78.2%
Blacks	314,248	49%	11%
Native American	29,166	5%	1%
Spanish	125,332	20%	4%
Oriental	23,338	4%	.8%
Other[b]	143,471	22%	5%
Totals	2,854,755	635,555	2,854,755

[a] Administration on Aging, Washington, D.C.
[b] Other, in this table, means participants who are non–English-speaking Europeans

with resident participation in congregate meal programs. This conclusion was drawn from observations of calendar or seasonal variations in frequencies of resident participation in a congregate meal program (see Figure 1). The study showed that residents participated more often and in larger numbers during Thanksgiving-Christmas and Easter holiday periods than during any other time of the year. These seasons are commonly festive, religiously significant, and characterized by parties, small intimate group activities such as family gatherings, decorative meal planning, and other kinds of specially planned programs. These findings suggest that carefully planned leisure activities before, during, and after meals can help to induce more participation by ethnic elderly in congregate meal programs.

A Note on the Concept of Ethnic Group

The meaning of ethnic group (Kitano, 1974; Watson and Maxwell, 1977) is two or more families with a common national origin. These people manifest a common race and a relatively distinct tradition of beliefs, values, and rules for social behavior that are found more commonly among members of the kinship system than among nonmembers. According to Goode (1974, Note 3), an ethnic group in an urban area is the nearest analogue to a relatively distinct culture in a pluralistic society.

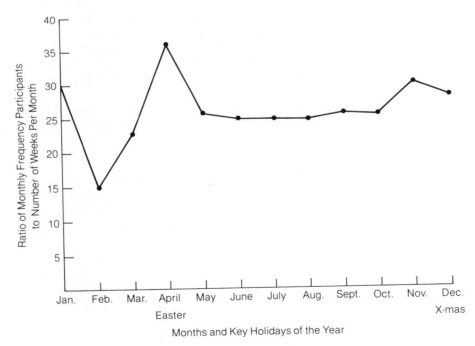

Figure 1   Monthly Frequency of Black Elderly Participation in a Congregate Meal Program during 1974. Source: Watson, Note 7.

So far as Watson's (1977, Note 7) findings apply to the relations between ethnic-group identity and mealtime preferences in general, the observed relationships between festive occasion, ethnic decor, and food consumption should hold in studies and planning of meal programs for other ethnic groups. For example, seasonal variations in the participatory behavior of Jewish elderly living in semi-independent housing facilities should show high frequencies of participation in congregate meals during Jewish holidays. Observations of Chinese, Japanese, Mexican American, American Indian groups, and so forth, may also show equivalent ethnic-related variations. Cross-regional and cross-class observations of black elderly and similar analyses within and between ethnic groups should provide even deeper insight into the social structures of mealtime behavior.

Recent research by Goode (1974, Note 3) helps to suggest at least one direction for further research in this area. Goode considers mealtime behavior a "group boundary marker." This idea is consistent with earlier findings by Whyte (1955). Tastes for certain foods, preferred decor for mealtime settings, and recreational conversation or music during and after meals are learned at an early age. Through family traditions in mealtime interactions with kin and close friends, ethnic customs are established and maintained through the socialization of successive generations of family and ethnic-group members. It is those ethnic-group customs for mealtime behavior expressed through relatively definite rules for kinds and preparations of foods, decor, co-participants, and other factors that help to substantiate Goode's (1974, Note 3) conception of mealtime as a group boundary marker. Given the importance of ethnic identity and the significance of ethnic decor in primary-group and surrogate settings where meals are served, future research on congregate meals for elderly people should focus more attention on the congruence among ethnic identity of elderly consumers, social structure of congregate meal programs, and actual participation of elderly persons.

Implications for Gerontology in Higher Education

Up to this point, the discussion has focused primarily on the need for more research on social, historical, developmental, and comparative ethnographic work in social gerontology. However, the substantive and methodological issues raised by research focuses are equally pertinent to gerontology programs in higher education.

In many disciplines and professions considerable attention has been focused in recent years on integrating minority content into curricula, education-related field-work experiences, and formal research activity. These developments have occurred in both established and new college and university programs in gerontology. However, the quality of instruction does not improve merely because there are new instructional programs. The efforts of educators to broaden their own and their students' perspectives on the field of aging and to deepen their understanding of human development and aging behavior are largely influenced by new insights gained through gerontological research and work in related areas of inquiry. Thus, a lack of research and insight in a given area, such as the comparative ethnography of aging behavior, limits the scientific knowledge that could be made available to enhance the educational activities of faculty and students.

Conclusions

All new emphases on minority content in gerontology in higher education should be accompanied by careful attention to the known cultural and behavioral differences of minority ethnic groups. The pitfalls associated with intellectually homogenizing minority elderly people are the same as those of stereotyping the aged in general. Both research and higher education in gerontology will be enriched by greater emphasis on historical and comparative analysis.

Without systematic research and carefully documented reports that yield definitive answers to the questions we have raised, speculative decision making will continue to dominate program planning and service delivery; and the results of subsequent planning and staffing of service programs—for example, in the area of congregate meal planning—will be equally uncertain for science, social policy, and the elderly.

Notes

1. Butler, R. N. *Our future selves: A research plan toward understanding aging of the Department of HEW.* Prepared by NIA/NIH, HEW, 1976.

2. Gemple, N. *Nutrition programs for the aged in a multiracial society.* Administration on Aging, 1973. Regional Office IX, 50 Fulton Street, San Francisco, CA 94102.

3. Goode, J. *The Philadelphia food project: A study of culture and nutrition.* Paper delivered at the Annual Meetings of the American Anthropological Association, Mexico City, November 21, 1974.

4. Marlowe, R. A. *Effects of relocating geriatric state hospital patients.* Paper presented at the 25th Annual Meetings of the Gerontological Society, San Juan, Puerto Rico, December 1972.

5. Pastalan, L. *Pennsylvania nursing home relocation program: Interim research findings.* Ann Arbor: Institute of Gerontology, University of Michigan, 1976.

6. Watson, W. H. *Stress and old age.* New Brunswick, N. J.: Transaction Books, 1979.

7. Watson, W. H. *Mealtime as social behavior: A study of a group of elderly black people.* Philadelphia, Pa.: Stephen Smith Geriatric Center, 1977.

References

Albanese, A. A. (Ed.), Bone loss causes, detection, and therapy. *Current Topics in Nutrition and Disease* (Vol. 1). New York: A. R. Liss, 1977.

Cannon, W. B. Voodoo death. In W. A. Lessa and E. Z. Vogt (Eds.), *Reader in comparative religion.* New York: Row, Peterson and Company, 1958. (Reprinted from *American Anthropologist,* 1942, *44,* 169–181.)

Double jeopardy: The older negro in America today. New York: National Urban League, 1964.

Durkheim, E. *Suicide: A study in sociology.* (John A. Spaulding and George Simpson, trans.) New York: The Free Press, 1951.

Howell, S. C., & Loeb, M. B. Income, age and food consumption. *The Gerontologist,* Autumn 1969, *9*(3, Part 2), 7–16.

Illich, I. *Medical nemesis: The expropriation of health.* New York: Pantheon, 1976.

Kalish, R. A., & Moriwaki, S. The world of the elderly Asian American. *Journal of Social Issues,* 1973, *29*(2).

Kitano, H. H. L. *Race relations.* Englewood Cliffs, N.J.: Prentice-Hall, 1974.

Lawton, M. P., & Yaffe, S. Mortality, morbidity and voluntary change of residence by older people. *Journal of American Geriatrics Society,* 1970, *18*(10), 823–831.

Leiberman, M. A. Relationship of mortality rates to entrance to a home for the aged. *Geriatrics,* 1961, *16*(10), 515–519.

Lindsay, I. B. *The multiple hazards of age and race.* Washington, D.C.: U.S. Government Printing Office, 1971.

Lipman, A. Ethnic and minority group content for courses in aging. In Seltzer, M. M., H. Sterns, & T. Hickey, (Eds.), *Gerontology in Higher Education: Perspectives and Issues.* Belmont, Ca.: Wadsworth Publishing Company, 1978, 223–227.

Lyman, S. *Chinese Americans.* Englewood Cliffs, N.J.: Prentice-Hall, 1971.

Moss, F. E., & Halamandaris, Val J. *Too old, too sick, too bad: A study of nursing homes in America.* Germantown, Md.: Aspen Systems Corporation, 1977.

Neugarten, B. L., & Havighurst, R. J. (Eds.). *Social policy, social ethics and the aging society.* Washington, D.C.: U.S. Government Printing Office, 1976.

Norman, J. C. (Ed.). *Medicine in the ghetto.* New York: Appleton-Century-Crofts, 1969.

Pinkney, A. *Black Americans.* Englewood Cliffs, N.J.: Prentice-Hall, 1969.

Slack, P. Disease and the social historian. *Times Literary Supplement,* March 8, 1974, 233–234.

Townsend, P. *The last refuge: A survey of residential institutions and homes for the aged in England and Wales.* London: Rutledge and Kegan Paul, 1964.

Watson, W. H. Aging and race. *Social Action,* 1971, *30*(4), 20–30.

Watson, W. H. The aging sick and the near dead: A study of some distinguishing characteristics and social effects. *Omega,* 1976, *7*(2), 115–123.

Watson, W. H., & Figgures, C. *An evaluation of resident participation in an evening meal program.* Philadelphia, Pa.: The Stephen Smith Geriatric Center, January 1975.

Watson, W. H., & Maxwell, R. J. *Human aging and dying.* New York: Saint Martins Press, 1977.

Whyte, W. F. *Street corner society* (2nd ed.). Chicago: University of Chicago Press, 1955.

Young, C. M., Streib, G. B., and Greer, B. J. Food usage and food habits of older workers. *Archives of Industrial Hygiene and Occupational Medicine*, 1954, *10*, 501–511.

Physicians Training in Geriatrics

Frederick G. Dorsey
Baylor College of Medicine

The training of physicians is usually thought of as undergraduate, graduate, and postgraduate—that is, the training in medical school, the training in residency programs in hospitals, and the continuing education programs by postgraduate medical schools or professional medical societies.

At the October 1976 meeting of the Gerontological Society, Senator Charles H. Percy reported the results of a questionnaire sent to all 114 medical schools in the United States, of which 87 replied. Three schools had established geriatrics as a specialty in their curricula: University of Health Sciences, Chicago Medical School; Arkansas College of Medicine; and University of South Dakota. Seven schools, including the University of Pittsburgh and Duke University, were viewed by their staff as very close to this goal. Only 10 of the 87 schools have a specialty in geriatrics, or were in the process of creating one. Thirty-five schools had other programs for research in gerontology in outpatient clinics or day centers for the elderly. The Gerontological Society has a Persons in Training Committee as a part of its Clinical Medical Section (Coccaro, 1977). Its first report listed geriatric training opportunities in the following schools: University of Arkansas-Little Rock; University of Connecticut, Health Science Center, Farmington; the Johns Hopkins University, Baltimore; Albert Einstein College of Medicine, New York; University of Pennsylvania School of Medicine, Philadelphia; Davis Institute, Denver, Colorado; University of Minnesota Medical School, Minneapolis; School of Medicine, State University of New York at Stony Brook; George Washington School of Medicine, Washington, D.C.; University of Wisconsin-Madison; and University of Wisconsin-Milwaukee.

There are several training programs in Canada, including School of Hygiene and Geriatric Study Center, Toronto; Research Projects and Fellows in Clinical Geriatrics, Winnipeg; Postgraduate Fellowships, Waterloo, Ontario; and University of Manitoba (Geriatric Clinical Teaching), Winnipeg.

Great Britain has ten chairs of geriatric medicine. The best known are Professor J. Brocklehurst, University Hospital of South Manchester; Professor A. M. Exton-Smith, University College Hospital, London; and Sir W. Ferguson Anderson, Strobhill General Hospital, Glasgow.

In November 1977, the U.S. Senate Special Committee on Aging, along with the National Institute on Aging, invited experts in aging to describe the programs in their countries. Representatives were from Scotland, Romania, U.S.S.R., Denmark, Czechoslovakia, the Netherlands, Israel, Japan, France, Norway, and Sweden. Although they were primarily interested in describing their research projects, it was notable that a number of professionals in each of these countries offer opportunities in postgraduate and continuing educational programs.

The American Medical Association publishes in its journal each year a list of the known continuing education programs in a number of fields, including geriatrics (Continuing Education, 1977). The 1977 listing includes 33 programs, usually of one to several days in duration, in Alabama, Colorado, the District of Columbia, Florida, Georgia, Hawaii, Illinois, Kentucky, Maryland, Minnesota, New York, Pennsylvania, Texas, and Washington.

Robert N. Butler, the first director of the National Institute on Aging, has made a number of reports concerning training in geriatric medicine (Butler, 1977; Butler and Speith, 1977). He says he is convinced of the necessity of having more geriatric medicine taught so that it might serve as a catalyst for the research that forms the framework of a good service-delivery system.

Joseph P. Freeman reviewed the catalogs of the medical schools approved as of 1970 (1971). He ascertained their curriculum content and staff appointments with respect to the subject of aging. There were 124 citations in 48 of the 99 catalogs, and there were 15 staff appointments under the headings of geriatrics or gerontology. His conclusion was that geriatric education had had little impact on the scholastic policies of the United States medical schools.

Leslie S. Libow has described in detail a full year's experience in a geriatric medical residency program at the Jewish Institute of Geriatric Care at Long Island Jewish Hillside Medical Center in New Hyde Park, New York (1976).

In October 1976 and again in March 1977, the American Geriatrics Society held a conference on geriatric education. The proceedings of this have been published in the November issue of the society's journal.

According to the Association of American Medical Colleges, 45 medical schools offered electives in geriatrics in 1976–77, an increase from the 32 reported in 1975–76. The 45 schools offered electives in geriatrics in the department of medicine (14), psychiatry (9), community health (6), family practice (3), surgery (1), other clinical services (10), and unspecified (2).

In 1972, the Information and Consultation Center was established by the American Geriatrics Society under the direction of William Reichel at the Franklin Square Hospital, Baltimore, Maryland. This organization has sponsored a large number of geriatric programs, and now approximately ten programs per year are accredited by the AMA for category I for physicians. A number of other institutions have devoted some effort to developing continuing-education programs in geriatrics, including, among others, the University of Wisconsin, Medical College of Georgia, Duke University, the Frederick D. Zeman Center in New York Center, the Philadelphia Geriatrics Center, and the New Jersey College of Medicine and Dentistry.

It is difficult to judge the extent of continuing education in geriatrics because many courses deeply concerned with geriatrics are not so labeled, and few faculties identify themselves with the specialty. For example, one university stated that although no courses are specifically labeled geriatrics, about 15 percent of the courses covered material of special interest to a physician or other health professional devoted to the study of the diseases of the elderly.

An example of recent developments in geriatric training programs is the announcement early in 1978 by the Veterans' Administration that it was initiating a fellowship training program in geriatric medicine at six hospitals in the VA system. A statement on research training needs prepared for the committee on a Study of National Needs for Biomedical and Behavioral Research Personnel for the Commission of Human Resources of the National Research Council, National Academy of Sciences, was made by the National Institute on Aging on February 10, 1978. The summary and conclusions are as follows:

1. The elderly population of the United States will more than double during the next 50 years.

2. This segment of the population consumes a disproportionately large fraction of health care costs.

3. The Congress has created a National Institute on Aging and has appropriated substantial increases in funding for research on aging. Future funding is likely to increase markedly.

4. There are abundant opportunities for launching an expanded research effort on aging.

5. The limiting factor is trained personnel.

6. Efforts are being made to define special mechanisms for supporting personnel development for research on aging, and special studies are being undertaken to identify personnel needs more precisely.

7. Assistance of the National Academy of Sciences/National Research Council Committee on the Study of National Needs for Biomedical and Behavioral Research Personnel is sought both in defining research and personnel needs and in devising suitable legislative authorities for training the necessary personnel.

References

Butler, R. N. Thoughts on geriatric medicine. *American Health Care Association Journal*, 1977, 3, 49.

Butler, R. N., & Speith, W. Trends in training in research in gerontology. *Educational Gerontology*, 1977, 2, 111.

Coccaro, E. S., Jr. Preliminary report of geriatric opportunities: Section on clinical medicine. San Francisco: Gerontological Society, 1977.

Continuing education programs (geriatrics). *Journal of American Medical Association*, 1977, 238, 739.

Freeman, J. T. A survey of education in geriatrics. *Gerontologist*, 1961, 1, 128.

Freeman, J. T. A survey of geriatric education: Catalogues of United States medical schools. *Journal of American Geriatrics Society*, 1971, 19, 746.

Goldman, R. Geriatric education at the undergraduate level. *Journal of American Geriatrics Society*, 1977, 25, 485.

Libow, L. S. A geriatric medical residency program. *Annals of Internal Medicine*, 1976, 85, 641.

Reichell, W. Proceedings of the American Geriatrics Society Conference on Geriatric Education. *Journal of American Geriatrics Society*, 1977, 25, 481.

Shock, N. W. *A classified bibliography of gerontology and geriatrics.* Stanford, Calif.: Stanford University Press, 1951.

Shock, N. W. Current publications in gerontology and geriatrics. *Journal of Gerontology*, bimonthly.

Special Committee on Aging, U.S. Senate. Report No. 95–88. Washington, D.C.: U.S. Government Printing Office, 1977.

Steel, K. Continuing education in geriatrics. *Journal of American Geriatrics Society*, 1977, 25, 492.

The Medical School and Interdisciplinary Geriatric Education

Noel D. List
University of Maryland-Baltimore

The inauguration of programs in geriatric medicine in medical schools meets with great resistance. This reaction is separate from the secondary resistance to geriatrics as a specialty and to the question of whether there is a sufficient body of knowledge that can be called geriatric medicine. In addition, the geriatric patient is already considered a part of the practice of many physician groups within medicine including family practice, general practice, and internal medicine. Therefore, a separate specialty in the medical school would create the beginnings of competition for this patient population. The resistance is further compounded by the autonomy of the departments within schools of medicine, and therefore, the diverse areas for teaching geriatrics have no coordinated effort.

In reality, the growing core of knowledge—the curriculum—as well as the development of faculty and personnel necessary for an integrated approach to geriatrics, is now in an early formulative stage. The attitude of students has been dulled or frankly negated by the lack of interest shown by the majority of role models in medicine who look upon the geriatric patient as the least important part of the practice.

This leads into the most difficult problem in geriatric medicine and its teaching in interdisciplinary settings, specifically in reference to the medical school. Given that we have a basic core of knowledge appropriate to a segment of our population and that we have individuals competent to teach it, there still exist problems with the acceptance of the composition of this core and with identifying the individuals inside and outside the medical school who are appropriate or necessary to the education of the medical student. The reason is that the core material stretches over multiple disciplines, including sociology, economics, dentistry, nursing, and other areas that are the province of other disciplines but that relate significantly to geriatrics. Curriculum organization in the medical school must deal with the appropriateness of integrating nontraditional and essentially nonmedical material into a program already constrained by the quantity of material and the limited time in which to teach it.

The problem then becomes the delivery of an education in an appropriate fashion and in a maximally effective way to a group of individuals who will be stimulated and will then utilize that material to meet medicine's obligation to the older population. As Senator Charles Percy said in October 1976 in beginning the hearings before the Special Committee on Aging of the United States Senate in New York City, "The medical profession must extend its blessing to all persons in all age groups in full understanding of the needs of the individual in each group" (Medicine and Aging, 1976:38).

We must deal with a group of problems ranging from economic considerations to psychosocial and ingrained attitudinal societal philosophies. The reality is that effective care depends on how medicine and the patient interact within the delivery system and how well interdisciplinary curriculum meets the need to deliver total medical care.

The five basic areas of interest and importance to bringing geriatric education into the curriculum of schools of medicine are curriculum, medical school isolation (insulation), context (psychological and physical settings) within delivery systems, attitudinal problems, and system capabilities.

Curriculum

Difficulties in developing a comprehensive curriculum involve several attempts to conceptualize the body of knowledge which is incorporated in "geriatric" medicine (Curriculum Development in Geriatric Medicine, 1976; Reichel, 1973; Harris, 1975; Rodstein, 1973; Libow, 1976). The question still being asked is, What is geriatrics? It must be admitted that a further need exists to conceptualize the body of knowledge to practice good geriatric medicine; this is not to overlook the problem of developing teachers and teaching skills and intra- and interprofessional interaction. The problem entails the amount and the nature of this material as well as its integration; fragmentation of this material into an amorphous educational delivery system; the lack of specific material in areas such as economics, politics, environment, and psychosocial aspects of aging; and the time-related competition in terms of department attitude toward the need for material to be incorporated into lectures and courses.

This problem has led many universities with medical schools to use electives at both the preclinical and clinical years to make multidisciplinary material available and to provide access to parts of the delivery system not usually used in the normal curriculum.

Geriatrics and Geriatricians

The question of geriatrics as a specific discipline seems to have superseded the evidence that caring for the elderly requires special training. It is generally agreed that we not only need to know the special physiology (therefore, a different presenting pathology) of the elderly individual but also need to have the ability to interact with a team of health professionals who will make recommendations relating to the social well-being of the individual.

The word *geriatrician* presents a problem to the profession. The argument is whether this individual, an identified specialist, is needed to teach geriatrics. The American Medical Association has specifically taken a stand against developing geriatrics as a specialty; it favors increased training within medical schools under a resolution adopted by the American Medical Association House of Delegates in June 1975 (Resolution, Adequate Training in Geriatric Medicine, 1975). The problem then is why should there be such difficulty in relation to the question of the teacher of geriatric medicine. This relates to the existence of a spectrum of medical clinicians, which range from the social gerontologist, who many colleagues feel is more a social worker, to the geriatrician, who may be represented by the superspecialized physiologically/pathologically-oriented internist.

General agreement exists that there is a need for interdisciplinary interaction and decision making as part of the care process; it, therefore, is a necessary part of the training process for individuals involved in medical care. Then too, the role of the geriatrician in the interdisciplinary-team approach is highly variable. It may be that the role model in geriatric education is a geriatrician within a medical school. This specialist may not be needed in the community, providing other specialties fill the gap. However, it would seem important that the role model—teacher, interprofessional interactor—be part of and necessary to geriatrics in the medical school.

The image of the geriatrician depends largely on the acceptance by the total academic and community medical environment. Prejudices of hospital staff are overt and range from the feeling that the geriatrician is not needed to competitive jealousy over the patients the geriatrician may take away. The time allocated to geriatrics within the curriculum and the emphasis placed upon it will have a great deal to do with the role and image of the individual responsible for geriatrics.

The Delivery System

Perhaps the most difficult problems with relation to teaching geriatrics are the methods necessary and the sites where they are carried out. Usually institutions of long-term care are adjacent to the major teaching hospital and the medical school, but sometimes they are at a distance. As the basic lecture portion of the curriculum, even at the time of preclinical training, relates to problems not essential to medicine (i.e., social, economic, agency problems, and so forth), access to these other agencies and care facilities is often necessary, especially for interdisciplinary teaching. This exposure is needed early to maintain interest and to cultivate those other disciplines that often participate in the care of the elderly even more than medicine. Do we then look for decentralized teaching involving nursing homes, senior citizen centers, housing projects for the elderly, churches, and so on? The obvious answer is that these must become a necessary part of the educational system and must be cultivated and developed. This should improve the quality of the education as well as total care delivery.

Attitudes and the Professional School's Location of a Geriatric Unit

It is obvious that the creation of interdisciplinary efforts affects the individual school's autonomy and, in a sense, its integrity, in turn affecting the context in which programs of geriatrics must evolve. This relates to the question of where geriatrics is taught and the nature of the courses. There is a great deal of controversy about whether the material should be integrated into existing courses or made into separate courses that specifically deal with the geriatric patient. It would seem that both required and elective areas should integrate natural human development with physiological and pathological changes over time and should incorporate those settings appropriate to integrating didactic and clinical material. These courses may be totally outside the medical school. It is also realistic to expect that the nature of the individual and of the department in which the care system develops will strongly affect this decision.

This leads to the problem of where within the medical school to locate a division of geriatric medicine or the teaching geriatrician. There are proponents for the placement of geriatrics in areas as diverse as the chancellor's office, the departments of preventive medicine, internal medicine, or family practice, or separate institutes and divisions. However, location plays less of a role in determining the success of a unit than the administrative support provided the unit. It would seem that the most successful existent schools have identified an individual as well as a medical school department in which to house geriatrics. In most universities there is a unified central development of geriatrics within one department, school, or other identifiable area. At least one university, the University of Maryland, has geriatrics as a component of the undergraduate campus, the medical school, the department of family practice, and the division of primary care of the department of medicine, and the department of preventive medicine. Geriatric activities in other schools have likewise developed in a decentralized manner. For the most part, this groundswell has been less effective than the identification and placement of the geriatric effort under one administrative department.

Summary

The geriatrician, in comparison to other specialists, suffers from problems of credibility, glamour, prestige, and specialty identification and from the reality that few top students and many foreign graduates become involved in the area. This is coupled with an immature delivery system, which is usually fragmented and in some cases intolerably poor or absent. The geriatrician works in a continuum of care necessarily involving inpatient and outpatient services. Since within each of these areas there are multiple levels at which care can be delivered and by any one of a number of specialties because it is an interdisciplinary program, the geriatrician must be multifaceted.

The communication failures, the lack of resources, and the diversity of knowledge and training coupled with the sometimes inordinate patient needs in terms of both social and medical resources lead to a system of failure with deep and longlasting frustrations. Add to this the problem of teaching students with negative attitudes toward the aged population, and the result seems an insurmountable hurdle. Teaching of understanding through identification with an individual who is perceived as a "doctor," who shows understanding for the problems of the total patient in context of society, and who can communicate with patients and gain their confidence, and who is perceived as being able to treat them should change the attitude from the problem and treatment of disease to the problem of the maintenance of health and total medical care. Further, delivery should be made by an interdisciplinary group functioning as a team in separate settings but integrated into the medical school.

The core of the problem is the need to answer the question, What are geriatrics and gerontology? This very formidable question engenders a deep desire to look at all of medical education and the need for an interdisciplinary approach to the geriatric patients in settings germane to interdisciplinary care.

References

Curriculum development in geriatric medicine. Chicago: Student American Medical Association, January 1976.

Harris, R. Model for a graduate geriatric program at a university medical school. *The Gerontologist,* 1975, *15,* 304.

Libow, L. A geriatric medical residency program: A four-year experience. *Annals of Internal Medicine,* 1976, 85(5), 641–647.

Medicine and aging: An assessment of opportunities and neglect. Hearing before the Special Committee on Aging, U.S. Senate, New York, October 13, 1976. Washington, D.C.: U.S. Government Printing Office, 1976, p. 38.

Reichel, W. New models in geriatric and long-term care. *Journal of the American Geriatric Society,* 1973, *21,* 259.

Resolution, adequate training in geriatric medicine. American Medical Association House of Delegates, adopted 1975.

Rodstein, R., et al. A model curriculum for an elective course in geriatrics. *The Gerontologist,* 1973, *13,* 231.

PART SIX
ISSUES IN EDUCATION FOR PRACTICE

Gerontology as a "multidiscipline" necessitates education and training in diverse subject areas at different levels of sophistication. Yet there are elements common to all approaches, as the five papers in this section illustrate. The authors describe career education in gerontology in settings as varied as associate degree, graduate level, and continuing education.

Practitioner Issues in Professional Training

Sheldon S. Tobin
University of Chicago

Whereas the biologist may be able to study the aging process without concern for the effects associated with cohort membership or produced by current historical time, this is not the case for the social gerontologist. Although in its strictest epistemological meaning, gerontology may not be the study of cohort or current historical effects, nevertheless, some of the questions most pertinent to practice issues focus explicitly on these effects. Consider, for example, the following questions: What explains the differences in how people age? What are the correlates of well-being among the elderly? Or, specifically in my own research: How does social interaction relate to life satisfaction among the elderly? What may help people age better? What services should we establish and policies should we develop to facilitate independent community living? How may an understanding of cultural differences help us develop services and policies that can meet the needs of all the elderly? Are the aging getting their fair share?

Thus, as we move from gerontology as a scientific enterprise in its most precise and narrow sense to gerontology as it concerns the well-being of the elderly and the specific practitioner issues, we shift from studying the process of aging to studying the elderly as a target group for social intervention. We become involved in measuring the current functional status of the elderly—their living arrangements and family interaction, their attitudes—and, of course, in examining how social programs and federal policies affect them.

The development of gerontology curriculum usually begins with designing two courses: one, on human development, to address the question of what we know about the process of human aging; and the other, on social aspects of aging, to address what the social influences on the elderly are. If the curriculum designer is a psychologist, he or she teaches the first course and recruits a sociologist for the other; if the designer is a sociologist, the second course becomes his or her responsibility, and a psychologist is recruited for the first. Unfortunately, curriculum designers seldom consider recruiting instructors from the biological sciences to teach the essential course in the biology of aging. This is certainly a difficult course to teach either to the novice social scientists or to beginning human-service practitioners, but it is, nonetheless, an essential course in a gerontology curriculum.

This type of curriculum building reflects a second issue—that is, an issue that goes beyond the distinction between content on the aging process and content on the social influences on the elderly. Although we may be academic gerontologists, we are not psychologists and sociologists and anthropologists and historians and political scientists. Gerontology is not itself an academic discipline; rather, it draws on the theory and operations of academic disciplines to answer its questions. As academic gerontologists, we are in the fortunate position of instructing those from the disciplines on how they themselves can become academic gerontologists. They only need to study the right questions. To the anthropologist, for example, you can say, "Study either how aging is similar in other cultures or how aging varies across cultures." Or to the historian say, "Study the early life-conditions for the current aging cohort or the treatment of the elderly in past times." And to the political scientist say, "Look at some political attitudes by age (explaining them by age, cohort, or current events), or study political organizations of the elderly." (See also Binstock and Shanas, 1977, and Birren and Schaie, 1977).

The academic gerontologist is foremost an advocate or practitioner in the higher-education setting (Tobin, 1973, and 1978). Recruiting (or, if you will, seducing) other faculty and playing deans or provosts for commitments are practitioner skills. All I have attempted to do is to clarify a few conceptual issues that will help you convert others in the academic world. Also convincing should be your arguments on the importance, or even the necessity, of curriculum content on aging in a world not only where we are graying but also where the impact of the graying has far-reaching consequences for every segment of society and certainly for the delivery of human services. Your arguments, however, may be far less persuasive to fellow faculty—who have previously accrued expertise and their own precious terrain—than to educational administrators. Yet convincing administrators is not a solution; it is only one step along the way in developing a committed and knowledgeable faculty. Too often programs are generated at top administrative levels with too few or no knowledgeable faculty in evidence. Certainly it appears more sensible to have one or more faculty members with the prerequisite knowledge before developing a comprehensive program. If no such expertise is present among the faculty, new faculty must be recruited.

This leads to a related issue: that is, the academic gerontologist may have great wisdom but too little knowledge of practice. This was true in my own case. Before I traveled across campus from the committee on human development, an academic department, to the school of social service administration, I thought I knew a great deal about human services. Only when I was socialized by faculty and students at the school of social work, however, did I gain any reasonable grasp of the delivery of social services. Yet, once humbled, I was prepared to affect the curriculum. Why? Professional practice with the elderly, I discovered, must be built on sound professional practice: The planner of social services for the elderly must know planning, the physician must know medicine, the lawyer must know law. "Thank goodness," I said to myself, "I don't have to 'own' the curriculum; but I must 'gerontologize it.'" The basic courses may, for example, need only incorporate aging into their content. In my academic setting the cliché is "human behavior must not stop at adolescence." The concept, of course, can be usefully extended to all curriculum content. For example, courses on psychotherapy must obviously include content on how therapy differs with elderly patients or clients. Let us not oversimplify the process. Spreading the gospel is not easy (witness the resistance of medical educators to attend not only to the elderly but also to the generic group of those with chronic illness), nor is it sufficient to incorporate aging only into standard curriculum offerings. Specific gerontology courses must be developed in both disciplines and in applied curricula.

In practice-oriented higher education, a further issue arises. Still to be exploited or developed are field experiences—sometimes called practica, or clinical settings, or clinical services. If you are educated in the disciplines, the problem of on-the-job experiences in human-service settings is a whole new game. One of the most difficult dilemmas I have had to confront in this arena is the contrast between the real world of practice and the ideal. Certainly at the graduate level we should teach both, but too often the available settings are far from the ideal. Early in this academic year, for example, directors of profit-making day-care programs began calling me for graduate students. The director would argue the importance of the day-care program and the need for trained personnel—incontrovertible arguments, of course. But my students have little to learn from a supervisor with no formal training in gerontology in a setting whose practice I often must question. Operators of proprietary nursing homes or recreation directors of profit-making high-rise buildings can be even more persuasive.

Our task, however, is not simply to provide the necessary personnel for the current diversity of practitioner settings. Academic gerontologists at the associate of arts level, at the baccalaureate level, at the graduate level— whether in social work, nursing, architecture, law, medicine, and so forth— must train practitioners who can transcend current practices. To be sure, our graduates must know the real world if they are going to transform it; moreover, they must understand excellence in practice even if it does not exist. To what extent our task is to stock the workforce of human services when the services themselves are, to say the least, fragmented and often dysfunctional is indeed a problem. Possibly our major task, as suggested by Robert Benedict, commissioner of the Administration on Aging, is to educate practitioners who can develop new social interventions. Training for changing the nature of practice, as well as educating our students to be "trainers of trainers," is indeed an ambitious goal but not an unachievable one. Maybe we should be less eager to spread the word to every campus and more eager to spread it to those campuses where there is a willingness to develop innovative and enriched programs capable of producing students who can transcend current practice, who can change its nature, and who can educate others to do likewise.

Yet another dilemma, apropos of training experiences in current practice, relates to how we value such experiences. The more we value activities outside the classroom, the greater the central predicament: If the best learning occurs on the job, then what is the reason for academic gerontology? Why not educate in the best of the liberal arts tradition, as well as impart the best of scientific knowledge, and leave practice training to the practitioners? "After all," to paraphrase one government official, "what do academics know about practice in the real world?"

This accusation cannot be taken lightly! To combat our antagonists and to diminish our naiveté we go forth into the real world. My going forth probably parallels your own experiences: board member of one voluntary social service agency; paid consultant to another and unpaid consultant to several others; chair or member of a few committees of the local Area Agency on Aging; and a member of the state advisory council on Title XX social services. Indeed, one day I realized that I was a practitioner too. Have I come out of the closet? Has the academic gerontologist in me been rightfully abandoned in my transformation to applied gerontologist, who can justifiably be called "a planner of services for the elderly" or "a consultant on programs for the elderly"? But just when I felt comfortable with my new status, I realized my shortcomings. "No," I said, "I am not capable of teaching the 12-week seminar on case management to supervising social workers and nurses who must assess and develop service plans for the frail elderly. I had better recruit the few outstanding practitioners in town. But," I added quickly, "I can help in the conceptualization of the training program." These words were uttered at a meeting of academic gerontologists and practitioners who had set about, under the auspices of the local area agencies on aging, to develop training programs for human services. My contributions were primarily in the initial stages, where I helped map out the terrain of human services, drawing distinctions between social services, physical health services, mental health services, and so forth. And then, in what is a common trick of our trade, I developed a two-axis grid with the areas of human services across the top (or X axis) and the level of person to be sensitized, educated, or trained along the side (or the Y axis)—ranging from policymaker to administrator to supervising personnel to direct service workers. To be sure, I was proud of my input, but the limits of my understanding were too obvious to all, particularly as we moved to develop curricula for various groups identified by their position on the grid. The practitioners in our group, some of the top practitioners in town, had already developed for their agencies training programs that could readily be adapted for personnel in other settings. All they needed was the wherewithal to do so. Housing the training effort at an academic institution certainly seemed sensible. We have the technology (classrooms, audio-visual equipment, cafeteria, and lodging, if necessary); we have the status; we can offer

CEUs (continuing education units or credits) or even a certificate with the school's name on it; and we can provide an academic lecture or two on the knowledge base for practice. Is my case overstated? Possibly. But too often the top practitioners are not faculty members.

Still faith in academia lingers on. Moreover, academicians in higher education are not only producers of new knowledge and disseminators of old knowledge, but obviously also educators of practitioners within academic institutions. Thus, it seems eminently sensible to encourage interchange among academic knowledge generators, academic trainers of practitioners, and practitioners in service settings. Indeed, each has a great deal to offer the others. The knowledge generators have the wisdom that comes only through scientific approaches to problems; the trainers of practitioners have the expertise and the mandate to educate the future workforce; and practitioners know the real world—the actual help-giving process for older people. Working in concert, the three highly skilled and well-intentioned sets of actors can synergistically add to each other's efforts without detracting from their own efforts. But can they work together? Obviously, they will be expected to work together in multidisciplinary centers on aging. Science and practice, however, do not mix as easily as some would lead us to believe. Indeed, when I was educated in graduate school to be a researcher, one of my mentors, when sensing my need to be relevant (the slogan of the 1960s), reminded me that there is little relationship between the yield from the study of scientific phenomena in the social sciences and its use in constructing social programs and policies. If there were, our approach to social problems would be dramatically different. Another example: recently I have questioned, as others have before me, how a scientific society, such as the Gerontological Society, can readily absorb the practitioner's world. It is more likely the other way around: the scientists will be absorbed by the practitioners. Yet the struggle goes on because it seems eminently sensible for the three sets of actors to interact and also because the payoff at this time is sufficient. That payoffs dictate directions taken by academic gerontologists, particularly given the constrictions in higher education, appears to be a reality.

The struggle is an important one: to develop curricula that enhance the world of practice and, thereby, the lives of the elderly. Unfortunately, we are engaged in this important task when the constrictions in higher education are both too real and quite painful. We—given what we do for a living—know only too well that higher education is not in the best of health. Fortunately, our individual and collective efforts can be particularly important in enhancing the health of higher education. Gerontology can and should be a stimulus for innovation and vitality in higher education.

References

Binstock, R. H., & Shanas, E. (Eds.). *Handbook of aging and the social sciences.* New York: Van Nostrand Reinhold, 1977.

Birren, J. E., & Schaie, K. W. (Eds.). *Handbook of the psychology of aging.* New York: Van Nostrand Reinhold, 1977.

Tobin. S. S. The educator as advocate: The gerontologist in an academic setting. *Journal of Education for Social Work*, Fall 1973, 9(3), 94–98.

Tobin, S. S. Social work: Gerontology in professional and preprofessional curricula. In M. M. Seltzer, H. Sterns, & T. Hickey (Eds.), *Gerontology in higher education: Perspectives and issues.* Belmont, Calif.: Wadsworth, 1978.

Vocational Education
and
Gerontology

Gamal Zaki
Rhode Island College

What is the relationship between vocational education and gerontology? What are some of the implications of this relationship? What is the role of vocational education in meeting education and training needs in gerontology?

To develop a data frame of reference for these questions, I conducted an experience survey. Qualified experts from both gerontology and vocational education were interviewed with unstructured and open-ended questions. During these interviews an attempt was made to define vocational education and gerontology broadly and to determine potential interrelationships. From this technique, three relevant areas of articulation were identified: curriculum development, vocational preservice and inservice education, and vocational adult training and education. For the purpose of this paper we discuss each area separately. The final part includes analysis and discussion of the findings.

Curriculum Development

Vocational education is based on early educational experiences. The study of enriching the K–12 curriculum with perspectives on aging, and death and dying, though important, is a new field. However, we must begin to educate during the early stages of development if we are to expect continued growth during the latter. Early attitudes may well affect later behavior.

Treybig (Note 1) studied the attitudes of children to the word *old*, selecting a sample of children aged three to six. In response to the question "What do you think *old* means?" three- and four-year-old children exhibited a strong tendency to reply with words or phrases indicating that *old* refers to something that should be discarded because it has deteriorated and is no longer useful. The following are typical responses for this age group: "Get rid of it," "Yukky and full of holes," "Throw it away," or "Don't touch it."

In contrast to the youngest children, the five- to six-year-olds tended to respond in a different way, reflecting perhaps a more developed ability to categorize. Most of the children said that *old* refers to some state of physical growth or an increase in chronological age. Typical of these responses are "It means when someone is going to die," "It means you are crooked and people can hardly walk," "Someone who's going to die but don't." When the children were asked, "Would you like to be old sometime?" the great majority replied negatively, rejecting the idea of being old. It is reasonable to expect that these early attitudes, perhaps deeply internalized, are important as partial determinants of later adolescent, young adult, middle aged, and elderly feelings about age and aging.

Another study, conducted by Harris and Associates for the National Council on Aging (Note 2), reflects the same thesis. Over 4,000 face-to-face household interviews were conducted. The sample included a representative cross-section of the American public 18 years of age and over. The results indicate that 45 percent of those 65 and over felt that they get "too little respect" from younger people. Surprisingly, the public under 65 seems more aware of the respect problem than the older public itself: A full 71 percent of the public 18 to 64 felt that people over 65 got "too little respect" from younger people.

While examining housing projects that accommodated elderly as well as newly established families (Note 3), I found similar results. It was evident that the two segments, the elderly and the families, existed in a very loosely integrated environment with minimal contact between them. Although 25 percent of the elderly indicated some relationship with the families residing in the project, only 16 percent of the families indicated that they had relationships with one or more of the elderly residents. As reasons for this isolation, the majority of the elderly indicated that they were usually harrassed, humiliated, and hurt by children and juveniles. As one elderly woman said, "What can you do? If you complain to the parents, they don't give a damn; and if you call the police, the kids will get you, and it becomes worse." Intensive research is needed in the area of attitudes toward the elderly in general.

Education about the processes of aging should start as early as possible; it should begin at kindergarten, not after retirement. Aging and death are integral parts of life and should be understood as such. As the policy statement of the 1961 White House Conference on Aging said, "Education for aging is related to each aspect of aging and is part of the lifelong learning process. Education for everyone about aging will influence community attitudes and actions with respect to aging problems. The initial stimulation of education programs for, and about, and by aging should be through institutions that have public responsibility for education, that in combination, have nationwide coverage and that have the confidence of all groups. These institutions are public schools, institutions of higher learning and libraries" (Note 4).

A review of literature indicates that although this statement was made years ago, little has been done. "While a considerable number of individual school systems have, in recent years, introduced some emphasis on education for aging below the adult level, no generally recognized pattern for elementary and secondary school systems has yet emerged" (Note 5).

The attitudes found in children, if not corrected, may well carry over into adulthood. Today we find many professionals and paraprofessionals who are directly responsible for services to the elderly and whose basic attitudes toward the elderly are based more on myth than on reality. There is evidence of this in service agencies, where one may observe a professional or paraprofessional treating older persons as children—scolding, controlling, supervising, condescending.

Two years ago, I was asked to review a proposal for standards of day-care centers for the elderly, a relatively recent phenomenon (Note 6). These centers are designed to provide needed services to older persons with physical, mental, or social impairment. The program serves the purpose of helping older persons with activities of daily living, and enables them to return home at night. While I was reviewing the proposal, I had a vague feeling that I had read the same material before. After much thought, I found that the proposal was in actuality a copy of the standards for licensing day-care centers for children. The only difference was that the word "elderly" was substituted for the word "child."

Similar to the K–12 curriculum, vocational education is suffering from an educational-cultural lag. In the broadest sense, vocational education schools prepare a cadre of paraprofessionals and technicians in different fields and for various occupations. A segment of the population they serve is the elderly. However, we have neglected to prepare students of vocational education to deal with this segment of our population. We need to re-examine the curriculum of vocational schools and investigate their function in serving the world of reality.

Some recommendations may help us alleviate these problems, as well as delineate the role for vocational education in this area:

1. The proposal of the 1961 White House Conference on Aging should be implemented: "Primary responsibility for the initiation, support, and conduct of education programs for older persons must be vested in the existing educational system, federal, state, and local, with active participation and cooperation of specialized agencies. A Division of Education on Aging should be established in the Office of Education immediately, to initiate supportive educational services for the aging. Similarly, all State Departments of Education should designate full-time responsibility to key staff for the development and implementation of programs in education for aging."

2. School districts should be encouraged to develop curriculum units introducing the young generation (K–12) to aging and its implications and ramifications. The main thrust should be on aging as an integral part of the life-span continuum.

3. High-school curriculum must include education in gerontology within appropriate course offerings, such as social science, biology, health maintenance, and home economics. Particularly important to the development of favorable attitudes toward aging would be the study of the later stages of the family life cycle and the analysis of attitudes toward the aged among students.

4. Career counseling should be provided to inform students of possible careers in gerontology.

5. Programs that bring the elderly into the schools and in contact with younger persons should be developed.

6. School libraries should collect books and other materials specific to gerontology.

7. School districts should develop inservice training opportunities for teachers to prepare them to develop units on adulthood, aging, death, and dying.

8. Vocational training should build into human services concepts aimed at sensitizing and familiarizing students with a view of aging as an integral part of the life cycle.

9. Existing vocational training programs that prepare people to work mainly or partly with the aged should be identified.

10. Inservice training opportunities in gerontology for instructors in vocational and technical schools should be provided.

11. Postsecondary institutions should identify the curriculum areas where gerontological awareness can be developed.

12. Teacher preparation programs should include units on adulthood, aging, death, and dying. All teachers, regardless of their area of specialization, should be required to include these units in their teaching plans.

13. Career-based practicum courses should be developed at junior colleges and four-year colleges to offer field experience to students in the area of gerontology.

14. The needs of minority elderly should be identified, and appropriate course content and practicum experiences should be designed to meet these special needs.

Vocational Preservice and Inservice Education

The concepts of preservice and inservice training and education have been variously defined. For our purposes both processes are defined as training and educational experiences aimed at: (1) developing awareness among practitioners of the need for upgrading their performance; (2) providing selected learning experiences to aid personnel in meeting changes and different patterns in their professional fields; motivating of individuals to gain competence to their vocations; acquiring new knowledge of skills; and (3) promoting better understanding of human needs and interpersonal relationships.

It is evident that preservice and inservice training and education fall in the domain of vocational education. However, the facts are often otherwise.

Institutions and agencies may conduct these training programs even though they do not have the necessary ability or skills. It is vital that we emphasize this distinction for policy planning and implementation. If federal funds for the expansion of vocational education become available, an adequate portion should be allocated for upgrading the performance of paraprofessionals through inservice training.

The lack of research, planning, and coordination of efforts in the area of preservice and inservice education and training impedes the success of these programs. In most cases, agencies and institutions do not have the expertise or capacity to implement these processes. This leads to the perpetuation of the same programs without the opportunity for experimentation and innovation.

The success of preservice and inservice training and education depends on the consent and support of employers and on the regulations developed by the different states. Licensing requirements should be very instrumental in promoting education in the field of gerontology.

The following recommendations will help us identify the role of vocational education in this particular area:

1. The personnel needs of programs in aging in the states should be assessed. Vocational training programs should be developed to meet those needs.

2. The states should take all measures to upgrade the educational and training levels of all personnel serving the elderly.

3. The states should develop minimum levels of gerontological training to be required for all those seeking employment in all aging-related occupations.

4. The states should require that those who do not meet the minimum requirements undergo remedial inservice training and education, which would be provided by their employers with built-in incentives for the participants.

5. Postsecondary institutions should make available continuing-education programs for preservice and inservice education and training programs to meet the mandate of the state.

Although the number of programs to meet the needs of the elderly has increased dramatically, the number and quality of personnel trained to meet those needs have not. Many people who are currently employed to deliver social and health services to older people have not had the opportunity to engage in academic study of the processes of aging. In many cases, paraprofessionals in the field of servicing the elderly are not required to have pertinent qualifications before employment.

The literature is replete with examples illustrating this problem. Gubrium and Ksander (1975) studied reality orientation (RO), a form of therapy that is supposed to be an efficient way of reducing the symptoms of senility in institutionalized elderly. Reality orientation sessions were conducted by nurse's aides acting as instructors, and were attended by four or five patients as students. Instructional materials included an RO board listing the name of the institution, its location, the date, day of the week, and state of the weather; and a cardboard clock was used to teach time keeping. A session normally began with drills by the aide. The aide asked attending patients to read the board one by one and then quizzed them on its contents.

Reality orientation may be valid in theory, yet there is often a discrepancy between what should happen theoretically and what actually takes place. The inherent danger in reality orientation is that it places the aide in a superior position and leaves much need for "parenting," thus furthering the eventuality that the older person is treated like a child.

Usually a certain amount of negotiation occurred before RO. The researchers observed that both patients and aides were often reluctant to participate in RO. Aides did RO because it was part of their jobs, but often remarked, "Look! Those who are alert are alert anyway and the senile ones stay senile regardless of RO." Or they said, "They each have their own little worlds and are happy. Why bother' em?" (Gubrium and Ksander, 1975, p. 143). Aides sometimes bargained with patients to get them to attend sessions, offering extra cigarettes, promising that they would not be asked too many questions. This reluctance of both patients and aides crushed the therapeutic value of RO before it ever had a chance. Instead, the aide performed RO according to instructions, and a comedy of human errors often ensued.

In one session the researchers observed, the aide asked about the state of the weather, pointing to the board that read "raining." The patient looked out the window and said, "It looks like the sun is shining kinda bright." The sun happened to be shining at the moment. The aide pointed at the board, questioned the patient again, bringing to her attention that it said raining. The patient at last said that it was raining.

Lack of vocational training for paraprofessionals plagues institutions for the elderly. We must be aware that most states require no vocational standards or training requirements for aides or attendants working with the elderly. This is unfortunate, because paraprofessional contacts may be the most frequent and most important contacts an elderly institutional resident may have.

As of late 1976 (*Occupational Outlook Quarterly*, 1976: 4–5), well over 1 million people held positions in the field of aging. An increase in the number of jobs serving the elderly seems likely for several reasons. First of all, the elderly population itself is growing, and those who are most in need of supportive services are becoming ever more numerous. By the year 2000, the number of people over 75 years of age will be much higher than it is today. This age group is the most vulnerable to the physical and social stresses that come with aging; it is the group most likely to suffer from low income, poor health, or social isolation. In addition, women and blacks are increasing as a proportion of the elderly. Thus, the groups that are the most vulnerable are the ones increasing the fastest.

In addition, public awareness of the elderly is growing. Public attention to the elderly over the past decade or so has produced an outpouring of public and voluntary efforts, many highly imaginative and truly effective. Pressure to expand and improve these efforts is not likely to abate. A major survey of attitudes toward the elderly (Harris, 1975) showed that 81 percent of the American people believe that tax dollars should be used to help support the elderly.

Finally, many needs of the elderly are not being met. Despite the resources, both public and voluntary, that have been channeled into programs serving the elderly, the unmet needs of older Americans are enormous. The current network of programs and services is not accessible to all who require help. Existing systems for health care, social services, and income support are not designed to meet the needs of all, or even most, of the elderly. Intended largely for the poor, these programs cannot readily accommodate people of modest means, much less those at the middle-income level. In many communities, especially in small towns and rural areas, no assistance is provided for the old, apart from that given by neighbors and friends. To extend timely and effective aid to all the elderly who need help will require a considerable expansion of programs and activities—and commitment of sizeable funds.

New and innovative ways of meeting older people's needs are being developed and tested. For example, demonstration projects are under way in a number of communities to strengthen resources for home care, thus helping old people remain in their own homes as long as possible. Widespread adoption of many programs depends on the availability of funds. In future years, as public concern is translated into program support, it is likely that many new jobs will be created in the field of aging.

Vocational-Technical Adult Education Programs for the Elderly

Education courses offered for the elderly tend to be few in number and poor in quality. If we are to provide meaningful adult education for the older person, it must be tailored to meet the needs of that person. Currently we expect the elderly to fit into our mold, to meet our expectations.

Education should never be equated with schooling. Education is a lifelong process. It should enhance the growth of personality and help the individual enjoy a satisfying, meaningful life. It is erroneous to believe that learning takes place only within the classroom in a highly structured atmosphere. This is the real challenge for adult educators. The elderly are demanding more relevant and meaningful educational opportunities. We educators need to provide programs in second careers, in preretirement and postretirement. Older persons have had enough of basket weaving and cake decoration.

The population of the "young old," as defined by Bernice Neugarten (1974), is large and diverse. Three people in ten are over 45 years of age, and they constitute an immense potential market of education consumers. Included in this group are the homemaker returning to the employment marketplace either by choice or circumstance, the early retiree looking for new or second careers, and the individual going through a midlife transition and seeking counseling, training, and education to support changes in self.

In general, educational and training opportunities for the elderly are limited and programs are inadequate, noninnovative, and not geared to meet the actual needs of the elderly.

McClusky (1973) observes that we find older persons gravely deficient in formal schooling and participating little in adult educational activities even though they are fully capable of learning and they are in a world of dramatic change where learning is important and where the rewards of learning are potentially great. McClusky asks, "How can we more nearly match their need to learn with a better performance in learning?"

The answer probably lies somewhere in the realm of motivation. It is my hypothesis that in general older persons do not perceive education as relevant to their interests and needs. This point was repeatedly confirmed in the community discussion groups held throughout the country in preparation for the 1971 White House Conference. Instead of thinking of education as a thing apart or as a decorative option, it should be regarded as a principal component of all the services designed to meet the necessities of living. Specifically, education should play an important role in producing, maintaining, and protecting health and income. It should also be a basic element in solving problems of housing, the use of legal services, in the adjustment to change of relationships in the family, in community organization, and so forth. In short, education should be regarded as a program category to which all other aspects of living in the later years should be related. In this sense it would become an "umbrella" for working in and comprehending the field of aging as a whole.

Gartner (Note 7) relates education for the elderly to work:

For the great number of Americans over 65 years of age, meaningful work is a central activity, whether or not an income support system is needed. Human services work, helping others, is particularly suited to many older persons. This type of work calls for education and training for those who had worked in different areas. College programs should be developed for older workers engaged in second careers, with credits granted for life experience, work experience, and previous learning, in order to sharply decrease the length of time required for a degree; entry points into education or careers should not be limited to prescribed age groups but should be open to those of all ages. Unlike the traditional picture, the growing pattern will be for people to be engaged in a variety of activities throughout their lifetimes. School and work should be seen as operating in tandem and not sequentially. Of course, efforts to combine work and study are not new. What is new is the concern for adults as well as for youth, the use of various equivalency devices, and the particular interest in human services jobs.

Sack (Note 8) emphasizes the educational implications of the changes in the characteristics and demography of the older population. In about 20 years there will be an identifiable group of 55- to 75-year-olds (15 percent of the population) who, compared with the same age group today, will be relatively homogeneous as a result of earlier retirement, prolonged better health, and increases in education level, expectations, political activism, and purchasing power. To meet the needs of this emerging age group, programs must be developed that offer a wider variety of options that enhance life. To be considered are lifelong educational experiences through sabbaticals and retraining, preretirement education beginning early in life, opportunities for community participation and services, and choices of alternative life styles and communal living arrangements.

Vocational adult education, in its broadest sense, can be a vital dimension of the life experience of adults in general. The following summary recommendations may help us understand the role of vocational adult education in gerontology:

1. "Education is a basic right for all age groups. It is continuous and henceforth is one of the ways of enabling older people to achieve a full and meaningful life. It is also a means for helping them develop their potential as a resource for the betterment of society" (Note 9).

2. The states' departments of education should conduct educational-needs assessments and investigate the possibilities of funding programs to meet these needs.

3. To encourage citizens to take advantage of postsecondary educational opportunities, the state should consider the possibility of reducing the tuition for citizens above 50 years of age. This is essential to the development of second-career programs, new visions programs, and so on.

4. Vocational counseling and placement services by the elderly should be explored. Many elderly, now or previously involved in industrial, commercial, and service occupations, are willing to offer their services and expertise to others in educational institutions. They constitute a wasted human resource. Further, the states should study the possibilities of recruiting retired technicians and paraprofessionals from industry, commerce, and service agencies to work as aides in vocational education institutions.

5. To encourage citizens 50 years old or over to participate in educational activities, we should consider retroactive credits for life experience, based on evaluation of the applicant's portfolio. The classroom experience is not the only method of instruction. More independent studies should be available to this group of citizens.

Notes

1. Treybig, D. L. *Language, children, and attitudes toward the aged: A longitudinal study.* Paper presented at the 27th Annual Meeting of Gerontological Society, Portland, Oregon, October 1974.

2. Harris, L., & Associates. *The myth and reality of aging in America.* Washington, D.C.: The National Council on the Aging, 1975, p. 65.

3. Zaki, G. *Hartford Park housing project, evaluation and assessment.* Washington, D.C.: U.S. Department of Housing and Urban Development Grant, 1969, pp. 21–23. (Monograph)

4. *Education and aging.* White House Conference on Aging. Washington, D.C.: U.S. Department of Health, Education and Welfare, Special Staff on Aging, 1961, p. 5.

5. Jacobs, H. L. Education for aging in the elementary and secondary school system. In S. Grabowski & W. D. Mason (Eds.), *Learning for aging.* Washington, D.C.: Adult Education Association, 1975, p. 86.

6. Zaki, G. *Summer consultation program.* Washington, D.C.: Gerontological Society, 1974, Appendix 2, p. 2.

7. Gartner, A. *The older American.* Presentation at the Annual Southern Conference on Gerontology, Gainesville, Florida, 1969.

8. Sack, A., et al. *Planning for the emerging young old.* School of Social Services Administration, University of Chicago.

9. *Toward a national policy on aging.* Proceedings of the White House Conference on Aging. Washington, D.C., 1971. (Final Report)

References

Gubrium, J., & Ksander, M. On multiple realities and reality orientation. *The Gerontologist*, April 1975, *15*(2), 142–145.

McClusky, H. Y. Education and aging. In *A manual on planning educational programs for older adults.* Department of Adult Education, Florida State University, 1973.

Neugarten, B. L. Age groups in American society and the rise of the young old. *Annals of Political and Social Sciences*, September 1974.

Occupational Outlook Quarterly. Washington, D.C.: U.S. Department of Labor, Bureau of Labor Statistics, Fall 1976, 4–5.

Design and Implementation of an Associate Degree Geriatrics Curriculum

Dan Cowley and Barbara Porter
Wayne Community College

The field of human services is beginning to function as an integrated system, or a network, much like a television network. Geriatrics services, for so long unwanted stepchildren, are rapidly becoming integral parts of the larger system. Territorial disputes, such as those that followed from Freud, Skinner, and Rogers, are fading into the historical tapestry, taking with them nature-nurture controversies, debates of innate goodness versus innate evil, and other disciplinarian arguments.

As the person is seen more and more as a varied and complex whole, with varied but interrelated problems, difficulties, and needs, the human services system is attempting to pool its resources to respond more adequately. Similarly, older people are being seen as needing more than just a place to rest until they die. Their basic needs are seen as more similar to than different from the needs of other people.

The emergence of an articulate interface between the person and the environment through behavioral interactions has created the need for a new level of human services worker, both in kind and in degree. For example, mental-health technicians are now fitting in between professionals and aide-level workers in mental hospitals, mental-retardation centers, and mental health centers. These middle-level workers are functioning in new roles, such as advocate, liaison worker, services broker, behavior manager, peer counselor, and in other roles. Their primary role has emerged as the worker to whom clients can go to have their needs met—directly or indirectly—from the beginning to the end of the human services experience.

The changing human services system, while reflecting changing attitudes and values, also influences and changes attitudes and values. As changes in the larger system change geriatrics services, and vice versa, the need for a new type of geriatrics worker emerges. A geriatrics technician is needed to fill the gap between highly trained professionals and undertrained and untrained aide-level workers. The older adult needs some one person to turn to in order to insure that his or her complex and varied needs are met. Even though such a worker needs essential knowledge and skills, perhaps attitude is most important in getting the job done—a fresh attitude that sees the older person as a whole.

Background

Located in Goldsboro, one of four major human services centers in North Carolina (broadly defined as locations for mental hospitals, mental-retardation centers, vocational rehabilitation facilities, alcoholic rehabilitation facilities, and correctional centers), Wayne Community College pioneered in developing technician-level allied health professional programs, including nursing programs at the associate degree, practical nurse, and nurse's aide levels, and dental programs for dental assistants and dental hygienists.

There was a natural flow from allied health training into mental health training, and eventually, human services training. Every community college in the state had to demonstrate the need for the mental health associate program through a community needs assessment. After demonstrating the need, the college had to obtain approval of its curriculum by the North Carolina State Board of Education, and the State Department of Community Colleges had to demonstrate that there was no competing program in the local geographical area. These three steps are necessary to begin any new curriculum in the state system of community colleges and technical institutes.

Likewise, continuing programs must also meet three requirements. The college must be able to recruit ample numbers of new students each year; the college must be able to get jobs for its graduates or show that most graduates are able to find employment; and the salary and duties of graduates must be commensurate with the training. The mental health associate program was so successful on these three counts, and community need so strong, that Wayne Community College developed an alcoholism technician training program and soon after a geriatrics technician training program.

With the rapid growth of human services related programs, the college created a department of human services and added two new curricula to the three already in existence. These new programs consisted of a one-year human services worker diploma curriculum and a two-year A.A.S. degree curriculum in human services technology.

Concurrent with these developments, a joint state committee was developed, and it recommended core curriculum approaches to human services and mental health training. As a result, Wayne Community College implemented the human services worker curriculum as the required first-year core curriculum and as the prerequisite for admission into each of the four associate degree programs in human services, mental health, alcoholism, and geriatrics. Also, several courses were identified as "core" requirements in all second-year programs. All other second-year courses consisted of specialized training specific to each curriculum.

Curriculum

The human services worker one-year diploma program, which also serves as the core curriculum for all two-year degree programs, consists of a variety of courses aimed at acquiring knowledge, developing skills, and changing attitudes. These courses cover grammar, composition, technical writing, introductory psychology, sociology, and human services; human relations training and group processes; and interviewing, counseling, crisis intervention, activities, behavior disorders, human growth and development, social issues and problems, and other survey courses.

Second-year courses included in the geriatrics curriculum, and considered core to all degree programs in human services, include learning and behavior, behavior management, marriage and the family, reading and research, seminar, and cooperative work experiences. Specialty courses in mental health technology concentrate on basic health-care knowledge and skills, behavior modification techniques, and individual and group counseling skills necessary for working in mental hospitals, mental-retardation centers, and mental health centers. Specialized training for alcoholism technology students focuses on alcoholism education for the public and public-school audiences and counseling techniques for working with alcoholics in groups and in their families. Second-year courses in human services technology are flexible and geared to individual students who wish to pursue a higher degree, with emphasis placed on college-transfer level courses relevant to particular university departments.

During the second year, geriatrics students enroll in many courses of specialized study in addition to core courses. The geriatrics curriculum encompasses many areas and includes classwork instruction in the following: introduction and orientation to gerontology, sociological aspects of aging, mental disorders associated with aging, the psychological and physiological aspects of aging, death and dying, aging in a contemporary society, activities coordinator for the aged and infirm, and geriatrics seminar. Courses range from one to five quarter hours of academic credit, and many have from two to four laboratory hours in addition to classroom hours. Students must complete 118 quarter hours of course work to qualify for graduation.

During any given quarter, students may elect to enroll in the cooperative work experiences in order to broaden and enhance their theoretical knowledge. The cooperative work experience program affords students an opportunity to accumulate at least 440 hours of practical work experience in community geriatrics programs, and it increases the likelihood of job placement upon completion of the program.

Faculty

The department of human services and the geriatrics technician program attempt to train interdisciplinary, generalist workers at the middle level of the professional helping services. Students are exposed to an educational training model that is somewhat interdisciplinary, somewhat multidisciplinary, and somewhat transdisciplinary. The program is interdisciplinary to the extent that students are exposed to faculty from other departments, divisions, and disciplines, including social science, the humanities, allied health, and physical health. For the most part, these faculty function in a "purist" role; in other words, they teach sociology classes as sociologists. There is little ongoing interaction among these various instructors that might affect their disciplinarian purity.

From a teamwork approach, the core faculty of the geriatrics program is multidisciplinary, when a psychologist, a social gerontologist, and a rehabilitation counselor work closely together in weaving student experiences in separate courses into a common fabric. To the degree that these faculty do not pay close attention to each other's disciplinary boundaries or "turf," and to the degree that they cut across such superficial and arbitrary lines and boundaries of professional territoriality, they are transdisciplinary. Observations of the behavior of program graduates on the job indicates that this model has a degree of success in producing interdisciplinarian generalists. Even though the program does not embody a pure model of inter-, multi-, or trans-disciplinism—which might be more or less advantageous—the staff prefers an "impure" model.

When considering all full-time departmental faculty, full-time faculty of other departments, part-time faculty, adjunct faculty, and consultants, the average geriatrics student is exposed to persons with every type of educational credential—M.D.'s, Ph.D.'s, M.A.'s, M.S.W.'s, B.A.'s, and A.A.'s. These faculty come from many disciplines, educational institutions, geographical locations, work backgrounds, and philosophical positions. Whatever the generic attitude and method of human services and geriatrics services, geriatrics students are exposed to it.

Students

The geriatrics program actively recruits high-school graduates, middle-age persons, and workers from other disciplinary fields who are seeking new job skills because of changes in the labor force. No discrimination is made on the basis of age, race, or sex, and minority groups such as the elderly and the black compose a representative proportion of students accepted into the program.

Students enrolled in the program are very heterogeneous on such variables as race, sex, age, and religion, but very homogeneous on commitment and dedication to working with and for the elderly. There is no economic stimulus to encourage students to enter the geriatrics technology program, only desire, commitment, and dedication to work with elderly persons.

Prospective students for the geriatrics program are primarily recruited through the media and by the college recruitment officer. In addition, employers in agencies providing services to the elderly often recommend potential students and help arrange work-release time for their class attendance. Students presently working within the system are usually lower-level geriatrics workers who are seeking upward mobility on the career ladder in geriatrics and gerontology. Late-afternoon and evening classes are offered for day-shift workers who cannot arrange to attend classes during the regular college hours.

Admission to the first year of the geriatrics program is open. The only requirement is a reading level appropriate to the written materials in the program. Persons scoring below the acceptable reading level on an entrance test are encouraged to enroll in remedial courses offered by the college. Once the requisite reading skills are acquired, the student may reapply for admission into the human services program.

Students successfully completing the human services core curriculum may apply to the geriatrics technology program for the second year of their training. Fifteen students are accepted into the program, based on relative cumulative grade point average during the first year and the recommendation of the department chairman. This policy allows students nine months to demonstrate their capability to perform acceptably.

Attending Wayne Community College full-time costs approximately $100 per quarter. Financial assistance to cover college expenses is available through various programs, such as the Work-Study Program and Basic Educational Opportunities Grants. Other sources of funds are state vocational rehabilitation, Social Security Administration, and the Veterans Administration. Students in the Geriatrics program receive no financial assistance or stipends from the grant that funds the program.

Agencies

In the local area there are numerous programs and agencies serving the elderly. The geriatrics technology program works very closely with them in coordinating course design and implementation with the needs of the elderly in the community. The agencies, through their support of the cooperative work experience program, provide the student with a learning environment for acquiring and practicing new skills. In addition, the community agencies serve as a source of adjunct faculty to supplement the college's geriatrics staff.

An advisory committee, composed of representatives from all levels of the geriatrics service system in the community, works with the college staff in evaluating the geriatrics program to insure that the curriculum properly reflects geriatric needs and offers quality education. The advisory committee also reviews and evaluates the progress of the program every six months to determine whether the program is meeting its goals and objectives. The community is surveyed once each year to determine the impact of the training program on the local delivery system of services to the elderly.

Upon completion of the geriatrics technology program, graduates work in a variety of settings, such as geriatrics units in institutions for the elderly retarded and mentally ill, in nutrition programs, as activities coordinators for rest homes and nursing facilities, with area councils of aging, and with regional councils of aging. Graduates are placed through the job placement service of the college, by the program coordinator, and through students who have had the opportunity to display their skills to potential employers through field practicums and cooperative work experiences. The cooperative education director, who arranges the work placements, is often contacted by employers with job opportunities.

Future

If the past is a valid and reliable predictor of the future, then the success of mental health technicians during the past ten years should predict a successful future for geriatrics technicians. The need for competent workers at middle levels has been well documented for the past quarter of a century. Predictions for increased service delivery needs of older persons for the next quarter of a century are already legion. If the futurists are at all accurate in their prophecies, then the next immediate era will be the age of human services and human resources development.

Developing Inservice and Preservice Models for Paraprofessional Training in Aging

Glorian Sorensen
Augsburg College
and
James Tift
St. Mary's Junior College

Few training programs are offered to meet the specific training needs of the paraprofessional working with older adults. Therefore, it is often found that the training of those who work directly with the elderly does not provide them with sufficient tools to fully understand the concerns of the older adult. Our model of inservice and preservice training for the paraprofessional seeks to fill this gap.

The content areas of this training model are intended to provide the participant with a basic understanding of aging processes and the particular needs of the older person. Through the use of active learning techniques, exercises, and simulations, the learner is taught how to be effective with the older adult in a variety of work situations. The content areas of the training model include: myths and realities of aging; social, psychological, and physical changes in the aging process; communication skills and building helping relationships; death, dying, and grief; intimacy and sexuality in old age; adjusting to the nursing home; and community services and resources for the elderly. These methods and concepts are detailed in our training manual, *Meeting the Psychosocial Needs of the Older Person* by Tift and Sorensen (Note 1). The training program based on this model is cosponsored by the Program on Aging at Augsburg College and by the Aging and Human Development program at St. Mary's Junior College in Minneapolis, Minnesota.

Inservice Perspective

Paraprofessional personnel are working with older adults in numerous settings, such as nursing homes, neighborhood groups, churches, settlement houses, and other community agencies. Very often these people have little training in working with older adults. To meet this need, Augsburg College's Gerontological Human Relations Training Program has developed an inservice training model to provide a learning experience directly and immediately applicable to work. Such relevancy increases the participation and involvement of the learner.

The training program is designed to be offered on site at individual nursing homes or community agencies. An advantage of on-site training is that one is working with an already cohesive group close to their situation. The training program is scheduled around the availability of the participants. For example, a series of eight one-and-one-half-hour weekly sessions has been found to be most convenient for nursing-home nursing assistants and housekeeping, dietary, and maintenance staff. For community groups, an all-day seminar may be more appropriate. Groups trained under this model have included congregate dining site coordinators, parish workers, homemakers, home health aides, volunteers, drivers, and advocates. The ease of transporting this training program has been demonstrated by offering it in a wide variety of work situations.

From the experiences and results of implementing the model, we may draw a number of generalizations about the elements that combine to make a successful inservice program.

Institutional Base This training model has been developed at a four-year private college, which is located in the center of a large metropolitan area. Other educational institutions with a strong community involvement, such as vocational-technical schools or community colleges, may also find it successful. A supportive educational environment, which is sensitive to and ready to serve community needs, will be most helpful to the search for funding. Community-based organizations such as community mental health centers could also use the training models.

Publicity Program development depends, of course, on the demand for training. Initial publicity may be gained through general mailings. Both nursing-home administrators and inservice training directors, who are most likely to be familiar with training plans yet often lack the authority to approve implementation, should receive relevant information. All letters should be followed by a phone call to answer questions and discuss program details. Similar approaches are used with other target groups.

After the program's initial contacts, word of mouth may become the primary source of new training activities. Participants and other staff at former training sites quickly tell other facilities about effective programs. Also, a support network in the community will distribute program information. For example, county welfare workers often work closely with nursing homes and organizations, and are usually eager to bring news of various training possibilities into these facilities.

Planning Each nursing home and organization is unique because of its individual type of staff and clients. For example, differences have been noted among the staffs of inner city, suburban, and rural nursing homes. The level of care offered by a nursing home will create different training needs. And the nature of the service, the educational background of the participants, and the location of community programs will cause differences in training content and methods. For this reason, the program must be planned specifically around the individual training site. Staff who will participate in the training are included in this planning process to incorporate their ideas and gain their support. Administrative input to and support of any training program are also imperative. Collaborative planning of content, methods, and time structure will create a program more relevant and useful to the staff. This planning process also allows the trainer to become familiar with the setting and to develop a rapport with staff.

Implementation For the effective use of active learning methods, the trainer should limit the class size to no more than 40 and, for discussion purposes, to no less than 12. Since many of the participants may be unaccustomed to the formal, traditional classroom settings, care should be taken to create a comfortable, informal atmosphere that will encourage learner participation and free interchange. Throughout the one-and-one-half-hour session or the all-day workshop, varied teaching methods are used to keep things moving. Role play, discussions, and simulations may be used along with audio-visual material and some lectures.

In some situations, it may be necessary to include an incentive for regular attendance, such as awarding a certificate.

Audience The training model has given rise to the possibility of changing the status of the paraprofessional. Often it is pointed out that there is a high turnover rate among nursing assistants or community homemakers. The low status and power of these positions certainly provide no reason to remain with them. Developing close personal relationships with the older person is often the only reward in these low-paying positions. Involvement in a training program may act as a way of raising staff morale if the paraprofessionals are given tools to do their jobs more effectively. The program coordinator or trainer may also become an advocate for these paraprofessionals, who are often eager to provide effective, caring services but, because of understaffing and poor supervision, may have neither the time nor the skills to do so.

Administrative involvement in the training program, especially in nursing homes, is vitally important because administrative support is necessary if the paraprofessional is to be paid and encouraged to attend inservice training. Staff members may be learning ways to improve the quality of care they offer, yet without the time allowance and reinforcement to use these skills, training may produce frustration due to impotence. Trainers working in the institution are also in a position to educate administrative and professional staff members regarding ongoing implementation of the skills and understanding acquired by paraprofessional staff during the training program.

Evaluation An ongoing evaluation of the variables involved in the program's success, such as geography, finances, experience, and work incentives that affect the attendance rate, provides data that can best distribute the training and resources available. For example, a pretest/posttest questionnaire can provide credible evidence that the training program does affect the paraprofessional. This evidence, in the long run, would offer substantial testimony that the program is producing a positive, meaningful outcome and is achieving its long-term desired outcome to increase the quality of service and the meaningfulness of life for older adults.

Funding Until recently, the training of nursing-home staff members has not been a high-priority expenditure. If state departments of health and welfare reduce or contain training programs by making it difficult for nursing homes to be reimbursed for training, they will jeopardize the continuance of any special training programs. As training programs become a requirement, however, it is more likely that funds will be allocated; otherwise, it may be necessary for training programs to find support outside the state system. To reduce the cost, the training-program sponsor should attempt to coordinate efforts with other educational institutions, as well as with consumer groups within the community.

Implementing this type of inservice training program will likely increase awareness of the need and demand for such training. There are growing numbers of people working with the elderly, and often those in the most direct contact with the elderly are the least trained. In-depth training programs may be developed to follow up the original training. Training may be offered to additional target groups, such as day-care workers, foster-care families, and custodial-care providers. A model for training of trainers may serve to broaden the impact of a program. Families, as well as older adults themselves, are interested in understanding the changes involved in the aging processes.

Preservice Perspective

A need also exists for education in a classroom setting for those who are interested in working with the elderly but have had little background or experience. The Aging and Human Development Program at St. Mary's Junior College—a one-year, 45-credit, undergraduate certificate program—was designed to help meet this need.

A fairly extensive outreach effort and a needs assessment were undertaken to determine and document the need for basic paraprofessional training in aging. The data indicated that practitioners in the field strongly believed that such an educational program in aging was needed and would be enthusiastically received. The needs assessment data suggested that not only was training needed for practitioners who would be working with older people in institutional settings, but also such a program should focus upon education and training for practitioners who would be working with older persons in community settings such as high-rise housing, senior centers, nutrition programs, and day-care programs. The model for preservice education implemented at St. Mary's is based on these assessment data.

This program is a long-term classroom model of paraprofessional training in aging. As the *preservice* label implies, such a model is geared primarily for persons interested in but not now working with older adults. Many will probably be young students, some perhaps only recently out of high school. In addition, especially in community college settings, there is a growing number of "mature" students who may be reentering the workforce or contemplating a change from technical to human service oriented fields. Some students may have had brief exposure to the elderly (as volunteers, for example) and subsequently may make a decision to seek an educational program in aging to broaden their experiences, develop specific competencies, and increase their job potential.

The following sections describe some of the components of this model preservice training program in gerontology.

Publicity The methods of publicizing an undergraduate certificate program on aging may vary considerably depending on the size of the community, availability of possible linkages with other educational institutions, and range and type of programs for seniors offered in the community. Formal and informal contacts with local civic leaders and professionals in human service fields may prove helpful in publicizing a program on aging.

When used effectively, the media can inform the general public about the availability of a program on aging. A small article in a local paper on two consecutive Sundays resulted in over 100 telephone calls and inquiries by mail about the aging program at St. Mary's. A number of these individuals eventually applied and enrolled in the program. Spot radio announcements have also been used with varying degrees of success.

Once a program on aging has been established, its graduates are probably the best source of publicity. Another technique is the open house, which incudes a general description of the program, a slide presentation, and sharing of information by program graduates.

Planning a preservice educational program for paraprofessionals involves much more than the initial curriculum and program development. Even with careful and purposeful initial planning, educators will continually have to make major and minor revisions in the curriculum and program. Such areas as conceptual framework, program goals and objectives, and graduate competencies may need to be altered to reflect the realities of the students and the program. Some educators first design an aging curriculum and then attempt to identify program goals and objectives and graduate competencies that reflect the curriculum design. However, it often proves more useful to begin by analyzing what practitioners in the field of aging are doing and what makes them successful. Having taken account of the state of the field, educators can define program goals and objectives. Thus, curriculum planning and development flow naturally from practitioner input and identified program goals and objectives.

Implementation In a preservice educational program held in a classroom setting, it is important to apply a variety of teaching techniques to accommodate students who have a variety of backgrounds and learning styles. This training model uses three approaches. The first combines lecture and discussion in one of the three major aging content areas: sociology, psychology, or physiology of aging. In this traditional approach to learning, theory and concepts are stressed. The second technique is teaching and practicing skills in the classroom laboratory. Such skills might include advocacy, communicating with the elderly, how to assess physical or mental health, or how to find and use community resources for the elderly. Active learning techniques such as role playing and simulation may be used to demonstrate or practice skills. The third and perhaps most important component is the student field experience in an agency or institution serving older adults. Such field experience should vary during the year so that students have an oppportunity to interact with older adults and services in several community and institutional settings.

Evaluation Most educational institutions make some provision for evaluating both students and teachers. Students may be given the choice of a grading system for the lecture and discussion component of the program. A simple pass/fail evaluation system for the classroom laboratory and field experience may be most appropriate because of the type of learning experience each provides.

As with the inservice program, program evaluation should be ongoing. Both practitioner input and student feedback should be strongly encouraged and actively sought. In addition to overall evaluations from students, written evaluations and suggestions from both students and practitioners might be solicited. Practitioners in the field, including present and potential student field experience supervisors, might be convened as a group. Their ideas and recommendations concerning program planning and development may prove to be an invaluable evaluation tool.

Summary

The urgent need for education and training in aging at all levels and in a wide variety of settings is well demonstrated by the establishment and growth of an organization like the Association for Gerontology in Higher Education. This paper has described two approaches to helping meet the need for trained paraprofessionals in the field of aging, one inservice and the other preservice. It is important and essential to provide training for those working in the field of aging and for those interested in the field. The enthusiastic response to both levels of this training model in Minneapolis during the last few years has dramatically illustrated the need and demand for paraprofessional training.

Notes

1. Tift, J., & Sorensen, G. *Meeting the psychosocial needs of the older person.* (1977 ed. available from Program on Aging, Augsburg College, 731 21st Avenue, South, Minneapolis, Minnesota 55454) (1980 ed. in press)

A Multidimensional Approach to the Implementation of Gerontology in Graduate Schools of Social Work

Eloise Rathbone-McCuan
Washington University

The broad range of social services that are being provided for the elderly involves social workers. Their knowledge and skills provide assistance to the aged as individual clients and as members of families, groups, organizations, and communities. However, many social workers now in the field of gerontology received no specialized graduate training in gerontology. They have adapted and applied generic knowledge about individual behavior and societal and environmental forces, about neighborhoods and communities, and about social administration and policy development to aged clients and the elderly as a general population at risk.

Although there is a rapidly growing trend among graduate schools of social work to provide some knowledge about the particular needs of the elderly and the dimensions and dynamics of aging, only a few schools provide courses about the treatment and intervention methods particularly appropriate for alleviating the problems of older men and women. This paper focuses on master's level education in gerontology, and analyzes trends in social work education that influence the development of gerontology specializations. Also discussed are appropriate content for these specializations, approaches for organizing the content, and the development of a specialization at one school of social work.

Social work educators and educational administrators have many factors to consider in the course of planning graduate social work curriculum. Most important among these are:

1. Core knowledge—areas of knowledge essential to broad practice competence and at the same time appropriate as a foundation for specialized theory and method content

2. Curriculum organization—conceptual organization of general and specialized educational offerings in a coherent curriculum model

3. Faculty utilization—matching the expertise of academic faculty with the general and specialized teaching functions needed

4. Personnel selection—selecting new faculty to insure that faculty composition is adequate to provide coverage for both the general and specialized educational needs of the students

5. Student educational interest—effective and efficient means of providing a multidimensional curriculum to meet the various interests of students

Each of these factors influences planning, implementing, and delivering a specialized program in gerontology. Social work educators responsible for establishing gerontological components within their schools need to recognize how these central issues control the short- and long-range curriculum planning of a specialization.

The strength of a specialization in gerontology depends on the quality of the total curriculum. Gerontological expertise is no substitute for social work expertise. Monk (1975) cautions: "It becomes even more serious for social work if gerontological training is defined in a narrow categorical sense. Yet a gerontological component within the graduate curriculum should not be developed at the expense of our generic social work foundation. We train social workers first and gerontologists second."

There is a gap between the practitioner's concern for specialized gerontological education and the educator's desire for noncategorical education. Those in the field recognize that the number of elderly people requiring social work services is increasing and that more social service programs are being established to meet the needs of the elderly. Practitioners, students, and national and local professional organizations are all encouraging schools of social work to develop gerontology specializations. However, the graduate schools are still responding very slowly. Perhaps the single greatest incentive for them will be the increased availability of training funds in gerontological social work.

Schools of social work that have developed programs in gerontology have applied a variety of models. Two particular models, which represent opposite types of curriculum, will be discussed here. The first type occurs within schools of social work that have links with a large multidisciplinary gerontology center. These centers provide a central source of students and of educational and research activity in the field of aging. The advantages of this model are numerous, since the school of social work can maintain interorganizational affiliations that enhance both the school and the center. However, this model is not dominant because most schools of social work are at universities without large gerontological centers.

The second model is more common. A number of gerontological specializations have been developed within schools of social work without input from other departments or professional schools. Typically, one or several faculty members with interest and expertise in aging conceptualize a specialization and work to gain the support of their colleagues and administrators.

For a school of social work to advertise that it has a specialization in gerontology, the overall curriculum must contain a cluster of courses with integrated gerontology content that can be sequenced. These courses must be offered regularly and be available to students intending to "major" in gerontology as well as other students desiring to obtain general knowledge about old age and the aging process.

Structuring the gerontological component of the total curriculum may be approached from many perspectives. Unfortunately, there is an absence of useful guides in the gerontology and social work literature. One apparently viable model was developed by Carroll (1975) in an attempt to conceptualize an organizational scheme that could guide all types of concentration development in social work curricula. Her threefold model incorporated the specific dimensions of social problems, social units, and social technologies. If a fourth dimension is added, that of spheres of functioning, the model becomes useful for conceptualizing a gerontology specialization curriculum.

Spheres of functioning account for the major areas of functioning that are subject to change throughout the aging process among individuals and subgroups of the elderly population. The social problem dimension accounts for the range of societal problems that may have different consequences for the elderly. The social unit dimension takes into consideration the spectrum of units that may be appropriate for social work intervention. The dimension of social technology specifies the range of methods, activities, and techniques that may be used to affect spheres of functioning and social problems within the parameters of specific social units.

The curriculum of a gerontology specialization manifests varying degrees of integration with different components of the larger curriculum. Gerontology faculty are in a good position to identify possible linkages with other specific offerings. Too often, social problems are incorrectly perceived as unrelated to the aged population. For example, courses on substance abuse and alcoholism rarely cover the problems of older abusers. However, the elderly are among the high-risk groups in relation to the overuse and misuse of prescribed drugs. Alcoholism is becoming increasing prevalent among older people, yet seminars on the topic rarely cover the problems of older abusers. The gerontologist could assist the specialist in substance abuse or alcoholism to introduce appropriate gerontological content.

A school of social work cannot plan and implement a gerontology specialization unless certain conditions are met: (1) support from the full-time faculty for the development of specializations in social problems or populations at risk; (2) more than one specialization, all with similar conceptual frameworks; (3) at least one full-time faculty member to act as coordinator and thus provide the necessary intellectual, educational, and administrative leadership for the specialization; (4) support from the administrators of the school and the university; (5) a group of students committed to specializing in gerontology; and (6) an appropriate range of field experience opportunities with competent supervision.

The gerontology specialization at the George Warren Brown School of Social Work, Washington University, is structured as a cluster of required, sequenced courses and elective seminars for students specializing in gerontology and other students who want knowledge and skills in the area. The school has three other specializations based on populations at risk: women, children, and families. A common conceptual framework is being explored to systematize the roles of these specializations in the overall social work curriculum. The specialization coordinators work together to develop mechanisms for creating interspecialization programs and service projects.

The school is conducting a project to design, implement, and evaluate an interspecialization program that trains students in the mental health of older women. The general aim of this project is to prepare social work students to assume professional roles in treating and preventing the mental health problems of older women. In addition, the project provides educational opportunities for social work graduate students in other specializations to increase their recognition and understanding of the mental health problems of older women.

Before the project was formed, students in the two specializations (gerontology and women) interacted little, and neither group was receiving educational content that sensitized them to the particular needs of older women. The biases of mental health professionals, which influence the treatment of and access to mental health service by both aged and women, were not conceptually connected.

Developing curriculum for interspecialization is one of the greatest challenges to faculty. It has been necessary for faculty and instructors to design content that helps students assess the mental health needs of older women and find ways of developing field practicum opportunities for the students. The latter task has been difficult. Few psychiatric or mental health service settings provide treatment for the elderly. Most of the mental health care provided by social work practitioners occurs in institutional settings, and the nonprofessional mental health service programs for women have devoted little attention to outreach for older women.

The lack of substantive knowledge and skills required to serve this at-risk population has forced faculty to develop knowledge through expanded roles in mental health research, community consultation, and actual program development. Plans are now being made at Washington University for the social work trainees to experience structured interactions with different subgroups of older women, including aged black women living in public housing in St. Louis, older female mental patients who have been discharged to permanent residency in nursing homes, older female alcoholics, and groups of aged widows.

Involvement with these different populations of older women will provide students with the opportunity to receive training in interpersonal, administrative, and policy-making skills for direct application to the mental health problems of older women. Each student trainee will have the opportunity to use skills in direct practice, community development, administration, and research.

Current patterns of service delivery do not encourage the integration of aging, mental health, and women's services. Gerontologists have not attended adequately to the range of psychological, social, economic, and health problems that differentiate older women from older men. Perhaps inadvertently, mental health practitioners of both sexes perpetuate sexism and ageism in therapy. Social work educators interested in women's mental health have for the most part forgotten older women.

The development of the core curriculum for this project has required the faculty in gerontology to expand the knowledge base of research on women, and the faculty in the women's specialization has had to become familiar with basic materials in social gerontology. The list of unanswered questions about practice with older women is growing, and many research and service projects are being planned. For the students and faculty in the project, the goal of service innovation has become a major educational objective. This is a concern shared by all those involved in this gerontological and women's educational experiment, and efforts in this area will help to increase the relevance of this project as a national model for training social workers in the mental health of older women.

Building a gerontology specialization as part of a graduate social work program is one example of educational innovation that may improve the quality of services to older Americans. A careful balance must be maintained in order not to abuse the innovative opportunities now possible in the field of gerontology. A specialization in gerontology should represent more than a popular educational development. Meeting the current and future social service needs of the elderly is of great importance. Gerontology social work educators should not take their tasks lightly. They are educating the professionals who must be qualified to meet these needs upon entry into practice.

Acknowledgement The training described in this paper is sponsored in part by NIMH Grant. No. IT21MH1990.

References

Carroll, N. K. Areas of concentration in the graduate curriculum: A three-dimensional model. *Journal of Education for Social Work*, Spring 1975, *11*, 3–10.

Monk, A. A conceptual base for "second generation" programs in gerontology. *Journal of Education for Social Work*, Fall 1975, *11*, 84–88.

PART SEVEN
CURRICULAR AND INSTRUCTIONAL METHODS

The expansion of gerontology throughout higher education presents opportunities for the use of varied didactic approaches. But these opportunities also raise questions of what we should teach about gerontology and how we should teach it. Curriculum and instruction are inseparable, and our concepts of gerontology education must incorporate both. The first two papers in this section consider the larger issue of how to select content and instructional methodologies, and the last paper illustrates the application of concepts.

What Should We Teach?
Content Validity in Designing Curricula
in
Gerontology and Geriatrics
for
the Education of Health Professionals

Vicki A. Zoot
University of Illinois-Medical Center

Curriculum planning is decision making: How do we determine what to include and what to eliminate? The criteria for such selections should reflect the relationship of course content to desired outcome—that is, it should be content-valid.

Historically, questions of content validity in education have been asked of test design, whereas curricular planning has been based on the opinions of content experts. Recently, however, educators planning curricula have been asking questions about content validity. This issue is of particular concern in health professions education because it is assumed that such curricula are based on known standards for the competent health professional (physician, nurse, pharmacist, dentist, occupational therapist, medical social worker, dietitian, etc.). Implicit in the notion of competency itself is the additional assumption that we know what a competent health professional should do, know, or value in practice. Thus, the practice domain must be delineated if we are to plan a content-valid curriculum.

Designing and implementing gerontological and geriatric content in the curricula of the health professions require attention toward what outcomes should be achieved and what goals and standards the future practitioner should meet. We must define the health professional who is expert in geriatrics. We must ask: What content is essential to make the health practitioner competent to care for older adults? Further, which components are identical in several professions and which are unique? Fitting curriculum to the answers to these questions makes the curriculum content-valid.

In geriatrics and gerontology, one can find many answers to the question of what to teach but no answers to the question of why. We need research data on which to base curricular decisions—and that need is as urgent as the need for the curricula themselves. A curricular decision made without evidence is an opinion. Such a decision is a value judgment, one based on possibilities ranked on the basis of what the decision maker thinks is important.

Why is it so important to know what to teach? Educational philosophers, such as Marler (1975), tell us that the study of epistemology has perpetually dealt with attempts to validate knowledge claims. Kliebard (1977) suggests the "possibility that the question of what to teach cannot be answered" and that "the value of the question . . . may lie in the issues it generates." Hughes (1962) disagrees, saying that "it is necessary to act without waiting for certainty." Tanner (1975) seconds the motion: "Forget the theoretical problems and get on with the job."

Possibly the questions are unanswerable, but they must be asked. Those of us in health professions education are faced with an enormous responsibility: The public assumes that we graduate competent students. If we make the claim that we will graduate a health professional expert in gerontology and geriatrics, then this professional will be expected to carry out the actions necessary to caring for older adults. This responsibility weighs heavily on the educator. In the health professions, we cannot assume that we are developing competence if we have not yet identified what competent performance is. If we have not identified and confirmed by research what it is that a health professional must understand, do, or value, we cannot be comfortable with our curricular choices or assume that they are correct.

John Bryant (1969) says: "An essential step in designing educational programs for health personnel is to develop a close understanding of their roles . . . an understanding in operational terms of the actual situation in which they will have to work, the kinds of problems they will have to solve, the kinds of tasks they will have to perform."

Perhaps what I am suggesting should lead to a competence-based approach to curriculum development in gerontology and geriatrics. McGaghie, Miller, Sajid, Telder, and Lipson (Note 1) say of competence-based medical education: "Competency-based curriculum in any setting assumes that the many roles and functions involved in the doctor's work can be defined and clearly expressed. It does not imply that the things defined are the only elements of competence but rather that those which can be defined represent the critical point of departure in curriculum development."

Looking to the future when gerontological and geriatric content will undoubtedly be included in national boards and licensing and certification examinations, I cannot suggest with confidence which domains must be included in such tests. It is widely recognized that professional schools "teach to the boards," but I do not know that the content taught to pass such examinations is what the health professional must be able to do to perform competently.

The validation of domains of expertise would inspire such confidence, however. These domains of expertise are areas of professional performance that systematic research of the practice has identified as critical to competent practice.

Content validity has largely been an issue in the construction of tests (Risley, LaDuca, and Madigan, Note 2). The test designer has been asked to demonstrate that what is actually being tested is, in fact, what is claimed is being tested.

We determine what to test in the first place by deciding what to teach. There is—or there should be—a direct relationship between our educational goals and our determination that we have reached those goals. Thus, content validity in test design depends on content validity in curricular design. Content validity in curricular design means that we are teaching what we claim we are teaching—or, more significant for health professions education, that we are producing the kind of individual we claim we are producing: a competent geriatric practitioner.

There are many ways for the content validity issue to enter the curricular arena. The first and broadest might be expressions of concern about gerontology in general curricula. If education is truly preparation for life, all school curricula should contain required courses in the entire continuum of human development, including the study of aging.

At the level of health professions education, if systematic research demonstrated that all health professionals cared for older adults, then all curricula that claimed to prepare health professionals should include mandatory studies in gerontology and geriatrics. Only then could such curricula claim to be content valid.

Clearly, all educators who have recognized the absence of gerontology and are working to include it in professional curricula have expressed concern about content validity, although they may not have identified it as such. Indeed, validity helps answer some of the questions a curriculum developer must ask. These questions are:

Should gerontology be taught? Gerontologists are bombarded ad nauseam with population and health care statistics. It is enough to say that because of data to support the validity of its inclusion in health professions curricula, there is justification for teaching it.

Whom should we teach? Systematic study would identify those health professionals that care for older adults. Some methodologies would also demonstrate the relative proportion of practice time spent in such care. Once such documentation has been made, any health professions curriculum so identified that continues to omit a required foundation in gerontology and geriatrics would not be content valid.

When to teach? Results of health-professions education research indicate that attitudes are formed early in professional socialization. These data suggest that a content-valid gerontology program espousing goals of positive attitude formation would begin on day one of professional school and continue to build throughout the total educational program.

What should be taught? We do not know for certain, but we could find out. We could expect to discover an identifiable core of essential content similar across professions and bodies of content unique to particular professions. We also must recognize that we must first identify and then specify not only what a student should know and value but also what a student should be able to do with and for older adults. Consequently, in the absence of documentation, a curriculum designed only on the basis of the opinion of a content expert would not be valid. Nor would it be valid if it concerns itself only with what the student should know or value upon its completion. Finally, if biological and physiological research reveals that many health care needs of older adults are a result of normal developmental decrements over time, a curriculum in which content draws only from a pathological, disease-oriented model would not be valid.

How to teach? Systematic analysis would probably demonstrate that many health professionals are involved in caring for older adults and that many of them are attempting, with varying degrees of success, to work together. It would follow that students who are expected to work together should be educated together. Therefore, programs that educate students totally in isolation from other professionals instead of incorporating some interdisciplinary learning experiences would not be content-valid programs. Additionally, no professional program can realistically expect its students to learn everything they need to know in the allotted time. Consequently, we would hope to train students to approach their lifelong learning needs in an independent, self-paced manner with emphasis on problem solving rather than information retrieval skills. Thus, a lockstep curriculum that does not facilitate self-directed learning or include the deliberate development of problem-solving skills would not be valid.

Where should we teach? We should be teaching clinical geriatric care in those settings where older adults seek out and receive such care; that is, in doctors' offices, ambulatory-care centers, acute-care hospitals, long-term care facilities, and the homes of older adults. If systematic analysis demonstrates that the majority of older adults receive health care in the community, then a program that limits itself to teaching health professions students in an acute-care hospital would not be a valid program. Nor would a program be valid if it adds a unit in geriatric study with clinical experience exclusively in a nursing home.

The literature on content validity in curriculum design is very limited. A computer search revealed only one appropriate citation from vocational education (Jacobs, Note 3), a significant finding.

In Peddiwell's *Saber-Tooth Curriculum* (1939), New-Fist, the educator, probably does the pioneering research on content validity. He looks around and observes the skills needed for survival: fish-grabbing-with-the-bare-hands, woolly-horse-clubbing, and saber-tooth-tiger-scaring-with-fire. New-Fist then proceeds to design and implement his curriculum; that is, to teach fish-grabbing, woolly-horse-clubbing, and saber-tooth-tiger-scaring. The rest of the story deals with the difficulties of revising the curriculum once it was recognized as no longer valid; in other words, formative evaluation. For educators who have already designed and are implementing programs in gerontology, research may reveal either that they are correct in their choices or that they are teaching an equivalent to woolly-horse-clubbing, which is inappropriate for survival in the real world of practice. Most educators, however, are probably at the stage of development where they must follow New-Fist's example and observe systematically what it is they must teach before designing the curriculum.

Hilda Taba (1962) mentions content validity in her now-famous book, *Curriculum Development*. She says:

Selecting the content, with accompanying learning experiences, is one of the two central decisions in curriculum making, and therefore a rational method of going about it is of great concern (p. 263). . . . There has always been more to learn than any student could learn in the time at his disposal. . . . Criteria are needed for assurance that temporary needs and feelings of urgency will not overwhelm other basic functions of education, that omissions will be considered as carefully as additions (p. 265). . . . Criteria can be applied realistically only to the extent that diagnosis reveals the particulars of a given situation (p. 267).

Finally, what will undoubtedly be the pioneering statement on content validity in health professions education comes from Risley et al. (Note 2) in a paper titled "Assessment-Focused Approach to Curriculum Revision." The statement says in part:

Validity of curriculum receives little attention. . . . The impact of behaviorism on curriculum can be seen in performance-based teacher education, the behavioral objectives movement, the widespread use of task analyses, systems approaches to curriculum design, and so on. All share one feature in common: the validity of curricula derived from them relies exclusively on an association with some universe of skills and knowledge deemed to be pertinent, usually by expert consensus. In measurement this relates to content validity. The test blueprint, typically a subject matter-cognitive process matrix, is a procedural demonstration of content relatedness. Matching instruction to, say objectives, produces a similar relatedness, or "curricular content validity". . . . Curriculum development or revision rarely adheres to procedures for content validation. Yet it would appear that the definition of "content universe" with explicit boundaries and an associated methodology for sampling that content is as necessary for curriculum as for measurement (p. 7). . . . If we conceive of curricula as producing trained, certifiable individuals (say, "teacher," or "occupational therapist"), then such professionals can be likened to theoretical networks in which are embedded an array of skill, knowledge, and attitude constructs, frequently aggregated as competence. For validity claims to be supported, the validity of these constructs and the network must be demonstrated (p. 8).

To summarize, curriculum validity appears to be: (1) the congruence of the curriculum with the *documented* needs of the real world; (2) the similarity between the graduate we claim to produce and the one we actually produce; and (3) the correspondence between our programs and the construct we are attempting to operationalize.

The idea of doing research to validate curriculum is not new. Bobbitt first suggested it in 1912 and again, as a member of the Committee on the Economy of Time, in 1915. He said: "Find out what people who are living and working successfully need to be able to do and just what information and skills they need." Although the committee relied heavily on consensus, Bobbitt himself used both survey methods and activity analysis (Tanner, 1975).

Methods used to identify valid curricular domains include: task analysis, practitioner surveys, observation studies, critical incidents, expert consensus (e.g., the Delphi method), chart audit, and the Professional Performance Situation Model (PPSM). All of these research methodologies have been and are being used to identify or validate content domains in health professions education. The purpose of this paper was not to discuss each of them in detail, but rather to suggest procedures which might be considered for research studies.

Gerontology is a very exciting field to be in at this time. Those of us beginning work now are reaping the rewards of the many years of hard work by those who have preceded us and led the way. Admittedly, curriculum implementation cannot wait for answers to all of the questions this paper raises. However, once we have acknowledged the need for research studies, we are in a position to incorporate them into plans for formative evaluation as well as into long-range plans for sophisticated research designs. The results of such studies could have profound impact. They could move curriculum development in gerontology and geriatrics from axiology alone to axiology and epistemology—from valuing alone to valuing and knowing. In so doing, they would contribute significantly to growth in gerontology in higher education.

Notes

1. McGaghie, W. C., Miller, G. E., Sajid, A., Telder, T. V., & Lipson, L. *Competency-based curriculum development in medical education: An introduction.* Geneva: World Health Organization, 1978. (Public Health Paper No. 68).

2. Risley, M. E., LaDuca, A., & Madigan, M. J. *Assessment-focused approach to curriculum revision.* Paper presented at the Annual Meeting of the American Educational Research Association, San Francisco, April 1976.

3. Jacobs, A. A. The content validation and resource development for a course in materials and processes of industry through the use of MASA experts at Norfolk State College. *Research in Education*, September 1976. (Final Report) (ERIC Document Reproduction Service No. 122053)

References

Bryant, J. *Health and the developing world.* New York: Cornell University Press, 1969.

Hughes, P. Decisions and curriculum design. *Educational Theory*, July 1962, *12*, 187–192.

Kliebard, H. M. Curriculum theory: Give me a "for instance." *Curriculum Inquiry*, 1977, *6*, 257–281.

Marler, C. D. *Philosophy and schooling.* Boston: Allyn & Bacon, 1975.

Peddiwell, J. A. *The saber-tooth curriculum.* New York: McGraw-Hill, 1939.

Taba, H. *Curriculum development: Theory and practice.* New York: Harcourt Brace & World, 1962.

Tanner, D., & Tanner, L. N. *Curriculum development—Theory into practice.* New York: Macmillan, 1975.

Suggested Bibliography

Andrew, B. J. Validation by task analysis. *Conference on extending the validity of certification.* Chicago: American Board of Medical Specialties. March 1976.

Broski, D., Alexander, D., Brunner, M., Chidley, M., Finney, W., Johnson, C., Karas, B., and Rothenber, S. Competency-based curriculum development: A pragmatic approach. *Journal of Allied Health*, Winter 1977, *6*, 38–44.

LaDuca, A., Engel, J. D., and Risley, M. E. Progress toward development of a general model of competence definition in health professions. *Journal of Allied Health*, Spring 1978, *7*, 149–156.

LaDuca, A., Madigan, M. J., Risley, M. E., & Grobman, H. *Application of a model for definition and assessment of competence in health professions.* Paper presented at the 14th Annual Conference on Research in Medical Education, Washington, D.C., November 1975.

McClelland, D. C. Testing for competence rather than for intelligence. *American Psychologist*, 1973, *28*, 1–14.

Mehlinger, H. D. Four perspectives on curriculum development. In J. Schaffarzick & D. H. Hampson (Eds.), *Strategies for curriculum development.* Berkeley, Calif.: McCutchan, 1975.

Menges, R. W. Assessing readiness for professional practice. *Review of Educational Research*, Spring 1975, *45*, 173–207.

Page, E. B., Jarjoura, D., & Konopka, C. D. Curriculum design through operations research. *American Educational Research Journal*, Winter 1976, *13*, 31–49.

Peterson, C. J. *Development of competencies in associate degree nursing: A new perspective.* New York: National League for Nursing, 1978. (Pub. No. 23–1707)

Stamper, J. H. Curriculum development: Assessing education needs. *Journal of Allied Health*, Winter 1978, *7*, 42–48.

The Application of Nontraditional Education Techniques to Gerontology Instruction

Betsy M. Sprouse
University of Wisconsin-Madison

In higher education, and particularly in gerontology, there is a growing need to expand the scope of educational programs to reach all interested people. One way to accomplish this expansion is by using what have been termed nontraditional education techniques in teaching both traditional and nontraditional students. The terms *traditional* and *nontraditional* have been used in many ways to describe students of various ages and learning styles. In general, traditional students are those who attend college full time immediately after high school, or those between the ages of 18 and 25. The nontraditional student is over the age of 25, has returned to college or started college after a hiatus, is studying full or part time, and may also be working full or part time.

One group with special educational needs in gerontology includes professionals or paraprofessionals in the field who want to enhance their skills with additional information about aging. Typically, these are not full-time students at higher education institutions, yet institutions can and should reach out to meet their learning needs. Colleges and universities can provide these outreach programs with minimal effort and resources and still meet the educational needs of their on-campus students.

Many nontraditional educational techniques have been in existence for some time; they are now receiving increased attention as the trend toward individualized education grows (Baskin, 1974; Commission on Non-Traditional Study, 1973; Cross, Valley, and Associates, 1975; Gould and Cross, 1972; Milton, 1972). Educators are now formally acknowledging that learning takes place in different ways for different people, and what people learn is more important than where or how they learn it. Although many institutional constraints still exist, colleges are gradually going to incorporate new forms of teaching and learning and new ways of certifying that learning. Nontraditional education is one way in which higher education institutions can simultaneously serve both campus-based students and the growing body of continuing learners and can perform a public service as well—that is, providing education about aging.

Nontraditional Techniques in Gerontology

Correspondence Instruction If a college has a correspondence study unit, it is not difficult to adapt campus-based courses on aging for correspondence instruction. Information is available in many places to assist educators with this process (see Baskin, 1974; Cross et al., 1975; Dressel and Thompson, 1973). In 1976, 51 colleges and universities in the United States and Canada were offering 99 correspondence courses in gerontology or closely related areas (Lumsden, Sprouse, and Hartley, 1976, Note 1).

Many campuses with correspondence study units allow undergraduates to apply course credits earned through correspondence to degree programs. Even at colleges without correspondence study units, it is possible to use correspondence materials with campus-based students who are interested in individual independent study with faculty members.

Self-Instructional Materials These materials (usually in the form of manuals such as Rich and Gilmore, 1972) can be used by both on- and off-campus students, as well as on the job by professionals. Generally they are more flexible than standard textbooks, for they incorporate self-pacing and immediate feedback on responses given by the learner. Another advantage is that self-instructional materials do not require any administration or supervision by an institution.

Television Courses Courses on television have been of three types: those broadcast over commercial or public television; closed-circuit videotapes or live programs; and closed-circuit live talkback programs. The first type is available to the general public; the other two are generally offered on cable television systems and in the classroom to on- and off-campus students. All of these vehicles have utility for educational programming in gerontology, although the practitioner has the easiest access to commercial, public, and cable television programs. However, educational institutions can increase the utility of classroom television programs by widely publicizing the range of programs available and by easing entry to these programs.

Cable television has other potentials for gerontology education. In some communities, cable television stations allow viewers and citizens to produce their own videotapes, using equipment borrowed from the station, which the cable stations then broadcast. Obviously this method can increase the range of programming in gerontology education for professionals and for the general public (see Voegel, 1975).

Radio Courses Although radio programs are also usually available to the general public, programming for special audiences can be done through universities or their extension divisions. Semester-length courses are usually not offered on the radio because of the time involved, but "minicourses" on aging can be adapted to this medium.

Cassette or Audiotape Courses Courses offered through audiotapes are becoming increasingly popular because of their convenience and portability. Students can use them anywhere they have access to a tape recorder and any time they wish. Audio tapes in combination with printed, illustrated materials can be particularly effective.

Videotape Courses Courses on videotape are being used in classrooms and on television. Videotapes, like audiotapes, have great flexibility, but their use is somewhat restricted by the equipment needed to run them. College and public libraries and public schools can play an important role in making videotape equipment more accessible to students and practitioners.

Courses by Telephone Extension programs at many colleges are using the telephone to connect learners (individually or in groups) with campus-based faculty. Because of the time it takes, the telephone is generally used to supplement independent or correspondence study courses or to present material and incorporate discussion around minicourses.

Independent Study Independent study activities are numerous and diverse, and range from the very formal (independent study degree programs) to the very informal, such as teaching yourself woodcarving (Berte, 1975; Dressel and Thompson, 1973; Houle, 1974). Most of us engage in independent study in one form or another (Tough, 1971). The issue of concern, however, is how to award credit for, or otherwise acknowledge, the independent study people have done in a certain field. Within an educational institution, independent studies in gerontology can be conducted under the supervision of a faculty member and can incorporate any number of traditional or nontraditional methods.

Computer-Assisted Instruction Using computers to assist in the teaching of courses limits somewhat the way in which material is presented. But, as with self-instructional materials, this technique has the advantages of time flexibility and immediate feedback on answers. However, the disadvantages of limited equipment and cost of computer time may outweigh the advantages for off-campus students.

Time-Shortened Courses Semester-length courses can be offered in many ways that make them more accessible to full-time professionals. A three-credit course generally requires 40 hours or more of class time; but the hours can be compressed into evenings, weekends, weeklong blocks of time in the summer, or into any variation thereof. Typically, "commuter colleges" for part-time students offer courses only in these "nontraditional" hours.

Proficiency Examinations Proficiency examinations come in several forms, but the best known are College Level Examination Program (CLEP) and College Proficiency Examination Programs (CPEP). In the main, these examinations cover the traditional liberal arts areas (Meyer, 1975). Credit earned by taking this type of exam can be used in degree programs by both on- and off-campus students.

Although proficiency examinations are very formal and standardized, they can be applied to the study of aging. The Regents External Degree Program—a series of degree programs administered by the state of New York, based on the completion of proficiency examinations—is exploring the possibility of developing college proficiency examinations in gerontology.

Credit for Life Experience People interested in gerontology may have had many types of life experience related to aging, such as caring for an aged relative, recording oral histories, or writing fictional accounts of aging. These experiences could be academically accredited, but there are problems in validating and evaluating them (Keeton, 1976: Meyer, 1975). A project called the Cooperative Assessment of Experiential Learning, a cooperative effort of the Educational Testing Service and colleges and universities concerned with the process, validation, and utilization of information on assessing experiential learning for credit, is working to eliminate many of these problems.

Credit for Work Experience Matriculated students may receive credit for internships or field experiences without difficulty, but it is harder for professionals to be awarded credit for the types of experiences they have had on the job. Again, the problems lie in documenting and assessing activities unsupervised by the educational institution. However, gerontological work experience can greatly enhance an individual's sensitivity to and knowledge of the aging process. Credit for this experience, or exemption from other courses, should be incorporated into degree programs.

Learning Contracts Learning contracts have great usefulness for both on-campus and off-campus students. The student can take full responsibility for determining what is to be learned, how it will be learned, when it will be learned, and how it will be evaluated. The contract is made with a faculty member who serves as a learning resource. The learning contract is a more structured form of independent study (Berte, 1975).

External Degrees External degree programs are valuable opportunities for people who want to pursue a college degree while working full-time or meeting full-time family responsibilities. Generally, these programs do not require campus residency, except perhaps for a limited term. The curriculum is adapted to the life and learning styles of adults with enough flexibility that students can complete the degree program in approximately the customary length of time. The study of gerontology can be incorporated into an external degree program as a major, a minor, or a series of elective courses (see Sprouse, Note 2).

Continuing Education Units (CEUs) Many short-term training and continuing education programs in gerontology are being offered for CEUs. These programs may or may not include an evaluative component, but the principal value of awarding CEUs lies in documenting attendance, experience, and, it is hoped, knowledge. Also some multidisciplinary gerontology programs, such as those at the University of Alabama, San Francisco State University, and soon the University of Wisconsin-Madison, are offering courses or certificate programs in aging, which can be taken either for credit or for CEUs.

Community-Based Educational Centers "Learning Centers" can be created by educational institutions or cosponsored with other organizations, such as public libraries, to provide off-campus students with centralized collections of resources in gerontology. Frequently, these learning centers incorporate many of the nontraditional approaches described above, such as videotape courses and computer-assisted instruction.

Conclusion

The aim of this discussion has been to expand the concept of gerontological teaching and learning methodologies. Many of these approaches have been around for a long time, and with the increasing number of part-time students and independent learners, educators and educational institutions can better meet the learners' needs by using nontraditional methods more. These approaches do require time to adapt the traditional curricula; they also require the commitment of human, fiscal, and material resources. But with the growing need of practitioners for information about aging and the decrease in the number of full-time, traditional-aged students enrolling in college, higher education is being forced to acknowledge and adapt to the learning needs and patterns of nontraditional learners. The opportunity now exists to make this adaptation a creative and rewarding learning experience for both educators and their students.

Notes

1. Lumsden, D. B., Sprouse, B. M., & Hartley, D. W. *Catalog of U.S. and Canadian correspondence instruction on aging*, 1976. (Available from

B. M. Sprouse, Institute on Aging, University of Wisconsin, 425 Henry Mall, Madison, Wisconsin 53706.)

    2. Sprouse, B. M. *Project report on external degrees in gerontology.* Albany, N. Y.: New York State Office for the Aging, 1975. (Available from the author, Institute on Aging, University of Wisconsin, 425 Henry Mall, Madison, Wisconsin 53706.)

References

Baskin, S. *Organizing nontraditional study.* San Francisco: Jossey-Bass Source Book Series, 1974, *4.*

Berte, N. R. *Individualizing education by learning contracts.* San Francisco: Jossey-Bass Source Book Series, 1975, *10.*

Commission on Nontraditional Study. *Diversity by design.* San Francisco: Jossey-Bass, 1973.

Cross, K. P., Valley, J. R., & Associates. *Planning nontraditional programs.* San Francisco: Jossey-Bass, 1975.

Dressel, P. L., & Thompson, M. M. *Independent study.* San Francisco: Jossey-Bass, 1973.

Gould, S. B., & Cross, K. P. (Eds.) *Explorations in nontraditional study.* San Francisco: Jossey-Bass, 1972.

Houle, C. O. *The external degree.* San Francisco: Jossey-Bass, 1974.

Keeton, M. T. *Experiential learning.* San Francisco: Jossey-Bass, 1976.

Lumsden, D. B., Sprouse, B. M., & Hartley, D. W. Correspondence instruction for the professional development of practitioners in the field of aging. *Educational Gerontology,* 1977, *2,* 5–13.

Meyer, P. *Awarding college credit for noncollege learning.* San Francisco: Jossey-Bass, 1975.

Milton, O. *Alternatives to the traditional.* San Francisco: Jossey-Bass, 1972.

Rich, T. A., & Gilmore, A. S. *Basic concepts of aging: A programmed manual.* Washington, D.C.: Administration on Aging, 1972.

Sprouse, B. M., (Ed.). *National directory of educational programs in gerontology.* Washington, D.C.: U.S. Department of Health, Education and Welfare, Administration on Aging, 1976.

Tough, A. *The adult's learning projects.* Ontario: The Ontario Institute for Studies in Education, 1971.

Voegel, H. *Using instructional technology.* San Francisco: Jossey-Bass Source Book Series, 1975, *9.*

Teaching an Aging Policy Course through Issue Confrontation

Thomas D. Watts
The University of Texas at Arlington

Teaching an aging policy course through the use of issue confrontation means giving students an opportunity to investigate, analyze, and argue various issues in aging policy. This approach involves thoroughly scrutinizing one or more points of view on a policy issue and presenting them in an analytical, scholarly way to convince an audience of their merits.

It is not a debating exercise; rather, it is an issue-oriented, issue-explicating activity. For example, one student might argue the case for mandatory retirement policy, and another student against such a policy. Often the same student will argue both sides of the case—a particularly valuable analytical and educational experience. Some students choose to argue a point of view they do not personally entertain—a fact they may wish to make known to the class.

The philosophical assumptions of this kind of educational approach rest on an inquiry method of instruction, the importance of philosophical and ideological concerns in aging policy, and social policy on aging and social policy in general conceived of as the outcome of confrontation of various points of view. The educational goal of this kind of educational exercise is to develop analytical thinking, critical capabilities, and an ability to appropriate and defend value positions and judgments—in short, the ability to defend a stated position or point of view.

What follows are an explication of the above philosophical assumptions and educational goals and a general discussion of the use of this approach in an aging policy class.

Classes that spend a major portion of their time presenting, classifying, and supporting opinions, hypotheses, and points of view on issues are characterized as inquiry classes (Massialas, Sprague, & Hurst, 1975). The earmarks of the inquiry class include an open climate of discussion, the consistent use of ideas as the center of thought and action, and the application of facts to support hypotheses. This setting differs from a traditional classroom, where discussion may not be greatly encouraged and where facts and conclusions are conveyed rather than investigated. Discovery is a key element in the inquiry approach to learning. Students who actively participate in the learning process, who discover on their own previously unperceived links among data, values, and ideologies, find ways to steadily improve their intellectual development.

The inquiry approach is anchored firmly in the notion of a democratic society. For a democratic society to function well, its citizens must be accustomed to independent, informed, and critical thinking. This was a central tenet in the educational philosophy of John Dewey (1916), and it continues to be of seminal concern today (Brock, Chesebro, Cragan, and Klumpp, 1973).

The inquiry approach emphasizes the importance of philosophical and ideological concerns in aging policy. Students are asked to direct their attention to the overriding philosophical and ideological questions about issues in aging policy. For example, inadequate income for the elderly is tied to the nature of income distribution in a capitalist society. The divisions of social classes in a capitalist society did not come about by accident. Hence, the ideological thinking of Karl Marx, Herbert Marcuse, Michael Harrington, and others becomes crucial to our thinking in this area. Indeed, one cannot properly address the major issues in aging policy without a direct and searching examination of ideology and, indeed, of social philosophy.

After many points of view on issues are heard, social policies are slowly "hammered out" over time. These points of view are expressed in newspaper editorials, letters to the editor, mass media in general, hearings of Congressional subcommittees, agency staff meetings, and many other areas. The extended debate on the merits and drawbacks of the Social Security System is an example of just such a continuing issue confrontation and national debate.

All of this is not to say that social policy formulation is only the outcome of the meeting of ideas. Social policy decisions are not made in the same fashion as judicial hearings. There are many other elements at work that have a strong influence on how the "debate" comes out: power, ideology, influence, special interest groups, values, and so forth. Still, the meeting of ideas or the confrontation of various perspectives and points of view on policy issues remains at the core of policy formation. How the debate or issue confrontation comes out strongly influences the policy that is formed. The inquiry method attempts to duplicate some aspects of issue confrontation.

The first of several goals in this kind of educational approach is the development of analytical thinking skills (Zeigelmueller and Dause, 1975). Legal education has had a long history of fine performance in this area, a performance level that may not have been shared by many of the human service professions or the emerging discipline area of gerontology. The ability to analyze current social issues in gerontology is directly related to the analytical capabilities of the students. Two ways to teach students to be more analytical are to help them acquire the fundamentals of analytical thinking and to engage them in analytical exercises of their own choosing.

The fundamentals of analytical thinking entail thorough understanding of the principles, of the differences between hypotheses and facts, of the role and necessity of comprehensive data collection, and of the inferences that can or cannot be drawn therefrom. Owing to the varied educational backgrounds that students bring to gerontology, one should probably not make too many assumptions about their knowledge of analytical thinking.

When undertaking analytical exercises, students choose policy issues in aging that they would like to investigate and analyze thoroughly. By using some aging policy issue as a testing ground, students can experience the satisfaction of engaging in a thorough analysis.

The second goal, the development of critical capabilities in the student, is related to the first. A student can learn scholarly criticism only by engaging in that process. Dewey's notion of learning by doing is a key concept here. Too often our educational system does not provide an avenue for experimenting with the student's critical faculties (Becker, 1967). Even so-called class reports, which are employed frequently in many courses, are not fashioned as truly critical exercises. Skepticism and criticism, cast not in a negative light but in a reflective, thoughtful, and positive light, are encouraged and fostered through the issue confrontation approach. Students are encouraged to criticize their own findings, their own position, even from the standpoint of the interest groups or citizens most adversely affected by the adoption of the policy stance they have taken.

The third goal is the ability to take and defend a stated position or point of view. Often educational practices can foster a situation where a student has never been called upon to defend a point of view and defend it well. Students in gerontology need to have the experience of staking out a position and arguing the case on behalf of that position.

Such an experience provides a good background for the future demands of a professional career. In most areas of gerontological administration and practice, and in most other areas of human services as well, professionals are called upon to voice and support points of view on particular policy changes. An example might be a professional on the staff of a senior citizens center who proposes in a staff meeting a new project designed to reach a previously unserved segment of the elderly population in that area. A persuasive argument with good supporting data will add to the likelihood of the project's adoption.

I have employed the issue confrontation approach successfully in classes on aging policy and have found it to be a fresh, interesting, and scholarly approach to the subject matter. Students as a whole seem to be more interested in an issue or problem focus. The traditional class report project often tends to be dull (except for the presenter, perhaps). With an issue confrontation approach, students are more engaged in the learning process, and certainly engagement can reap the considerable educational reward of increasing knowledge of aging and aging policies.

References

Becker, E. *Beyond alienation*. New York: Braziller, 1967.

Brock, B. L., Chesebro, J. W., Cragan, J. F., & Klumpp, J. F. *Public policy decision making: Systems analysis and comparative advantages debate.* New York: Harper & Row, 1973.

Dewey, J. *Democracy and education*. New York: Macmillan, 1916.

Massialas, B., Sprague, N., & Hurst, J. *Social issues through inquiry: Coping in an age of crisis*. Englewood Cliffs, N.J.: Prentice-Hall, 1975.

Ziegelmueller, G. W., & Dause, C. A. *Argumentation: Inquiry and advocacy.* Englewood Cliffs, N.J.: Prentice-Hall, 1975.

PART EIGHT
COMMUNITY-INSTITUTIONAL PARTNERSHIPS: BRIDGE OVER TROUBLED WATERS

A cooperative relationship between higher education and the community is essential to what we might call "effective gerontology." The two spheres are really one, and the tendency to separate them is inappropriate. The institution and the community must be able to recognize their mutual concerns and to work together to address effectively the problems and concerns of older Americans.

The first two papers of this section describe the progress of state offices on aging and a regional consortium of state units on aging in establishing joint efforts in governmental-educational gerontology. The third paper provides a higher education perspective on the aging network. This section concludes with an example of a cooperative community–higher education project.

Developing Aging Training Programs: Relationships between Higher Education and the Aging Network

Diane S. Piktialis
Massachusetts Department of Elder Affairs

The primary challenge for state units on aging has been to create interorganizational relationships and delivery structures to provide an integrated approach to training for the aging network. This paper analyzes the organizational aspects of establishing aging training networks under the state Title IV-A program in Massachusetts. Title IV-A of the Older Americans Act mandates, through institutions of higher education where possible, the development of short- and long-term training for those who provide social services to the elderly.

The initiative of the Administration on Aging (AoA) to support aging training has been based on one fundamental assumption: the existence of a cooperative partnership, or at least a working relationship, between government agencies and institutions of higher education. After four years of funding under Title IV-A, it is imperative to critically examine this assumption of aging–post secondary education linkages and to lay out both the barriers to and the paths for creative and cooperative training partnerships between the two sectors. The ultimate goal of these efforts is, of course, to train personnel to better serve the nation's elderly.

This paper is limited to discussing aging and higher education relationships from the perspective of a state unit on aging. Thus, the primary focus will be on that portion of Title IV-A funds allocated directly to the states.

Barriers to Cooperation and Coordination

Many constraints affect program planning and implementation at the state and area levels of training delivery. Two classes of variables affect these efforts: variables external to the network, and organizational constraints specific to the aging and higher education systems. The first area involves the history and mandates of the Administration on Aging and the wider organizational context of Title IV-A activities; the other entails organizational characteristics of the aging and of higher education institutions and the political milieu in which training is delivered.

External Barriers

The Vertical System   Historically, the Older Americans Act has defined mandates and provided funds for various programs. Much of the difficulty in developing and coordinating long- and short-term training through discretionary funds can be traced to AoA requirements for implementation, especially with respect to the portion of Title IV-A funds directly allocated to state units on aging. AoA's goal has been to use these funds to "gerontologize" higher education and at the same time to establish cooperative and productive relationships between aging networks and higher education networks for delivery of training.

Two major problems arise from these dual purposes. First, the two mandates often conflict. How can higher education be "gerontologizing" and "capacity building" while it is producing higher-quality education, research, and training? Second, how can the network be patient during early years of rapid growth and program development when inservice training and staff development are such pressing concerns? Although these issues seem somewhat theoretical, their constraining effect on aging training and education becomes clear when seen in the context of problems of organizational development and institutional change.

Organizational Development   AoA defined the mandates of the Title IV-A, Title IV-B, and Title IV-C programs but did not define the specific roles of either the aging network agencies or higher education in those efforts. Though the legislation mentioned general goals, it outlined no model of organization. More important, an established organizational base, a "network" so to speak, did not exist in most cases.

The term *aging network* has most often been more rhetoric than reference to reality. Only after many years and many millions of dollars are various local agencies, programs, and services funded under separate titles of the Older Americans Act achieving a semblance of cooperative efforts to serve older persons. Effective and efficient coordination of service delivery still seems to lie in the future. In most cases, higher education has even less of a "network."

In short, AoA has often operated from a model of rational planning that has little to do with the real world. As can be seen with many Title IV efforts, the relation between federal guidelines and the ability of agencies to implement these models is often dubious. To ignore these larger questions of organizational development and to consider only technical and program issues in training, research, and education will, even with the best intentions, bring only frustration and aborted projects.

Federal Guidelines and Funding Cycles

Other cooperation problems arise from specific AoA funding cycles, funding patterns, and guidelines for applications. These specific factors are: state versus higher education allocation, development of guidelines, national versus local impact, AoA funding cycle versus academic calendars, and limitations of project periods.

State Allocations As both long- and short-term training have become pressing concerns, the allocation of sufficient funds to training and continuing education for individuals providing services to older persons has become increasingly important. The greatest issue here is the percentage of funds allocated directly to postsecondary educational institutions under Titles IV-A, IV-B, and IV-C, and the Title IV-A awards to the states. Though this section focuses on the Title IV-A awards, it discusses the current overall pattern in terms of its implication for cooperation between the aging network and higher education in other Title IV-A programs as well.

Although AoA has strongly encouraged cooperation and coordination between state units on aging and institutions of higher education, funding patterns for various programs and services funded under the Older Americans Act have outstripped awards to the states under Title IV-A. As Miller and colleagues (this volume) note, the total allocation of all Older Americans Act programs rose from $217.8 million in 1974 to $508.75 million in 1978, an increase of 133 percent. In focusing only on the total discretionary fund allocations under titles IV-A, IV-B, and IV-C, one finds an increase from $16.5 million to $28.3 million, a rise of 72 percent. Finally, when considering only Title IV-A during the same period, one finds an overall rise of 78 percent, an increase from $9.5 million to $17 million. However, the figures obscure the lack of significant growth in Title IV-A allocations to state units on aging, which rose from $4 million to $6 million, an increase of only 50 percent, 28 percent less than the increase in all categories of Title IV-A funds (Note 1).

Increased Title IV-A awards to the states that have not kept pace either with the growing demand for inservice training and continuing education in the network or with growth in other AoA-funded programs create a significant barrier to cooperation with higher education. The states and other components in the aging network feel shortchanged when their Title IV-A awards are compared with those of postsecondary educational institutions. This is especially true when a large university literally a few blocks away may have a Title IV-A or Title IV-B award that exceeds a state's entire allocation for the year.

This constraint to working relationships is exacerbated by divergent program goals. Whereas a state must respond to seemingly unlimited numbers of demands for short-term training, a career training program or the educational activities at a university may have a long-term, generalized focus or may be geared to undergraduate and other preservice education and training. Although AoA's funding priorities may justify this in terms of "national significance" or long-term impact on personnel development for the aging network, both state and area agencies are hard pressed to view these institutions as "cooperators" in training. Even coordination of actual training activities is difficult, since grants for career training (Title IV-A) research (Title IV-B), and multidisciplinary centers (Title IV-C) to higher education institutions and others usually lack in the ability to meet the specific local needs of the aging network.

Development of Funding Guidelines A point of contention between states and higher education is the lack of state input into guidelines developed for discretionary grants to postsecondary education. Though state units may not always have significant training or research capability in their agencies, they do have a wealth of direct experience with programs and personnel serving the nation's older population. Yet these agencies are traditionally bypassed when funding priorities are determined for programs of "long-range" impact on the network. Insufficient input into guidelines often exacerbates already envious feelings toward educational institutions receiving large amounts of money. This often devastates good relationships with local institutions of higher education, especially when, to many in the aging network, the left hand doesn't seem to know what the right hand is doing.

Funding Cycles and Project Periods Another difficulty comes from state Title IV-A grant awards that are not geared to an academic calendar year. Even where a state may work closely with higher education in planning for meeting short-term training needs, Notification of Grant Award (NGA) for funds arrives at the state unit on aging no earlier than October 15. Since contracts often cannot be processed for at least another month, training must be deferred, often until late winter because of the weather. One of the best periods of training both for the network and higher education is lost. Working relationships often become strained, especially with those providing training for the first time.

Finally, the limit of state awards to one year with no mechanism for extension beyond the project period means that state units cannot really enter into long-term planning with higher education around inservice training needs of the network. Changes in AoA guidelines and priorities for use of funds may also interfere in continuity of these joint planning and delivery efforts.

Organizational Constraints

There are also many organizational barriers to developing interorganizational linkages between the aging network and postsecondary education institutions. This is a horizontal rather than a vertical system of organizational relationships.

Intermingling of Goals and Perspectives Historically, it has been difficult enough to coordinate program planning and implementation between institutions and agencies with common purposes. For example, the difficulties of area agencies on aging in coordinating services for older adults at the local level are proverbial. Cooperation and coordination are even more difficult where organizational goals and purposes diverge.

The main goal of postsecondary educational institutions has been to provide a full-time, undergraduate education to students of traditional college age (18 to 22). Although educational institutions are expressing a need to recruit new students to offset declining enrollments and a desire to relate more closely to the needs of the community, these goals have not been a high priority until recently. Whether higher education can assume a training role for the aging network by providing continuing and inservice education for practitioners remains to be seen (Peterson, 1976).

Of even more immediate concern are the communication problems arising from the different perspectives of these institutional spheres. Segmentation and specialization have been developing in education and service organizations (Etzioni, 1964; Prethus, 1965). One often hears practitioners accuse academic institutions of being "ivory towers" and "out of touch with reality." This view of education expressed in everyday clichés by people in the "real world" of business, industry, and government indicates a commonplace perception of organizational autonomy and a concomitant distrust of academe. Such a rigid separation of functions is an important obstacle in launching, directing, and coordinating broad-based programs in two ways. First, dissimilar goals and values create difficulties in communication and interaction. Second, the combination of divergent interests and seemingly similar goals generates conflict at the community level when practitioners and educators begin their joint plans and directions for training.

Bureaucratic Structures. Both postsecondary education institutions and social service agencies for elders are large bureaucratic organizations. Each has obstacles to developing interorganizational linkage in its internal structure. The turn-around time for completing a contract to an institution of higher education provides the simplest example. The contract must go through the internal channels of approval of both systems. In the interim, the individual parties involved can be frustrated and impatient with bureaucratic processes and with each other. The state training officer wants sorely needed and long-awaited training to be delivered. Training contractors or project directors want funds so they can get started before the momentum of planning is lost. Given these bureaucratic obstacles, it is not uncommon to hear individuals blame the red tape of other organizations for frustrating delays. Those of us who may be defensive about accusations of government bureaucracy have been surprised to find similar red tape, review, and signoff procedures as prevalent in higher education as in our own agencies.

Political Constraints

It would be naive in any analysis of the organizational aspects of planning and program development not to point out political constraints affecting implementation. Everyone who has been involved in program planning in any sector understands how easily internal politics can wreak havoc with the best-laid plans. Although political barriers are mentioned only in passing, their impact on cooperation between higher education and the aging network cannot be overlooked. More analysis of the politics of training, education, and research is sorely needed.

Even though these barriers are widespread, organizations and their environments do change. Certainly the growth of the aging network over the past decade is the best example of organizational development. But institutional change need not be fraught with conflict. Only when barriers to interorganizational cooperation and coordination are recognized and openly admitted can productive solutions to those problems be collectively developed. It is those mechanisms for facilitating cooperation between the aging network and postsecondary education that the next section will address.

Mechanisms for Cooperation

This section focuses on a two-year effort by the Massachusetts Department of Elder Affairs (DEA) to plan and develop a statewide training network to provide quality training to practitioners in gerontology. Through Title IV-A training monies and the planning and contracting process, the state agency involved substate planning and service areas (including local service providers) directly in the planning process with public and eventually private educational institutions. Steps were taken to establish and strengthen communication and interactive relationships between the various agencies working with the elderly and the educational institutions. Though the domains of educational institutions and aging agencies differ, they intersect at the specific area of gerontological education and human services training. The role of the state unit was to facilitate interorganizational relationships and delivery structures to provide an integrated approach to training.

Raising the Consciousness of Higher Education: The Beginning of Capacity Building In the early years, Massachusetts state agency policy was to use Title IV-A funds as seed money and as the first step to institutionalizing support for aging training and education. Most programs during the first period were intended to raise consciousness for and about aging rather than to actually provide skills training. The state training officer, on leave from a community college, had substantial knowledge of the state system of higher education. With that background, he began to develop a communications network between DEA and each college as well as between colleges themselves.

Through activist outreach, college presidents and academic deans were encouraged to incorporate gerontological curriculum within the regularly state-funded academic activities of the colleges rather than in continuing-education divisions. The development of ongoing relationships with these administrators was viewed as an important factor in creating a network for gerontological education among academic institutions. Constant communication was established between the state agency and project directors at the colleges. The overall effect was to establish administrative support for the programs and to begin to develop a mechanism of accountability from the grantees.

The leadership role played by the state unit on aging worked to alert institutions of their obligations to the changing populations. The result was to improve the program planning and proposal design in accordance with the educational needs of older people. It also stimulated ongoing commitments to this target population, indicating the value of explicitly conveying to the colleges what should be done regarding older people. The strategy of giving centralized direction to a statewide program proved successful in "gerontologizing" many institutions of higher education to make education for and about older adults an integral part of the educational process.

Building the Network In the early years, the state agency focused on the educational sector largely because federal and state program objectives called for building sensitivity to aging and capacities in gerontology in postsecondary institutions. Later efforts concentrated on aging service agencies and specifically on the problem of getting their planning input and participation in programs.

Because of this new focus and changes in federal regulations, the emphasis shifted from general education to training in the second year. Working through institutions of higher education, the state agency made its objective the delivery of advanced gerontological education and skill training to personnel working with elders.

A training focus required a rigorous and systematic way of assessing training needs and establishing priorities. Therefore, the state agency contracted for an assessment of Massachusetts' training needs and an identification of training properties by local program directors.

Conferences, institutes, and seminars previously limited to studies of aging processes and characteristics of the elderly or to consciousness raising were largely replaced with skill training, skill-related knowledge, and opportunities for practice. Trainers were encouraged to have their programs agency based and to support where possible the "learning by doing" and participatory techniques that have proven successful in adult training (Meyer, 1977). Early capacity building laid the groundwork and established educator-practitioner relationships that enabled program redirection.

At the same time, planning continued to address ways in which a network could be established to deliver training. The most important component of this strategy was to develop joint planning with aging agencies around training objectives at the state and substate level. The first step was formation of a state training committee to advise in the implementation of fiscal year 1977 Title IV-A training activities and to begin developing long-range training objectives. That committee was made up of delegates from all types of agencies in the aging network, and it met bimonthly during the year. It considered broad issues such as evaluation of current programs, identification of training gaps, and priorities for the next year's training plan.

The Department of Elder Affairs also attempted to develop a creative and productive partnership between educational institutions and network agencies at the local level. Extensive agency input was needed to establish the mutual trust necessary for developing relationships between those agencies and colleges. To cultivate trust, the state agency contracted for an independent evaluation of the Title IV-A training programs delivered by the various colleges and universities. Results of those evaluations were later made available to area agencies before the fall 1977 programs began in order to aid agency personnel in selecting appropriate training.

Representation at the substate level was built in through the Request for Proposals (RFP) process and through conditions established for all training grant awards. All proposals for Title IV-A funds were required to have a letter of support from the appropriate area agency or, in the case of an undesignated area, the local home-care corporation. Moreover, each Notification of Grant Award required formation of an advisory committee representing the appropriate area agency and other elder service agencies at the local level.

A new and major thrust of joint planning is to develop regional consortia of educational institutions and aging agencies. They will have two roles: training needs assessment by agencies, and resource identification and mobilization by the colleges. By developing these regional consortia into working groups, much of the needs assessment, planning, and recruitment can be accomplished at the local or regional level. The department intends to act as a facilitator to formalize these regional groups into working consortia and ultimately to move toward joint submission of proposals by educational institutions and aging agencies.

Conclusions

The institutional impact of the Title IV-A program was as important in developing a network as was the programmatic aspects of curriculum development and training content, though the two developed side by side. The institutional impact can be divided into four areas: (1) development of a contracting process for Title IV-A funds with clear, measurable objectives to assure accountability; (2) expansion of resources for the aging network through educational institutions; (3) attention to meeting generic skill needs and human service needs for the aging network; and (4) development of a growing organizational base for collaborative planning and training.

Though the Department of Elder Affairs is still far from able to meet all training needs through this developing network, much of its success to date can be traced to the strengths of centralized planning and administration. DEA's central role in managing training brought a statewide perspective to planning, needs assessment, and resource identification. Leadership provided by the state agency and the state training officer facilitated development of ongoing relationships with college presidents and academic deans. Outreach activities generated greater diversity in locations and programs, improved program planning and proposal design, and increased community awareness for and about elders and aging. In the final analysis, however, the success of this training program is due to collaborative efforts involving the participation of elder-service agencies and the educational community.

Service agency collaboration has also brought about the unintended result of opening channels of communication often severed through political conflict and competition for service dollars on the local level. Many trainers found that combining personnel from various types of aging agencies in training programs contributed to the cross-fertilization of ideas and to mutual respect.

Although this paper focused largely on successes, there were many localities where trust and collaboration did not occur and an effective training base did not develop. Clearly, much is to be learned in this area, and controlled attempts to train and evaluate are sorely needed.

Note

1. *Expenditure plan for use of (1) fiscal year 1977 training funds to support state and area level training activities and (2) fiscal year 1978 title III model projects funds to support state agency developmental activities for legal aide and nursing home ombudsman services.* Washington, D.C.: U.S. Department of Health, Education and Welfare, Administration on Aging, AoA-PI-77-13, March 5, 1977.

References

Ehrlich, I., & Ehrlich, P. A four-part framework to meet the responsibilities of higher education to gerontology. *Educational Gerontology*, 1976 *1*(3), 251–261.

Etzioni, A. *Modern organizations.* Englewood Cliffs, N.J.: Prentice-Hall, 1964.

Meyer, L. Andragogy and the adult learner. *Educational Gerontology*, 1977, *2*(2), 115–123.

Peterson, D. A. Educational gerontology: The state of the art. *Educational Gerontology*, 1976, *1*(1), 61–73.

Prethus, P. *The organization society.* New York: Vantage Books, 1965.

The Future of Older Americans: A Cooperative Approach

The Region V Training and Education Consortium:
Rick Miller, Jeanette Secret, Jack Loman, Wanda McKee, John Peterson, Sally Vaughan

As the training and education specialists with the six state units on aging in Region V (Illinois, Indiana, Michigan, Minnesota, Ohio, and Wisconsin), we want to share our concerns for the future of older Americans and to suggest ways personnel in aging can cooperate to identify and solve problems. This paper is based on four assumptions. First, we are committed to implement the purposes and objectives as stated in Titles I and IV of the Older Americans Act of 1965, as amended. Second, quality training and education that proceed from sound research are major support systems in the effective delivery of services to older adults. Third, we must be responsive to the annual programmatic goals and objectives of service providers by supplying the specific training and education they need. Fourth, maintaining the support systems needed to keep older Americans living as independently as they can means finding better ways to cooperate with service providers and to coordinate our efforts.

With the above assumptions in mind, we discuss three crucial areas: research, funding, and coordination.

Research

We support and recognize the value of sound, quality research in the field of aging. As noted at the 1971 White House Conference on Aging, "Research, demonstration, and evaluation are basic tools by which a society produces the knowledge it requires to deal with the problems of its people and to improve the quality of life" (Note 1).

Many sophisticated research efforts are currently taking place in the biological, medical, behavioral, and social areas of aging. However, because the inquiries are widespread (both in public and private sectors), it is very difficult for practitioners in the field to be aware of the findings and to profit from them. We need a better system for retrieving these findings and an easier method of translating them into meaningful data for planners, administrators, trainers, and direct-service providers in the aging network. Such improvements could greatly increase the quality and relevance of programs and training.

For instance, we could profit greatly by knowing what findings had emerged from the many research, demonstration, and evaluation projects implemented by postsecondary educational institutions (e.g., *Cumulative Index*, Note 2). Knowledge of these findings is essential since research by postsecondary educational institutions, with their insistence upon academic excellence, will always have a dominant impact in this field.

However, we also need to know the results of the excellent inquiries being conducted by all levels of government agencies. One notable example at the federal level is the National Institute on Aging, whose research inquiries have the direct oversight of the Gerontology Research Center at Baltimore. Under the direction of Robert N. Butler, the NIA conducts investigations and inquiries at its four branches and laboratories in clinical physiology, molecular aging, behavioral sciences, and cellular and comparative physiology. Other governmental agencies currently involved in aging studies include the Veterans Administration, the National Institute of Mental Health, and the Health Services and Mental Health Administration.

In the private sector, the Gerontological Society, the Association for Gerontology in Higher Education, the Western Gerontological Society, the American Geriatrics Society, the Association for the Advancement of Aging Research, the Research Center of the National Caucus on the Black Aged, and others are all actively engaged in research in aging.

As previously noted, however, much of the research of these agencies is not always easily understood by the service delivery system. On more than one occasion, when the results of some particular research were received, the language of the report was unintelligible to many practitioners, yet the data could well have been very important to the aging network. Because of this, we agree with Kaplan (Note 3) that social policies, programs, and training are often not proceeding from a scientific base. Sensing a great need for a stronger scientific base for our actions, we join O'Brien (Note 4) in asking, "Is there any way to apply the techniques of systematic science to the uncontrolled settings of direct service programs?" Although several educators, such as Hickey and Spinetta (1974), Urban and Watson (1974), and Miller and Cutler (1976), have addressed this question, the issue remains unresolved. George Maddox, the 1978 president of the Gerontological Society, concurred with O'Brien when he wrote, "My concern is that our Society has not been vigorous enough in its devotion to basic research and to insuring that basic research findings are effectively translated in ways that will be useful to those who teach, advocate, and develop programs in behalf of older persons" (Maddox, 1978).

Yet some excellent efforts have been made to translate the sophisticated investigations of the researcher into meaningful data for the service provider. One of these is the Aging Research Information System (ARIS) developed as a part of a Title-IV Research Utilization Grant in 1972 in Austin, Texas (Note 5). With over 20,000 individual records in its computerized information storage and retrieval system, ARIS is designed to make available to the practitioner a large amount of research information. Another effort was conducted by the Southern Regional Education Board of Atlanta, Georgia, in 1972. Its report, "Translating Aging Research into Training" (Note 6) summarizes new information and knowledge, which had surfaced through project grants made under the Older Americans Act (as well as elsewhere).

Another way service providers can obtain relevant data is for practitioners, programmers, planners, evaluators, trainers, and administrators to share with gerontological researchers the information they feel would be helpful to better carry out their functions. The report "Older Texans: Research and State Policy" (1974) shows such successful interface activity.

The total field of aging is growing so rapidly that we need to stop frequently and evaluate the impact of past efforts. An excellent example is the evaluation of the Title IV-A Career Training programs sponsored by the Administration on Aging. Another aspect of evaluation research, with which we fully concur, is stated by O'Brien (Note 4). In speaking about the various authors that contributed to the seminar on evaluative research, O'Brien writes: "Each of these authors emphasized that, unlike the laboratory setting where externalities are incidental to the problem, evaluation research in real life settings requires critical attention be paid to the larger context within which a program is implemented, a treatment applied, or an impact measured. Basic to their model is the message that a sensible evaluation research design must take into account not only the service-client interface, but also the interorganizational arena and the larger community environment in which the program is lodged."

As we begin to broaden our horizons and think about the larger community environment where our programs and trainings are lodged, we realize the great value of research relative to the future needs of older people. We need strategy in our planning and service areas about what programs and services will be most appropriate in 5, 10, and even 20 years. Such future projections will give direction to the types of training necessary to help implement such programs and services. Thus, more inquiries about the future roles and needs of older Americans, such as those conducted by Neugarten (1975), Peterson, Powell, and Robertson (1976), Cohen (1976), and Palmore (1976), are needed. Even with the variables of future political, social, economic, and environmental forces, certain trends can be identified that will help the service delivery network keep pace with anticipated program and training needs.

There is an urgent need to set short- and long-range national priorities in the areas of research. As Kaplan (Note 3) states, "Despite the relative burgeoning of reports, studies, investigations, articles and volumes on gerontology, the goals for research have not been fully identified." Therefore, we recommend that the Administration on Aging take the initiative in establishing such priorities in full concert with postsecondary educational institutions, state and area agencies on aging, other federal agencies with similar programs, direct service providers, and older Americans themselves.

Funding

As state and area agencies on aging avail themselves of research data and as they plan for future needs, it becomes increasingly important that sufficient funds be allocated to the states to conduct inservice training and education for providers of services to older persons. Thus, this section will focus on the Title IV-A awards to state units on aging granted between 1974 and 1978, the period following passage of the Older Americans Comprehensive Services Amendments in 1973.

State awards have primarily emphasized the upgrading of the skills and knowledge of any person, paid or volunteer, who works with or on behalf of older people. From the beginning, the Administration on Aging has encouraged cooperation and coordination between state units on aging and postsecondary educational institutions, which has allowed high-quality short-term training and education (Note 7).

However, an examination of the funding pattern for the various programs and services funded under the Older Americans Act shows that the awards to the states under Title IV-A have not kept pace with other funded programs and services. For instance, in fiscal years 1974 through 1978, the total allocation for all Older Americans Act programs rose from $217.8 million to $508.75 million, a 133 percent increase (1977). During this same period, the total of the discretionary funds allocated under Titles IV-A, IV-B, and IV-C increased 72 percent, from $16.5 million to $28.3 million. Title IV-A alone increased from $9.5 million to $17 million, a rise of 78 percent, but the state portion of Title IV-A increased only 50 percent, from $4 million to $6 million (1978).

Yet from the inception of Title IV-A awards to the states, the means for meeting the demand for short-term training have been increased dramatically. One of the more important causes of this increase was the creation of area agencies on aging, a result of the 1973 amendments to the Older Americans Act. Since then, more and more people have been employed in such areas as administration, program development, planning, grantsmanship, evaluation, and training. A recent study (Klegon, Note 8) shows that only about 25 percent of service providers in the field of aging have had previous formal or informal training in aging. In spite of concerted efforts to train and educate personnel, we still find persons, such as clergy and lay religious workers, community health and mental health workers, and legislative personnel, not receiving the training they need to serve the older population as effectively as they could. Further, the start-up demands inherent in implementing the new program requirements under Titles V and VII Management Initiative Tracking System (MITS) and under Section 504 of the Rehabilitation Act have placed heavy demands on immediate inservice training. We, therefore, recommend that training awards to state units on aging be increased substantially in order to keep pace with increasing demands for short-term training in aging.

Besides increasing the amount of the awards to the states, we suggest separating these awards from the portion of Title IV-A awarded to postsecondary educational institutions. In this paper, we will call the state awards Title IV-A(1) and the remainder Title IV-A(2). Once Title IV-A(1) has been extracted, we recommend that it be changed from a discretionary grant to a formula grant with a multiyear funding cycle. There would be several advantages to these changes. Title IV-A(1) funding would remain more consistently available to the state units on aging. This would facilitate both short-term and long-range planning and ensure a long-term commitment from the Administration on Aging. Also, state units on aging would not be competing with postsecondary educational institutions for Title IV-A funds, thus promoting a more harmonious working relationship between them. As a formula grant, it would enable training dollars to be used beyond the project period. This is important, since unused portions of funds often are returned to the state unit on aging by grantees late in September. When this happens, there is insufficient time for such funds to be reallocated properly before September 30. This extension of time also would be important in states such as Minnesota where area agencies on aging are not authorized to sign training contracts until after January 1, which means that since training cannot take place until after the contracts are signed in March or later of each year, there are only nine months or less of each fiscal year to hold training workshops. If the awards to the states remain discretionary grants under Title IV-A, we recommend that such awards be extended 90 days beyond the present September 30 expiration date.

Another of our concerns related to funding is the Title IV-A(1) Notification of Grant Awards (NGA), which arrive at state units on aging no earlier than October 15. We ask that the NGA be received by the states no later than September 1. This change would alleviate difficulties in the present arrangement. Since states cannot release or spend Title IV-A(1) funds until the NGA is received, and since it takes at least four weeks to process the NGA and issue checks to contractors, funds cannot now be disbursed until mid-November for training that was scheduled earlier. Thus, contractors must either carry such expenses in their own accounts (and some do) or defer all training events until the check arrives (which some also do) and lose one of the best time periods for workshops. Neither alternative is desirable.

We have several suggestions related to the AoA guidelines that spell out both the amount of funding allocated to each state as well as the parameters within which the states may distribute funds for meeting inservice training needs.

Our first suggestion is concerned with the late arrival of this document at the state units on aging. In the past four years, the Expenditure Plan for Use of Title IV-A Training Funds to Support State and Area Level Training

Activities has been received no earlier than March 11. Since the planning and proposal writing process is already well under way by that date, any changes in anticipated funding or in the guidelines for implementation of funds create a great deal of work for the entire aging network. We ask that such guidelines be in our hands by December 31 of each year. From that day on there is a tight schedule (at both the state and area agency levels) for proposal writing, for review and comment on the proposal, and for establishing the Training and Manpower Development Plan for the state. With the plan due at the regional office by August 1, and with printing, review, and public hearings, any new rules and regulations for the implementation of this plan must be integrated hastily.

Another problem is that because the guidelines arrive as a previously unseen document, either we have to live with the changes or we have to ask for exemptions from certain portions. Therefore, we ask to give input to the Administration on Aging on the formulation of these guidelines well before they are final. A draft copy sent out early in the fall would afford the principals a chance for review and comment. These principals should include representatives of state units and area agencies on aging, of Title VII nutrition projects, and of postsecondary educational institutions.

Because area agency and nutrition staff give a considerable amount of time to administering and implementing their Title IV-A(1) training contracts (including the development and writing of specific training proposals), we recommend that up to 8 percent of the total award to such agencies be allowed for administration expenses.

Finally, we recommend that the Administration on Aging allow up to 10 percent of the Title IV-A(1) awards to be identified as a contingency fund to meet unexpected training needs. This would enable us to more easily meet priority training demands that arise after the plan has been approved and the funds committed. A contingency fund is far more appropriate than sending in an amendment to the existing Training and Manpower Development Plan, since an amendment means canceling previously planned training that is legally bound under contracts. Under the present system, unexpected needs for training cannot be met until the following fiscal year.

Coordination

Historically, coordination of planning and program implementation efforts among various agencies and institutions with common vested interests has been uneven at best. However, with funding at a premium and needs at a maximum, we feel that the various components of the aging network can ill afford the luxury of "doing their own thing." We would like to share some of the ways training and education have been coordinated between Region V personnel and state units on aging, among the six states of the region, and within a particular state's aging network.

In 1974 the Administration on Aging directed that a symposium be held in each of the ten regions in the nation (Note 9). The purpose of these symposia was to bring faculty members and others who would be offering courses funded by state Title IV-A(1) awards together with regional and state agency staff to foster better coordination and cooperation. Out of the Region V symposium, held in February 1975 at Ann Arbor, Michigan, several examples for coordination emerged that could well serve as models adaptable for implementation elsewhere in the aging network.

First, the Region V Training and Education Consortium was formed. It comprised the Training and Education Specialist from each of the six states in the region, and it was funded by 2 percent of each state's Title IV-A(1) award. Aided by consultant Robert O. Washington, currently dean of the College of Social Work at Ohio State University, and by the staff from the Region V office in Chicago, the consortium immediately established six training and education goals for the region. The activities of the consortium began in August 1975 with a regional workshop on evaluation and data collection. To this training came the consortium members and the consultant, plus the program analysts of the state units and area agencies on aging. This workshop was followed two months later by an educational workshop on program evaluation process and findings in the development of training. Educators from postsecondary educational institutions in the region participated fully in this event. A significant outcome of this workshop was Washington's *Program Evaluation in the Human Services* (Note 10). Also, at this workshop, the need for regional training in advocacy was identified. Thus, in January 1976 the consortium held a workshop on this subject attended by area agency, nutrition project, and state agency staff and by educators from postsecondary educational institutions. Subsequently, Robert O. Washington was funded by the consortium to write *Evaluating Training Programs in Aging: A How-To Manual* (Note 11).

Following a meeting of the consortium in July 1976 to evaluate its past training activities, a regional workshop was held for educators, area agency and nutrition project staff, and state trainers. Training needs at all levels of the aging network within the region were identified and placed in priority. As an outcome of this process, nutritionists from all six state units on aging assembled for intensive training. Another outgrowth was a two-day, in-depth workshop on Title V of the Older Americans Act and Section 504 of the Rehabilitation Act. Yet to be conducted by the consortium are workshops on Title V (follow up), staff development, Title VII supportive services, program planning and development, and interstate training of specialists with common needs. We plan to hold a second symposium similar to the Ann Arbor 1975 symposium.

Another result of the Ann Arbor symposium was that all six states initiated efforts to work more cooperatively with the postsecondary educational institutions within their bounds. The highly structured and successful program implemented in Ohio offers a model for cooperation and coordination.

In September 1975, a three-day meeting, "Dialogue: Academia and Administration," was held in Ohio, attended by 14 area agency directors, 13 representatives of postsecondary educational institutions, and state training and education specialists. As a result of this dialogue, the Ohio Network of Educational Consultants in the Field of Aging was formed. Under the leadership of Jerome Kaplan, Mildred Seltzer, Harvey Sterns, and Carol Fought, this network of 24 educators has successfully demonstrated the coordination that can take place between academia and state and area agency administration in local community planning efforts, needs assessment, review and comments of Title IV-A(1) training proposals, and the teaching of short-term training workshops.

All the training and education specialists in Region V are committed to increasing and strengthening coordination and cooperation among all components of the training network within the region and within the individual states, for we can attest to the benefits that accrue to all.

Summary and Recommendations

For the aging network to cooperate better in the future, we recommend the following ideas.

1. Efforts should be increased to find more effective ways to identify and translate the results of research into useful data for programs and training.

2. A national policy on short- and long-range priorities for research in aging should be established.

3. Title IV-A awards to state units on aging should be increased, changed to a formula grant, and allocated for at least two years at a time.

4. Notification of Grant Awards for Title IV-A awards to state units on aging should arrive no later than September 1 of each year.

5. Principals who are affected by the guidelines for implementation of Title IV-A(1) training should be afforded the opportunity to give input to their formation. Also, such guidelines should arrive no later than December 31 of each year.

6. Up to 8 percent of Title IV-A(1) awards should be allowed for administrative expenses.

7. Up to 10 percent of Title IV-A(1) awards should be identified as contingency funds.

Notes

1. *Toward a national policy on aging—proceedings of the 1971 White House Conference on Aging.* Washington, D.C., 1971, 2, 93.

2. *Cumulative index of AoA discretionary project grants, 1965–1976.* AoA-IM-76-87, September 7, 1976.

3. Kaplan, J. *A perspective on policy for gerontological research in Ohio.* Position paper prepared for the Ohio Commission on Aging, 1976.

4. O'Brien, J., & Streib, G. (Eds.). *Evaluative research on social programs for the elderly.* U.S. Department of Health, Education, and Welfare, 1977, 1–2. (Pub. No. [OHD] 77-20120)

5. *Aging research information system.* Aging Research Utilization Report, Texas Governor's Committee on Aging, Austin, Texas, 1974, No. 1, p. 3.

6. *Translating aging research into training.* Southern Regional Education Board, December 1972, 1–44.

7. *Expenditure plan for use of (1) fiscal year 1977 training funds to support state and area level training activities and (2) fiscal year 1978 title III model projects funds to support state agency developmental activities for legal aide and nursing home ombudsman services.* Washington, D.C.: U.S. Department of Health, Education and Welfare, Administration on Aging, AoA-PI-77-13, March 5, 1977.

8. Klegon, D. *Manpower and the field of aging.* A report to the Ohio Commission on Aging, Scripps Foundation Gerontology Center, Miami University, Oxford, Ohio, 1977, p. 14.

9. *Support of regional symposia for faculty and others conducting courses in aging under state agency training grants.* ROM-74-20, May 22, 1974.

10. Washington, R. *Program evaluation in the human services.* Cambridge, Mass.: Schenkman, 1975.

11. Washington, R. *Evaluating training programs in aging: A how-to manual.* Center for Advanced Studies, School of Social Welfare, University of Wisconsin, Milwaukee, 1976.

References

Cohen, E. Comment: Editor's note. *Gerontologist,* 1976, *16*(3), 270–275.

Hickey, T. & Spinetta, J. Bridging research and application. *Gerontologist,* 1974, *14*(6), 526–530.

Maddox, G. A society devoted to research on aging. *Gerontologist,* 1978, *18*(1), 5.

Miller, E., & Cutler, N. Toward a comprehensive information system in gerontology: A survey of problems, resources, and potential solutions. *Gerontologist,* 1976, *16*(3), 198–205.

Neugarten, B. (Ed.), Aging in the year 2000: A look at the future. *Gerontologist,* 1975, *15*(1:2), 1–40.

Older Texans: Research and state policy. *Aging,* 1974, *18*, 233–234.

Palmore, E. The future status of the aged. *Gerontologist,* 1976, *16*(4), 297–302.

Peterson, D., Powell, C., & Robertson, L. Aging in America toward the year 2000. *Gerontologist,* 1976, *16*(3), 264–269.

217 million for AoA carried in HEW-Labor appropriations bill. *Aging,* 1977, *3*, 277–278.

78 funds for new projects: Where to find them at AoA. *Supportive Systems,* 1978, *3*, 22.

Urban, H., & Watson, W. Response to bridging the gap: Alternative approaches. *Gerontologist,* 1974, *14*(6), 530–533.

The Role of Higher Education in the Aging Network

Betsy M. Sprouse
University of Wisconsin-Madison
and
Harvey L. Sterns
The University of Akron

The preceding papers by Piktialis and by Miller, Secret, Loman, McKee, Peterson, and Vaughan have raised some important questions and concerns about the aging network and the relationship between higher education and state units on aging. This paper discusses some of those same questions and concerns from an educational viewpoint.

In and among all the points about cooperative relationships, training needs, and Title IV-A funding allocations, some broader issues need to be addressed. Why have higher education institutions become involved in short- and long-term training in gerontology? What is their role in the aging network? What is the responsibility of the higher education institution to the state with regard to training? How have the states been using their Title IV-A allocations, and what are the long-range impacts of these actions? What are the responsibilities of the states to their subunits and to higher education with regard to training?

Higher Education and the Aging Network

The aging network by definition is composed of agencies and organizations that receive funds through the various titles of the Older Americans Act. Through overuse and misuse of this term, it has been interpreted to apply to only those agencies receiving Titles III, V, and VII funds. Higher education institutions are truly members of the aging network, since they may be receiving funds under Title IV as well as Titles III, V, VII, and IX. Perhaps many of the relationship problems between higher education and state agencies that

Piktialis cites have arisen because she and others conceive of the relationship between higher education and the aging network as one between two separate networks rather than one between members of the same network.

The role of higher education in the aging network is most often to provide short- and long-term training. Colleges and universities have assumed this role for a variety of reasons: in response to national or local community manpower needs, as an outgrowth of faculty and student interests, under pressure or suggestion from state units on aging, in response to the availability of training funds, or in an attempt to build up falling student enrollment figures. The institutions that will still be providing quality training 20 years from now will likely be those who entered the field for the first two, or similar, reasons.

As closely related as higher education institutions and state units on aging are, some distinct differences emerge in discussions of gerontological training and research. Higher education has traditionally concerned itself with long-term education, training, and research, although it can also provide short-term training. The resources of state units on aging are well suited for coordinating and funding short-term training. Within an interactive relationship, higher education institutions and state units on aging can both check and balance each other's activities and can work cooperatively on joint programs.

Responsibilities of Higher Education to States

In their roles on aging network members and as training providers, higher education institutions have certain responsibilities to state units on aging and their subunits.

As members of the aging network, educators must establish their credibility in the world of practice. The ivory tower versus real world arguments that Piktialis cites are unfortunately too often true, but they can be resolved. One reason for this gap relates to Miller and colleagues' point about poorly translated research results. Educators must make greater efforts to relate both research and training efforts to "real-world" needs.

As training providers, higher education institutions must clearly be responsive to expressed and perceived training needs. Yet the role of higher education in providing short-term as well as long-term training creates some of the problems in the relationship between higher education and state agencies. Colleges and universities providing gerontology education must do so in response to long-term, national personnel needs (however they can best be forecast). At the same time, state units on aging are calling upon higher education to respond to immediate, local personnel needs. Some colleges can meet both needs; others cannot. Perhaps what is needed is a reconceptualization of "training" and of how higher education can respond to local personnel needs in different ways. This idea is explored in the following section.

State Title IV-A Programs

Both Piktialis and Miller et al. refer to Title IV-A allocations as a bone of contention between state units on aging and higher education. State units on aging receive Title IV-A funds from AoA for personnel development and in-service training, which they either retain, divide among their subunits, or contract out to higher education or other trainers. Higher education institutions may receive Title IV-A funds directly from AoA for career training, or they may receive Title IV-A training contracts from the state unit on aging. Because of these two channels of funding, higher education institutions are likely to have a larger share of the Title IV-A funds. The statistics cited by Piktialis and Miller et al. show that in 1974 the states received 42 percent of Title IV-A money but in 1978 they received only 35 percent. Presumably, higher education and other trainers received 65 percent.

Admittedly, this division does seem disproportionate. But we must look beyond the statistics and address the more important issues. It's not who gets how much money, but rather who has what resources to provide what services. The fact that state units on aging and their subunits contract out most of their Title IV-A allotment may indicate that other organizations, such as higher education, have more or better resources to provide training.

One alternative to Miller and colleagues' suggestion of dividing the Title IV-A funds into state and education allotments (which would probably do little to reduce competition) is to reconceptualize how Title IV-A funds can be used for personnel development and inservice training. The aging network associates personnel development with workshops and conferences, which tend to be only a day or two long with few follow-up programs. Given the high turnover in volunteers and paraprofessional and professional staff in agencies, trainers often find themselves conducting a workshop on basic aging to a group of practitioners who have all been hired since the previous basic aging workshop three months before. It's little wonder that it is difficult to observe and measure the long-range impact of conferences and workshops.

Personnel development can be much more than workshops. For example, in January 1978, the Wisconsin Bureau of Aging and its Training Advisory Committee defined five channels for the expenditure of the state's share of Title IV-A funds. These methods can be used jointly or separately to meet personnel development needs in transportation, health care, legal services, and so forth. The five methods to be used in Wisconsin are:

1. Training programs. These include workshops, conferences, and serial noncredit or continuing education credit courses leading to certification.

2. Local leadership development. This tactic aims to develop expertise in local communities through invitational workshops, technical assistance, or expert consultation. Trained local leaders then become providers of training or technical assistance.

3. Educator and staff development. That is, "training the trainers."

4. Technical assistance. State unit on aging staff, educators, gerontology students, and other experts will provide on-the-job, expert consultation on program planning, development, and evaluation.

5. Material preparation and dissemination. Information packets and how-to manuals will be prepared by either the state unit on aging or the higher education institution for distribution to appropriate practitioners.

In Ohio, a sixth method is used; namely, tuition stipends are available from the area agencies on aging for community professionals to take credit courses at local colleges and universities.

A similar approach to personnel development is reflected in the AoA fiscal year 1978 guidelines to states. They suggest that Title IV-A funds be used for educational resource development, staff development, training and continuing education, and technical assistance. The point is that the traditional workshop may not be the best use of Title IV-A money, from the point of view of either the state unit on aging or the higher education institution. Clearly, there should be a marriage between state units on aging and higher education. At the least, they can live together while awaiting the final outcome.

Responsibilities of States to Their Subunits and to Higher Education

In the sometimes precarious relationship between state agencies and higher education, each has responsibilities to the other. Those of higher education have been suggested earlier. The state's responsibilities lie in the area of directing and guiding manpower development.

In relating to higher education, the state unit on aging should be able to provide the trainers with fairly accurate and comprehensive assessments of current and predicted training needs in its state. As difficult a task as this is, it does allow for long-range planning of training programs. The state unit on aging should also be willing to share its long-range planning materials with educators, whether they are directly related to training or not.

The states also have the responsibility to effectively use their "review and comment" options on federal grant proposals submitted by higher education institutions. What is too often a routine signoff procedure can and should be an excellent opportunity for the state units on aging to influence federal discretionary grants and to shape the nature of future grant proposals.

With regard to their subunits—generally defined as area agencies on aging, local offices on aging, nutrition projects, senior centers, and so on—the state units on aging should assume the responsibility for establishing a mechanism to convey the research and training needs perceived by the subunits to higher education institutions. Miller et al. cite the need for more sharing of information between local practitioners and higher education, yet it is impractical for each college in a state to survey all agencies and organizations in the state each time it develops a research or training proposal. The more that state units on aging can act as clearinghouses, the more effective the flow of information will be.

One example of a cooperative approach between higher education and a state unit on aging can be found in Ohio—the Ohio Network of Educational Consultants in the Field of Aging, which is still in its developmental period. Each area agency on aging appoints an educational consultant and an alternate from qualified educators. These appointments are approved by the consultant's educational institution and the Ohio Network's membership committee. Each area agency has a local education committee (of which the consultant is a member), which plans training for that area. Educational plans for each area are then reviewed by the network as a whole and the Ohio Commission on Aging training staff. Each area's educational plan becomes part of the area agency plan.

The Ohio Network undertakes a number of statewide training programs on its own, using the talents and resources of its members, and inviting national experts when appropriate. The Ohio Commission on Aging plans and conducts its own training program, carried out by commission staff, which is reviewed by the Ohio Network. Thus, each partner in the training experience has an opportunity to review and comment on the other's plans. The final approval of training activities rests with the Ohio Commission on Aging and becomes part of the state plan. This approach, although far from perfect, presents an example of dynamic and constructive cooperation.

Summary

There is no denying that higher education institutions and state units on aging have often acted at cross-purposes, either out of a sense of "protecting turf" or simply because of lack of communication. Yet the time is past due for accepting the fact that both are members of the same aging network, a network that cannot function effectively without internal cooperation. It is also time to look beyond the financial issues to resources and capabilities. Higher education institutions and state units on aging both have roles to perform. Some can be performed in partnership, whereas others are best done separately by mutual consent. The effective development of the aging network will surely come to rest on a cooperative and mutually beneficial relationship between higher education institutions and the state units on aging.

Problems and Issues in Multi-Agency Programming: A Case for University Involvement

Robert Deitchman
The University of Akron

It is hoped that the issues presented here will provide information to those who have had difficulties in planning, implementing, and evaluating multipurpose community centers for the elderly. The purpose is to delineate both the needs for interagency cooperation and some of the potential problems in implementation. A model is discussed from the premise that the university should be active as a community resource in research, training, and coordinating service delivery.

The problems and abuses of meeting the support needs of older adults are many and well documented. Many practitioners have pointed out that the present system for delivery remains somewhat insensitive, inadequate, and punitive. At the National Caucus on the Black Elderly a number of symposium presenters, including the author, were much concerned that the current support systems for the elderly seem oriented toward one common denominator—dependency.

Many new problems have increased the pressure to find a solution. The one most emphasized is the obvious increase in size of the population of those 65 and older. Another is that older adults account for a significant percentage of health and drug expenditures.

The present system does not appear to be geared to handle the support needs of our older adults. We are concerned with the delivery of care, using external support systems based on a quality of life index, be it in a community-based facility, in the home, or in institutions. The concern should be for developing support systems that include health, economic, and social components. Current services seem to center around just "nutritional" or "medical" needs. A more effective approach to human support systems needs to start from a total-person approach. Current problems stem in part from the fact that at state, local, and federal levels there are at least a dozen separately funded programs, most of which are uncoordinated and are designated to fund specific needs areas. The result is a maze for both those who receive the services and those who provide them. The programs are designed with known gaps, and in many cases the benefits of one program negate the benefits of another. Not only are eligibility requirements inconsistent, but also they are inappropriate with regard to their base requirements.

A philosophical approach that gives equal weight to the medical, social, economic, psychological, and cultural needs of the older adult must be developed. The support services should enable older adults to remain independent and in their own homes as long as they choose. The support services should have the following characteristics:

1. Programs should continue for as long as they are needed. Too often a program is made available for only a short period of time, and as older adults respond to it, the funding is stopped or the service terminated.

2. The programs must have ready access. An alternate to multipurpose centers is neighborhood programs within walking distance for most residents.

3. There must be a way to assess the individual needs of the older adults at the center. The older adults themselves must have input into the ongoing programming.

4. A strong evaluation component needs to be developed along with the programs.

5. The facilities should be built to meet the needs of the older adult. Many centers are esthetically pleasing, but the older adults' activities are located in less than accessible areas.

6. Services should be appropriate for the population they are serving. We have witnessed over and over the sheer folly of trying to fit people into prepackaged, predetermined programs.

7. There should be a definite movement away from territoriality and duplication of services. The university could coordinate the activities of a variety of service agencies without competing in the direct delivery of services.

8. The overall quality of services needs to be made more uniform. However, it is important to point out that quality of service does not mean that all older adults in a county should be eating the same meal at the same time.

To best serve the needs of the older adult population in the development of a multipurpose center, the university can use individual expertise from as many disciplines as possible, stressing the overall enhancement of the older adult's physical, social, and emotional well-being.

Identifying basic needs is the first step. At a minimum, meeting these needs may require transportation services, counseling and mental health services, visiting nurse/homemaker service, health services, recreation activities, nutrition education, diagnostic and assessment services, speech and hearing services, and exercise programs. Obviously, no single agency can handle all the services. An alternative is to coordinate as many agencies as possible.

The next step in developing a model that is interdisciplinary and multi-agency based and that uses the university as a community resource is to identify available resources. These resources can be broken down into a variety of categories: (1) state and local (community and mental health facilities, health departments, welfare departments, Title VII nutrition programs, area agencies on aging, meals on wheels, departments of recreation); (2) voluntary groups (Retired Senior Volunteer Program, Service Corps of Retired Executives); (3) religious groups; (4) educational institutions (community colleges, universities, public library); (5) foundations; and (6) federal departments (Department of Transportation; Department of Health, Education and Welfare: Health Services Administration, Social Rehabilitation, Administration on Aging; Housing and Urban Development).

One model that may be useful in illustrating this approach was developed by The University of Akron and the Akron Metropolitan Housing Authority (AMHA). AMHA has recently completed the construction of a community center located adjacent to the Edgewood Community. The Institute for Life-Span Development and Gerontology of The University of Akron, in cooperation with AMHA, is programming the center for both community needs and as a practicum training site for undergraduate students.

The multipurpose center approach provides several advantages for the university. First, whereas community service does not in and of itself enhance the educational institution's development, the approach does provide an atmosphere for direct multidisciplinary interaction that not only allows but also encourages development in new directions by those involved. Second, students are provided a greater scope of training than would otherwise be possible. For students in fields without disciplinary identity, a multipurpose center setting provides direct interactions with specialists in a variety of areas. Third, a multipurpose center can be used as a direct research site. The range of research orientations can include program evaluation, needs of the older adults, and theoretical questions to be tested in the field.

The Edgewood Community Services Center caters to the needs of the older person and the preschool-aged child. The day-care program serves children in two broad categories: those whose parents are in employment-related circumstances, and children with special needs met by a developmental preschool program. Programs for older adults provide health-related social service activities that are now being funded by the area agency on aging. These include a midday meal and activities and special shopping trips in cooperation with the Young Men's Christian Association.

To the university, this special community project, with services and activities for preschoolers and older adults, provides a training and research facility. This center is a service provider to minority low-income older adults.

The interaction between the community and the university is demonstrated by the range of services provided at the Edgewood Center. The health-related services and their providers include: modified exercise—the department of physical education, University of Akron; speech and hearing—the department of speech and hearing, University of Akron; counseling—various departments at the University of Akron and the Case Western Reserve, human services department; dietary—Title VII YMCA Nutrition Program; shopping—Title VII YMCA Nutrition Program; well-baby clinic—public health services. The social-related services include: arts and crafts—Title XX, Summit County welfare, student participation; movies—Akron Public Library; reading—department of speech and hearing, University of Akron; religious activities—local community services; cooking classes—agricultural extension services; sewing classes—Family Life Care; and child-care center—Title XX. Financial and personnel assistance comes from the Area Agency on Aging; Administration on Aging (Titles IV-A, IV-C), Comprehensive Education and Training Act (Title I), Senior Workers Action Program (IX DOL), Summit County Welfare (Title XX), and Akron Metropolitan Housing Authority.

Community programs attempt to help meet human needs and to increase success in coping with problems and needs, whether they are perceived or not, real or not. The older adult or child is part of a family network, and we must tap into that network. This network is frequently ignored when working with the older adult. The professional in a multi-agency center will be working with problems that demand a variety of solutions.

An attempt has been made to present a model which serves the needs for interagency cooperation and communication, and to point out some of the characteristics of the services needed. The emphasis of the model presented is continuous and flexible support. It is apparent that given the basic services needed and the emphasis on individual need, no single agency can handle all of them. Models based on comprehensive knowledge of current services and multi-agency involvement can provide an effective way of meeting community needs.

I am suggesting that the university can play a primary role in developing adequate criteria for community programs. Within a university, a variety of departments can offer a variety of approaches to specific research, training, and service models.

Universities generally do not seek extensive input from professionals and community personnel who remain outside the usual departmental structures. A multidisciplinary service model can serve to bring in these individuals from a variety of areas both within and outside the university as consultants and resources for department needs.

Multidisciplinary community-centered programs present the university with a challenge to learn from the outside world. The impact of community involvement will be stressful. Language, values, and goals for education will be different for each participant and also for each university department. Another tension is the artificial difference between community and departments.

However, the variety of individuals involved will form a new problem-solving relationship. The cost of being a member of such a group is in trying to cope with the uncertainties of group goals and the ambiguities involved in crossing over a variety of disciplines.

The multidisciplinary environment increases our ability to solve some practical problems and develop new research approaches. From the university's point of view the major benefit is that both undergraduate and graduate students will adopt a professional identity that is not self-centered.

PART NINE
LIFE-SPAN LEARNING AND COMMUNITY APPROACHES

Historically, constrictive notions of adult human development have typified the self-concepts of older people and the community's response. The five papers in this section describe the concept of life-span learning, and show how educational programming in this area relates to both community concerns and to older adults. The issue of developing special programs for the elderly as opposed to integrating the elderly into existing programs is addressed, as is the issue of the responsibility and accountability of the educational institution to older adults.

Personal and Cognitive Development across the Life Span

**Harvey L. Sterns
and
Shirley Mitchell
The University of Akron**

One of the most stimulating social challenges confronting educators is to help individuals "get in touch with" their personhood through lifelong learning experiences. Personhood may be defined as a learned lifelong developmental process; it is the continuum of life from birth to death in which one is encouraged to develop one's potential to the fullest regardless of chronological age.

The individual may obtain personhood in many ways. Maslow speaks of personhood in his work on self-actualization and needs. Of special interest to educators is Maslow's concept of the need to know, which is as basic a need as physical, security, or belongingness needs. Certainly, the need to know, with its sequential frustration-gratification-frustration process, is an important mechanism in motivation (Maslow, 1954).

For Maslow, as well as Erikson (1950, 1963), development progresses along the continuum of personhood into the later years, which are potentially rich in wisdom and self-actualization. Educators need to help facilitate the attainment of lifelong personhood with its concomitant wisdom and self-actualization.

Rather than life-span personhood approaches, human development patterns are all too often stereotyped as rigid, age-specific structures that begin and end with dependency. The very labels of infancy, childhood, young adulthood, middle age, and older adulthood, because of their age-specific connotations in our society, limit the individual's development. Even classic approaches, such as the developmental tasks of Havighurst (1948, 1952, 1972), which have been a real contribution to developmental psychology, perpetuate age-graded expectations that may no longer be appropriate.

In life-span psychology, the meaning of chronological age has come under serious question. Birren (1964) suggests the need to specify the dimensions of biological, psychological, and social aging, each related differently to chronological age. Schaie (1965) and Baltes (1968), in their developmental models, call for consideration to be given to the time when the study was conducted, to the specific generational membership of the age groups, and to the role and importance of environmental impact on the changing development system.

Students of the life cycle have given much thought to the biological timetable of human development, using such concepts as maturation, age, and stage as major dimensions in mapping significant changes. Much attention has been given to the sociohistorical context and to the development of concepts for mapping change in the social environment as they affect the way an individual lives life.

The sociohistorical perspective of the life cycle has not yet received systematic treatment. Studies often search for universal sequences of psychological personality changes that are comparable to, if not paced by, the maturational timetable (Erikson, 1950, 1963; Havighurst, 1948, 1952, 1972; D. J. Levinson, Darrow, Klein, M. H. Levinson, and McKee, 1974; Levinson, 1977a, 1977b) rather than for sequences of personality changes that reflect historical and social events as well (Gubrium and Buckholdt, 1977; Hultsch and Plemons, 1979).

Neugarten and Datan (1973) point to the need to consider three dimensions of time: chronological, social, and historical. The dimension most often used is life time (chronological). Many people have viewed the life cycle as a series of orderly changes from infancy through childhood, adolescence, maturity, and old age, with the biological timetable governing the sequence of changes in growing up and growing old. Yet chronological age does not accurately measure physical or psychological development; individual differences must be taken into account, as well as specific cultural differences.

Social time refers to the dimension that underlies the age-grade system of a society, which does not necessarily follow biological timing. It is important to recognize that separate cultures instill different age expectations and status. Chronological age itself does not determine age status; rather, it simply signifies the biological potential for systems of age grade and age norms that form individual life cycles (Neugarten and Datan, 1973).

Behavioral scientists have advanced the concept of historical time as they have recognized the importance of the timing of major historical events in the life of the individual. Cohort analysis was originally developed by demographers to relate life time to historical time. A cohort is a group defined by the period of birth. The relationships between life time, social time, and historical time vary for each cohort.

All societies divide life time into socially relevant units and thus transform chronological time into social time expressed in age-grade systems.

Every society has a system of social expectations regarding age-appropriate behaviors, which are internalized (Kimmel, 1974; Neugarten and Datan, 1973). Age norms and age expectations give individuals an idea about the timing of their own development. Our society has many expectations that may be appropriate or inappropriate based on our age. However, this kind of analysis points to the potential tyranny of age expectations, especially in the later life period, when society has developed incorrect and inappropriate belief systems.

Using a social phenomenological approach, Gubrium and Buckholdt (1977) question the assumption that life inherently cycles in some ordered or progressive fashion. They question some of the traditional approaches to life change, which have emphasized research identifying the characteristics of persons in various stages and then locating the mechanisms that either hinder or facilitate movement. Gubrium and Buckholdt focus on "what ideas are held about the advance of life, how do people use these ideas to construct and control each other's lives in terms of time, and how do they come to think and talk about movement from one life stage to another. The 'truths' about life change become what people believe and say about it and how these beliefs and such talk accomplish human development" (1977: viii).

Research data and belief systems, scientific as well as popular notions, can set severe limitations on our expectations about the potential for cognitive and personal development. Birren and Woodruff write: "The concept that development ends with biological maturity is fallacious. Differentiation continues until death, and education should have an important role in helping individuals to meet the challenge of developmental tasks throughout the lifespan" (1973: 334–335).

The stimulating challenge for educators, then, is to help people of all ages overcome the problems of restrictive age stereotypes (Baltes and Willis, 1978; Schaie and Willis, 1978).

Cognitive Development

A major problem that must be overcome is the false stereotypes regarding intelligence and learning abilities of adults and older adults. Intelligence implies both a potential and an actual ability. In practice, however, we deal with measured abilities. Traditional global measures of intelligence such as IQ have been found to be ill suited to developmental analysis. A multidimensional approach to intelligence is useful since dimensions (factors) of intelligence differ in their developmental functions over the life span (Baltes and Schaie, 1976; Botwinick, 1967, 1973, 1977; Horn, 1970; Horn and Donaldson, 1976; Baltes and Labouvie, 1973).

A very good example is found in the different ontogenetic trends in fluid and crystallized abilities (Cattell, 1963; Horn, 1970). Fluid intelligence includes logical reasoning, associative memory, and figural relationships. It is measured by culture-fair perceptual and performance tests and by specifically developed tests of judgment and reasoning that have been considered relatively culture free. One major characteristic of fluid intelligence is that it leads to perception of complex relations in new environments. Crystallized intelligence is thought to result from all that a person has learned in a given culture. Crystallized intelligence includes verbal meaning (vocabulary), numerical ability, mechanical knowledge, well-stocked memory, and habits of logical reasoning. Crystallized intelligence is high on the subtests that are built into traditional IQ tests, such as vocabulary size, analogies, and classification involving cultural knowledge of objects and problems.

Research studies (see Horn, 1970; Horn and Donaldson, 1976) indicate that fluid intelligence exhibits a pattern that closely matches the growth and decline of biological processes, that is, a steady decline from early adulthood onward. Crystallized intelligence, which depends principally on learning and acculturation, is assumed to show an increase all through adulthood and only slight, if any, decline in old age. Thus, if we talk about decline in intelligence with age, we must ask what aspects.

Results from cross-sectional studies of traditional IQ tests, such as the Wechsler Adult Intelligence Scale (WAIS), have tended to show declines in intelligence from early adulthood. Botwinick (1967, 1973, 1977), in his analyses of a large number of cross-sectional studies using the WAIS, concluded that performance subtests exhibit a greater decline than verbal subtests.

Conclusions about general age decrements and different age functions have also been seriously challenged by the differences found between cross-sectional and longitudinal studies. Cross-sectional studies of intelligence produce age functions indicating earlier performance decrements. Longitudinal studies suggest maintenance and stability into late adulthood (Schaie and Strother, 1968; Jarvik, Eisdorfer and Blum, 1973; Baltes and Labouvie, 1973; Schaie and Labouvie, 1974; Schaie, Labouvie and Buech, 1973).

Schaie (1965) and Baltes (1968) both offer models that deal with the differences in cross-sectional and longitudinal results. The focus of their argument is that cross-sectional studies sample age groups from different generations (cohorts). Members of different generations may differ in their experiential background, education, health, and nutrition. Thus, differences between cross-sectional groups can be due to age or to differences related to membership in a specific generation. A good example here would be the great changes in education that have taken place in the last 70 years. Cross-sectional group differences could be due to differences in age or education or both.

Longitudinal studies use the same generation and test the same subjects on a number of occasions. Thus, changes must be due to aging or to some experience that occurs between repeated testings. Longitudinal studies of intelligence have found either no decline or a much smaller decline than was found with cross-sectional testing. What appear to be declines in intelligence may reflect changes in skills and environmental input emphasized by the culture over time.

It is relevant here that our cultural milieu has different expectations and demands for adults and older adults. Baltes and Labouvie (1973) point out that, in our culture, there is little reinforcement for good cognitive behavior for older adults. Changes in intellectual and learning abilities may well reflect lack of reinforcement and disuse. Recently, there has been considerable debate regarding whether cognitive decline in adulthood is a myth (Baltes and Schaie, 1976; Horn and Donaldson, 1976; Botwinick, 1977). Intervention strategies have been successful in modifying scores on intelligence and other cognitive tests (Sterns and Alexander, 1977; Sterns and Sanders, 1979; Labouvie-Vief, 1976; Labouvie-Vief and Gonda, 1976; Plemons, Willis and Baltes, 1978).

This raises the questions of what all this research means and what its relevance to real-life situations is. Clearly, the research studies call into question the popular notion of decline in intelligence with age. In summarizing this research, Atchley (1977) feels that age-related decline in measured intelligence probably has little to do with performance in everyday tasks. Unless there is an extensive decline in intelligence, such factors as persistence, responsibility, and group pressure may compensate for changes in intellectual functioning.

A similar kind of analysis can be applied to learning research in terms of differences in learning that result from generational change as well as from aging (Goulet, 1972). Learning refers to the acquisition of information or skills. Thus, improved performance on a given intellectual or physical task indicates learning.

A number of factors other than learning ability affect performance. These include motivation, speed, and physiological states and psychological sets. It is extremely difficult to separate the components of performance from learning. A major trend in learning research has been to investigate the nonlearning factors that vary systematically with age (Botwinick, 1967, 1973, 1977; Goulet, 1972; Arenberg, 1973; Birren, 1970; Eisdorfer, 1968; Falk and Kline, 1978).

Inferior performance in laboratory learning situations has been ascribed to the inability of older adults to respond in short intervals of time. Also there are age-related changes in the spontaneous use of mediative techniques that assist learning. Thus, a good deal of the decline found in learning in the laboratory may be in large part due to performance factors. Intervention strategies have been found to be extremely effective (Sterns and Sanders, 1979). Thus, although there are some declines in learning ability, much can be done to provide optimal learning situations. Performance factors may influence learning in the laboratory, but there is some question about how much effect this would have in the classroom situation. Birren (1964) indicates that there is little evidence to suggest a great deal of change in learning capacity over the major part of the life span. It would thus appear that little reason is given to suppose that adults and older adults could not benefit from extended periods of education throughout the life span.

The University as Facilitator

Ideally, the university should be a facilitator in increasing public awareness of the continuum of personhood through workshops and curricula developed specifically for lifelong learning. However, as Hechinger (1975:18) points out:

Traditional institutions have been slow to realize the potential of continuing education and to make the necessary readjustments to offer and reap the benefits of a movement of rapidly accelerating momentum. In addition to welcoming mature and even old people to their regular classes, American campuses will be called upon to extend their influence into former students' homes, lives, careers. Colleges may have to help employers, labor unions, civic organizations, medical and bar associations, and other agencies to create new academic patterns for lifelong learning; they ought to be able to tape and package courses for home study; they should, in other words, overcome their own static view of themselves as enclaves reserved largely for post-adolescent resident students to be visited for brief and rigidly defined periods of time.

A major thrust of two- and four-year colleges and universities and technical schools has become the training or retraining of adult students. Currently we are seeing a movement to make post-secondary education a center for the adults of our society. Services to adults of all ages include outreach activities aimed at bringing adults to campuses, counseling and guidance in employment, educational and volunteer opportunities, and information-referral activities designed to link adults with adult services, and continuing-education programs (see Ansello and Hayslip, this volume).

The movement away from education at specific points in the early part of the life span to education throughout the life span is supported by the growing numbers of adults enrolled in full-time, part-time, and evening programs. Birren and Woodruff (1973) and Baltes and Labouvie (1973) stress the need for education to become a lifelong endeavor. Education can facilitate the continuing development of the individual to meet the challenge of our fast-changing social and technical milieu. As leisure time increases for the individual, education must also be viewed as a very positive form of recreation. The growth of adult education over the last 50 years, with special emphasis on the two-year college, is discussed in the excellent review by Koos (1970). Many additional factors regarding motivation and attitude that perhaps play a decisive role in whether adults continue in educational endeavors must be considered.

Without a doubt, the challenge for educators to overcome social time stereotypes is difficult; age-grade systems are important parts of social time. Neugarten and Datan (1973) note that age-grade systems are "expression of the fact that all societies rationalize the passage of time, divide life time into socially relevant units, and thus can be said to transform calendar time (or biological time) into social time."

Birren and Woodruff (1973) believe that educators should focus on the development of affective experience and motivation rather than being concerned exclusively with cognitive skills. Hence, course content should be changed and methods such as small group discussions of personal experiences and attitudes should be attempted. Another recommendation by Birren and Woodruff (1973) is to aim strategies at altering negative stereotypes toward aging and the aged. Possible strategies might include some age integration of classes at all levels and training in life-span development at the elementary, high-school, and graduate levels.

One specific strategy suggested by Hechinger (1975) is to grant credit for proven practical experience. Hechinger believes that academic departments must show a greater readiness to let students work independently both on and off campus, citing the creation of Empire State College as part of the State University of New York as an example. Here mature students may complete many of their requirements by working at home, following academic outlines individually designed for them, and pursuing their studies with the aid of supervising tutors at conveniently located centers throughout the state. For an extensive discussion of adult education see Ansello and Hayslip, this volume.

Personal Change and Growth during Adulthood

Neugarten and Datan (1973) are concerned with adult behavior change and experiences. Ahammer (1973) thinks that the "rationale for seeking the prime source of adult behavior change in experience" is best expressed in Flavell's words: "If one could discount the nature of the organisms involved (for instance, that young children might be regarded as intrinsically more malleable than adults), one could argue that adulthood is the nearest thing we have to a pure experiment-in-nature for assessing the change-making power of experience alone, that is, relatively unconfounded by significant and directional biological changes" (Flavell, 1970: 250). Flavell's point that adulthood is undoubtedly the period of time in the lifespan where there is the most stability (in a biological sense) is well taken. Yet it appears questionable that "adulthood is the nearest thing we have to a pure experiment-in-nature for assessing the change-making power of experience alone," at least in a social sense. Such a statement seems to imply a freedom inherent in adulthood experience that Clarence Darrow so succinctly and facetiously contradicts: "The first half of our lives is ruined by our parents and the second half by our children." In other words, while one's adult experiences undoubtedly have change-making power, so also do the childhood experiences upon which adulthood is founded. Some questions therefore arise: Is it possible to separate the child from the adult? Is the child truly father to the man? How important is previously learned behavior?

Ahammer, like Darrow, also seems to recognize that adulthood is not necessarily a "pure experiment-in-nature." Past experiences and learning may indeed be exceedingly influential in one's continuum of personhood (1973:263–264):

Although one major argument of the present chapter is that systematic and significant behavior changes do occur in the adult years, a tendency seems to exist among adults to seek environments which support previously learned behavior. In this sense, people tend to choose marriage partners who are similar to themselves in a number of respects (e.g., regarding educational level, age, race, religion, ethnic origin, social class, values, interests, and personality variables) (Barry, 1970; Laws, 1971). Although the complementarity hypothesis is revived from time to time, the overwhelming part of evidence supports homogamy as a basic norm in mate selection (reviews by Barry, 1970; Laws, 1971; Tharp, 1963).

In short, Ahammer (1973) supplies evidence to contradict the old wives' tale that opposites attract. Apparently, most individuals build upon what they have learned from past experiences, especially those experiences in which they felt comfortable.

Perhaps one reason many people tend to cling to what they have already learned is the discomfort they may experience with new experiences. Ahammer discusses the discomfort that one may experience when meeting someone for the first time.

When people enter into new situations (new social environments, new social relationships), they bring with them behavior systems that have been maintained by particular stimuli in previous relationships. Since it is unlikely that the behavior of two interaction partners has been maintained by the same discriminative stimuli, relearning or new learning has to take place whenever two previously unacquainted people interact. That is, each partner probably will present stimuli to the other signifying information about appropriate responses which may differ from previously learned information with respect to this stimulus (Ahammer, 1973: 258).

Kimmel (1974) appears to agree with Ahammer (1973) as he discusses anticipatory socialization and resocialization. Kimmel defines anticipatory socialization as the "process of preparation for a change in role or status. It involves exploring the new norms and expectations that will be associated with the new role or status once the transition is made" (1974: 69–70). Resocialization takes place "when the role or status is actually begun . . . in each socialization situation the individual carries part of his old self along with the new part of the self into his new situation" (1974: 70).

Whereas continuity with one's familiar past appears to be a "security blanket" for many persons, it may also eventually be the source of discomfort. Sears and Feldman (1973) discuss a crisis situation: "The dread prospect of 'settling down' then is the crisis. . . . Most people, especially the married ones, experience this period as one of 'finding themselves' in their working and married lives, gaining the confidence born of feeling no longer novices, and of the widening scope of life. . . . But the typical emotional difficulties in this phase may be embraced by the word disillusionment—whether with oneself, work, marriage or life in general" (p. 88).

Questions raised about identity and personal development are dealt with through special programming at some colleges and universities. Lifespan Planning: The Choice is Yours (Mitchell and Vegso, 1978) is one example of materials developed to facilitate answering such questions as, Who am I? Introspective exercises in small group settings provide women and men with the opportunity not only to address such questions but also to come to the comforting realization that they are not alone in their uneasiness—other women and men are also experienceing similar discomfort.

Choice is a key word in life-span planning workshops as individuals begin to become aware of who they are through introspective exercises and group interaction. Groups are led by trained, lay facilitators, who encourage participants to set aside stereotyped roles for a short time. For example, individuals who live the stereotype of parent, with its concomitant sacrifices, are asked to set the role aside to see who they are as individuals, to see the parent role as just one part of their lives. Emphasis is placed upon how people feel about themselves and their attitudes and dreams. Fantasizing is encouraged as a part of finding out who they are. Attention is called to the continuum of personhood with an emphasis upon the 40 or so years that may remain after the main responsibilities of the parent role have been met. Choice, needs, expectations, and decision blocks are key words. Other sessions include decision-making and assertiveness training.

Tyler (1972) predicts that a woman in the year 2000 will make decisions at various points in her life on the basis of the total picture, not just some narrow segment of it, as people often do now. Tyler believes such decisions call for integrating "self-knowledge" with a great many other kinds of thinking. For one thing, life-span thinking should be encouraged. It is not enough to consider what one wants life to be next year or the year after. Tyler says that we must somehow get the flow of time into our awareness; we must think the way a novelist or a biographer does, sensing direction of movement as well as the existing life pattern.

Sommers (1975) is concerned with sexism as one grows older: "Sexism is compounded as a woman grows older. Jobs are harder to come by, the dependency status increases; self-image deteriorates; health care goes from bad to worse; marriages flounder. For a large majority of older women, poverty is no longer on the doorstep—it moves in. Our society is not only permeated with sexism from top to bottom, it is also pervaded with ageism. This denial of personhood affects both genders, but women, already weakened by sexism are especially vulnerable" (p. 60).

Birren and Woodruff (1973) point out that the rate of social and technological progress continues to accelerate, and an individual can no longer be programmed for an entire lifetime by education in the first 20 years of the life span. Men, as well as women, appear to be asking themselves questions about midcareer changes and retirement planning. Such explorations can be part of each person's individual development.

Conclusion

The expectations we have about ourselves and other people come from our social and technical milieu. These expectations often limit our opportunities for personal and cognitive growth. Belief systems, scientific or cultural, change slowly, yet demands on the individual in a fast-changing society require a facilitating environment for personal and cognitive development. Educational institutions can play important roles in fostering individual development at all points in the life span, giving educators the chance to better understand the psychological and sociological perspectives of personhood. The challenge is to apply our new knowledge about growth potential at all points in the life cycle. Education has been and will continue to be a major influence in the growth of individuals and the development of personhood.

References

Ahammer, I. M. Social-learning theory as a framework for the study of adult personality development. In P. B. Baltes & K. W. Schaie (Eds.), *Life-span developmental psychology: Personality and socialization*. New York: Academic Press, 1973.

Arenberg, D. Cognition and aging: Verbal learning, memory and problem solving. In C. Eisdorfer & M. P. Lawton (Eds.), *The psychology of adult development and aging*. Washington, D.C.: American Psychological Association, 1973.

Atchley, R. C. *The social forces in later life*. Belmont, Calif.: Wadsworth, 1977.

Baltes, P. B. Longitudinal and cross-sections sequences in the study of age and generation effects. *Human Development*, 1968, *11*, 145–171.

Baltes, P. B., & Labouvie, G. V. Adult development of intellectual performance: Description, explanation, and modification. In C. Eisdorfer & M. P. Lawton (Eds.), *The psychology of adult development and aging*. Washington, D.C.: American Psychological Association, 1973.

Baltes, P. B., & Schaie, K. W. On the plasticity of intelligence in adulthood: Where Horn and Donaldson fail. *American Psychologist*, 1976, *31*, 720–725.

Baltes, P. B., & Willis, S. L. Life-span developmental psychology, cognitive functioning, and social policy. In M. W. Riley (Ed.), *Aging from birth to death*. Washington, D.C.: American Association for the Advancement of Science, 1978.

Birren, J. E. *The psychology of aging*. Englewood Cliffs, N. J.: Prentice-Hall, 1964.

Birren, J. E. Toward an experimental psychology of aging. *American Psychologist*, 1970, *25*, 124–135.

Birren, J. E., & Woodruff, D. S. Human development over the life span through education. In P. B. Baltes & K. W. Schaie (Eds.), *Life-span developmental psychology: Personality and socialization*. New York: Academic Press, 1973.

Botwinick, J. *Cognitive processes in maturity and old age*. New York: Springer, 1967.

Botwinick, J. *Aging and behavior*. New York: Springer, 1973.

Botwinick, J. Intellectual abilities. In J. E. Birren & K. W. Schaie (Eds.), *Handbook of the psychology of aging*. New York: Van Nostrand Reinhold, 1977.

Cattell, R. B. Theory of fluid and crystallized intelligence: A critical experiment. *Journal of Educational Psychology*, 1963, *54*, 1–22.

Eisdorfer, C. Arousal and performance: Experiments in verbal learning and tentative theory. In G. A. Talland (Ed.), *Human aging and behavior.* New York: Academic Press, 1968.

Erikson, E. H. *Childhood and society.* New York: Norton, 1963. (Originally published, 1950.)

Falk, J. L., & Kline, D. W. Stimulus persistence and arousal. *Experimental Aging Research*, 1978, *4*, 109–124.

Flavell, J. H. Cognitive changes in adulthood. In L. R. Goulet & P. B. Baltes (Eds.), *Life-span developmental psychology: Research and theory.* New York: Academic Press, 1970.

Goulet, L. R. New directions for research on aging and retention. *Journal of Gerontology*, 1972, *27*, 52–60.

Gubrium, J. F., & Buckholdt, D. R. *Toward maturity.* San Francisco: Jossey-Bass, 1977.

Havighurst, R. J. *Developmental tasks and education.* New York: David McKay, 1972. (Originally published, 1948, 1952.)

Hechinger, F. M. Education's new majority. *Saturday Review*, 1975, *18*, 14–16.

Horn, J. L. Organization of data on life-span development of human abilities. In L. R. Goulet & P. B. Baltes (Eds.), *Life-span development psychology: Research and theory.* New York: Academic Press, 1970.

Horn, J. L., & Donaldson, G. On the myth of intellectual decline in adulthood. *American Psychologist*, 1976, *31*, 701–719.

Hultsch, D. F. & Plemons, J. K. Life events and life-span development. In P. B. Baltes & O. G. Brim, Jr. (Eds.), *Life-span development and behavior* (Vol. 2). New York: Academic Press, 1979.

Jarvik, L., Eisdorfer, C., & Blum, J. *Intellectual functioning in adults.* New York: Springer, 1973.

Kimmel, D. C. *Adulthood and aging.* New York: John Wiley, 1974.

Koos, L. V. *The community college student.* Gainesville: University of Florida Press, 1970.

Labouvie-Vief, G. W. Toward optimizing cognitive competence in later life. *Educational Gerontology*, 1976, *1*, 75–92.

Labouvie-Vief, G. W., & Gonda, J. N. Cognitive strategy training and intellectual performance in the elderly. *Journal of Gerontology*, 1976, *31*, 327–332.

Levinson, D. J. The mid-life transition: A period in adult psychosocial development. *Psychiatry*, 1977(a), *40*, 99–112.

Levinson, D. J. Middle adulthood in modern society: A sociopsychological view. In G. DiRenzo (Ed.), *Social character and social change.* Westport, Conn.: Greenwood Press, 1977(b).

Levinson, D. J., Darrow, C. M., Klein, E. G., Levinson, M. H., & McKee, B. The psychosocial development of men in early adulthood and the mid-life transition. In D. F. Ricks, A. Thomas, & M. Roff (Eds.), *Life history research in psychopathology.* Minneapolis: University of Minnesota Press, 1974.

Maslow, A. H. *Motivation and personality*. New York: Harper & Row, 1954.

Neugarten, B. L., & Datan, N. Sociological perspectives on the life cycle. In P. B. Baltes & K. W. Schaie (Eds.), *Life-span developmental psychology: Personality and socialization*. New York: Academic Press, 1973.

Plemons, J. K., Willis, S. L., & Baltes, P. B. Modifiability of fluid intelligence in aging: A short-term longitudinal training approach. *Journal of Gerontology*, 1978, 2, 224–231.

Schaie, K. W. A general model for the study of developmental problems. *Psychological Bulletin*, 1965, 64, 92–107.

Schaie, K. W., & Labouvie, G. V. Generational versus ontogenetic components of change in adult cognitive behavior: A fourteen-year cross sequential study. *Developmental Psychology*, 1974, 10, 305–330.

Schaie, K. W., Labouvie, G. V., & Buech, B. U. Generational and cohort specific differences in adult cognitive functioning. *Developmental Psychology*, 1973, 9, 151–166.

Schaie, K. W., & Stroether, C. R. A cross sequential study of age changes in cognitive behavior. *Psychological Bulletin*, 1968, 70, 671–680.

Schaie, K. W., & Willis, S. L. Life-span development: Implications for education. *Review of Educational Research*, 1978.

Sears, R. R., & Feldman, S. *The seven ages of man*. Los Altos, Calif.: William Kaufmann, 1973.

Sommers, T. When sexism meets ageism. *Modern Maturity*, October–November 1975, p. 60.

Sterns, H. L., & Alexander, R. A. Cohort, age, time of measurement: Biomorphic considerations. In N. Datan & H. W. Reese (Eds.), *Life-span developmental psychology: Dialectical perspectives on experimental research*. New York: Academic Press, 1977.

Sterns, H. L., & Sanders, R. E. Training and education in the elderly. In R. R. Turner & H. W. Reese (Eds.), *Life-span developmental psychology: Intervention*. New York: Academic Press, 1979, in press.

Tyler, L. E. Counseling girls and women in the year 2000. *Counseling girls and women over the life span*, National Vocational Guidance Association Monograph, 1972.

Mitchell, S., & Vegso, K. 1978. *Life-span planning: The choice is yours*. Akron, Ohio: The University of Akron, 1978.

Older Adult Higher Education: Stepchild and Cinderella

Edward F. Ansello
University of Maryland
and
Bert Hayslip, Jr.
North Texas State University

The involvement of older adults in higher education has been made difficult by a number of access and process variables. The former include such factors as a youth orientation and a production mentality antipathetic to attracting large numbers of older adults to higher education. The latter include factors such as negative expectations of ability with age and insufficient or misinterpreted research on lifelong learning. Both reduce the meaningfulness, direction, relevance, and the very number of offerings for older adults.

Access Variables

Adults, especially older adults, have not always been welcome in higher education. Their years have made them suspect; surely they were infected with some intellectual disease—mental deterioration, rigidity, unteachability. The probability of successful intervention—to make them more like their younger counterparts—would be small. It was judicious, higher education assured itself, not to become involved.

For the young, however, the expectations were different, if no less myopic. The province of higher education was youth. Armed with the latest information, we injected our young with knowledge. As Cox (1978, Note 1) observes:

Until very recently in this country, the attitude, both on the part of the public and even more tragically on the part of the higher educational community, toward our mission was that education, higher education, was a one-time in-

oculation against ignorance which we administered to young people between the ages of 18 and 22. And once having been inoculated, they were guaranteed to be free of the awful disease of ignorance for the remainder of their lives, and that was the basis upon which most of what we did, most of our activity, most of our budgets, and most of our manpower and personnel was expended.

As such, higher education has been a youth ghetto with rites of admission (high-school diploma), of transition (daytime classes, sororities and fraternities), and of exit (proms, senior week) specifically linked to youth. One consequence of this youth orientation has been, ironically, the postponement of adulthood *because* of higher education. The availability of further education meant more and more years spent in preparation for a life role. Another consequence of this outlook has been the implication that higher education has little or nothing to do with those who have already chosen life roles—older adults. As a result, adulthood and higher education did not meet.

Some self-feeding arguments have served to support this youth orientation. One is the premise that the proper function of higher education is to prepare people to *do* something. In its basest form, this argument equates higher education with vocational skill preparation. More commonly, it is assumed that higher education functions to develop the person to be a better producer, whether a professor, a therapist, or a C.P.A. As Withall (1974) notes, "Our educative enterprise, at all levels, seems geared less to the cultivation of human beings and their humanity as *ends* in themselves, and geared more to nurturing people as *means* to production of goods and services."

Another self-feeding argument is that the proper function of higher education is to prepare people to *be* something. That is, higher education is concerned with no less than the full development of the individual, sometimes vertically, as in a thorough education in some discipline, sometimes horizontally, as in the broad classical education.

Proponents of each of these arguments have maintained, apparently successfully, that the older adult has little or no place in their definitions of higher education. Supporters of the first position point out that older adults have occupied vocational positions for some time and that, if older adults seek education to aid vocational transitions, the return on the educational investment in subsequent production would seem small. This argument has, until recently, kept large numbers of older adults away, especially from professional schools. Holders of the second position assert that the period for maximizing human potential occurs early in life, in the adolescent years, according to some, in the twenties or early thirties according to others. Regardless, the older adult is thought to be beyond the period of optimum intellectual functioning. The assumption of the deceleration or cessation of mental growth after adolescence has been a major impediment to adult higher education (see Sterns and Mitchell, this volume).

Given the emphases on production and mental growth and the recency of our awareness of how misunderstood the older adult's mental processes have been, higher education's orientation toward youth seemed logical at the time, and limiting the access of older persons to academia appeared justifiable. Such activity was consonant with processes of implicit socialization operating within the larger social structure. Past youth, one was increasingly expected to phase out of interactions with organizations. The theory of disengagement reified this expectation.

As far as older people were concerned, traditional higher education was of no interest to them, nor was higher education interested in them. Bortner (1974) offers this incisive summary:

Margaret Clark (1968) . . . found that those old people who gave up or did not have high levels of achievement motivation were better adjusted and had fewer mental health problems. She and Anderson (1967) also made that beautiful distinction between adaptation and adjustment in a developmental context. By contrast, Ahammer and Baltes (1972) found that the desirability of achievement is still high in old people despite the fact that the middle-aged and young saw the need for achievement as less typical of or important to old people. Could it just possibly be that there is subtle, culturally based prodding? Is it that, to become an adjusted old person, one has to learn not to be ambitious and that one must learn not to learn? They have the job of unlearning, but what to learn in order to give new activities and abilities a cohesive role character and definition is less clear.

For older adults seeking continued if nontraditional education, new learning was to be found in the part-time Evening College Movement (ECM). Because older adults were outside the "mission" of the institution, the ECM was often treated condescendingly by "true" educators, often barely tolerated. Speaking from experience, Cox (1978, Note 1) notes that the attitude of many academicians was:

Well, as long as it really didn't matter very much and as long as most of these folks didn't really earn real degrees, and as long as they really didn't get in the way and since most of it happened after dark and was hidden away from the light of day, and since after all they did perform such humane and important services for higher education, for academe, such as providing summer employment as well as additional income in the evening, and as long certainly as the twain didn't meet, continuing education in the Evening College Movement went along on its own.

Adult education, in this way, was separate but not quite so equal as in the pre-1954 days of racially segregated education. Older learners were, and often still are, only included in daytime classes on a space-available basis; if the institution had nothing to lose, then the older adult was taken in.

Recently, however, access problems for older adults would seem to have been resolved. Higher education has apparently seen the light. Adult education may be coming in vogue, but one has reason to suspect the motivation. "True" higher education—that is, oriented to the young—is in a tenuous state, with enrollments and degree-seeking applications declining along with the demographic base of younger people. The pressures to maintain institutional size and to support tenured faculty may encourage higher education to open its doors to older adults just for the tuition monies they can provide.

Commenting recently on the uncertain political and economic future of California's system of public higher education, Lindsey (1978:1) of *The New York Times* reported the views of Patrick Callan, director of the state's Postsecondary Education Commission. "He warned of the possibility of growing competition among institutions for fewer available students, a 'harmful' internecine battle for money and pressure to change a system that in the past has often resisted change. There are already indications of the kind of struggle he forecast—competition for older students considered necessary to offset the decline, between the state's universities and the community colleges and high schools. They have traditionally handled 'adult education' courses."

Process Variables

Allowing, even encouraging, access to higher education for older adults has little to do with the educational process they experience once they enroll. In operational fact, access and process variables function separately, though they share a common philosophical heritage. That heritage is the negative expectation of ability with age.

This equation of mental deterioration with age affects considerations not only of entrance into higher education for older adults but also of course offerings, subject content, classroom procedure, evaluation, and other material factors related to teaching. For example, in some cases, courses labeled "for older adults" will be outside the standard curriculum or will have a watered-down content or intellectual challenge.

Paradoxically, higher-education circles have underemphasized research on adult learning and abilities. Perhaps the lack of research reflects how much the association of age and loss has been ingrained; that is, the issue has not been a controversial, researchable problem. As Christoffel (1977, Note 2) underlines, "It is worthwhile to note here that the major agency supporting education research, the National Institute on Education (NIE), has no organized research program to study the demand for and needs of older adults in lifelong learning." Examining further the broad area of education for adults, she notes the generally inconsistent commitment by the government, the nation's chief potential sponsor of education and research on lifelong learning. For example, within the U.S. Office of Education's Community Service and Continuing Education program, which seeks to involve higher-education resources in continuing education to solve community problems, none of the authorized funds for the section on special programs for the elderly have been allocated. Likewise, the Office of Education's major program serving adults, the Adult Education (State Grant) program, has seen a decline in involvement with older adults since 1972. The percentage of total participation by people over 45 years of age dropped from 20 percent in fiscal year 1972 to 18 percent and 15 percent in fiscal years 1974 and 1976. A more precipitous decline in program participation came among those over 35 years: from 39 percent to 31 percent between fiscal 1972 and fiscal 1976.

It seems feasible that expectations of mental decline pervade not only the education providers but also potential recipients. Until recently, social scientists and educators have uncritically accepted notions of universal decline in many areas of adult cognitive function (i.e., intelligence, learning, memory, problem solving). The result, of course, is an unrealistic picture of what the older student can and cannot do. This jaundiced view is inculcated early in the educational life span and often becomes incorporated into the older person's self-concept, frequently leading to a self-fulfilling prophecy of a lack of interest in and an inability for continued growth in adulthood. Brubaker and Powers (1976) underscore the importance of the adult self-concept to the acceptance or rejection of stereotypical views of older persons. We know that expressions of intellectual function grow and decline differentially through the life span, challenging the view of loss with increased age (Horn, 1970, 1976).

What were previously viewed as genuine losses in cognitive ability can now be at least partially explained by what many gerontologists prefer to call *noncognitive* or *performance-related* factors (Botwinick, 1973; Furry and Baltes, 1973). These factors may mask genuine growth and may overestimate decline with age. Such variables include: fatigue (Furry and Baltes, 1973), lowered motivation for success on traditional tasks (Hulicka, 1967; Knox, 1977), the use of meaningless or irrelevant materials (Howell, 1972), lack of practice or unfamiliarity with task requirements (Baltes and Labouvie, 1973; Goulet, 1972; Wittels, 1972), lack of reinforcements in the environment that would facilitate the growth of competence in adulthood (Baltes and Labouvie, 1973; Labouvie-Vief, 1976), and other factors. Pointedly when these noncognitive or performance-related factors are accounted for through experimental strategies, increased cognitive performance is found with older adults. Hultsch (1969), Hoyer, Labouvie, and Baltes (1973), and Meichenbaum (1974) demonstrated improved older adult performance after using, respectively, mnemonic devices in free-recall learning tests, practice and reinforcement in speeded tasks, and a self-instructional training program in problem-solving tasks.

Researchers have turned away from a model of adult development emphasizing irreversible decrement to one that accepts the reality of some loss with age but, nevertheless, assumes that such losses can be compensated by appropriate intervention strategies (Schaie and Gribbin, 1975).

This shift in the view of the older learner has had little impact in continuing and adult education. Few educators have concerned themselves with the nuts and bolts of applying the research on adult learning and cognition. These data have not been widely reflected in the design of programs for the older learner. Hultsch (1977) argues for a contextual, ecologically valid approach to aging and learning, one that would reflect a nondecremental position on age changes in performance. This more "organismically oriented" (Reese and Overton, 1970) approach toward adult learning has been evident in the recent concern for more humanistic (Wass and West, 1977), andragogical (Meyer, 1977) adult education. This view values the life experiences, uniqueness, and creative ability of the individual. It considers the person's feelings about what he or she is learning as well as the process of learning. It emphasizes self-education based on a respect for the diversity of possible environments for personal development and productivity (Cohen, 1977). It stresses the personal meaning of education, for example, as a vehicle for coping with problems relevant to the satisfaction of needs of the older learner. Wass and West (1977) observe that the need to feel adequate, to fulfill and develop oneself, may be even more important to the older person, who has been given negative societal attitudes toward aging that frustrate self-actualization, than to the younger adult or adolescent.

That higher education has not attended to such concerns is evidenced in the research on older adults and their values concerning education. Daniel, Templin, and Shearon (1977) found that students aged 60 and over viewed education along a social-cultural orientation rather than a vocational-monetary one. Reasons for continuing their education ranged from "to learn more things of interest" to "to meet interesting people" and "to improve my social life." March, Hooper, and Baum (1977) found over two-thirds of those sampled from various senior citizen groups to be uninterested in attending university classes. Many felt lifelong learning can occur outside the classroom, that "living is learning." Whereas Graney and Hays (1976) obtained results suggesting otherwise, March et al. (1977) failed to support the thesis that "education begets education." In their study of people aged 62 and over, however, Graney and Hays (1976) did find that those who were not interested in taking classes lacked information or were misinformed about course offerings and the intellectual and learning capacities of older persons. These findings suggest that current education programming for older adults is out of step with the need and value orientations of the present cohort of older persons.

Regarding higher education and older adults, Hultsch (1974) suggests that we have tended to take an interventionist approach modeled on making older people more like their younger counterparts.

I would suggest that, in the case of interventions into the aging process we have focused largely on the goals of culture rather than the clientele. It is probably reasonable to suggest that our culture views aging as a process of decrement and deprivation. Aging is seen as synonymous with physical and intellectual decline, personal and social inadequacy, and economic and cultural deprivation. Even given an optimistic position concerning the modifiability of these decrements, such a view of aging has led to an emphasis on alleviation as a goal with the behavior of young adults as the criterion of optimum functioning. Again, the assumption has been that the behaviors exhibited by older adults are dysfunctional while those exhibited by younger adults are functional. Schaie (1973) has argued cogently that it is just such a view of aging that has, in fact, been causing a major share of the problem. He concludes that we cannot change the behavior of the aged until society changes its view of aging. This leads to the suggestion that the target of interventions should be young adults and particularly middle-aged adults who are usually the decision-makers in our society. At the very least, it is time to consider the goals of the clientele as we develop intervention programs. It is no longer reasonable to label older adults as relatively deprived and proceed to develop

programs to alleviate this condition. It is worthwhile to note that early child-
hood education fell exactly into this trap. In this field there are significant
efforts under way to involve the clientele, particularly parents, in the interven-
tion process (Peters, 1973, Note 3). To date, gerontologists have made little
effort in this direction.

At this point in our development, we can conceive of higher education as an intervention into a system. It has tended to intervene in a manner collaborative with the self-feeding system that minimized and frustrated continued human development through the lifespan, that is, by limiting access and by subscribing to educational and research processes substantiating the assumption of cognitive inability with age.

To be an effective, needed intervention for older adults, higher education must not do certain things. Older adult education should not intervene to make the performance of older persons more like the performance of younger. This, as Hultsch (1974) notes, is the concept of "relative deprivation," and it assumes that the behaviors of older adults are dysfunctional. Nor should older adult education attempt to perpetuate the equation of competence and productivity employed so frequently as the model of higher education for traditional (18 to 22 year old) students. This mentality seems especially inappropriate when ascribed to older adult education.

In a related vein, Canestrari (1974:52) says:

In my experience with basically intact but anxious elderly patients, I am less impressed with the importance of whatever changes have taken place in cognitive functioning as compared with the clearly stated and often heart-breaking statements about feelings of worthlessness and a sense of uselessness. From a clinician's point of view, what becomes striking is that the problem is not rooted in old age but in the life style and personal orientation which is developed during the course of the life span. The at-risk population, from my point of view, are the individuals whose worth is linked to concepts of mastery in the external world and whose orientation is basically obsessive-compulsive in nature. Small failings in capacity become magnified in such individuals with consequent depression and anxiety. The middle-aged population of today may show greater proneness to this process than today's elderly who were reared in a more leisurely environment and whose own contact with the aged was probably not as contaminated by current values.

Instead of intervening to relieve relative deprivation or to perpetuate the production mentality, adult higher education should intervene to assert its place in the self-developmental lifelong learning process (Sterns and Mitchell, this volume). It should attempt to modify the notion that competence is defined by productivity. It should shift its focus to include personal-affective target behaviors as well as the cognitive. As Looft (1973) observes, such an attitude change requires elevating the importance of such skills as introspection, interpersonal relations, emotional expressiveness, and other affective behaviors. This task is made more difficult by the fact that older adults have already internalized our cultural bias toward cognitive activities in education.

This shift in attitude can, of course, be accomplished with effort. Older adults would seem, in yet another underestimation, to have far greater internal locus of control than attributed to them. In one case (Driver and Ansello, 1975, Note 4) lower (more internal) Introverted-Extroverted Attitude Scores were found among institutionalized elderly in Virginia than among a separate study's undergraduate sample at the University of Maryland.

Given at least the likelihood of substantial internal locus of control among older people, we might ask ourselves if the adult higher education "offered" them is compatible with self-direction, self-control, and self-decision-making. Could this be one reason why, as March et al. (1977) found, so many older people stay away from higher education? What role does the clientele play in fashioning the intervention processes and content of adult education?

In addition to being compatible with self-direction and self-control, adult higher education must also foster self-developmental processes. Monge (1974) states that "educational intervention . . . must be aimed at assisting individual adults in coming to some optimum degree of understanding of self and society consistent with the satisfaction of the needs of both." Such understanding would require teaching aimed at the cognitive and the affective-emotional processes of the older adult. It would assist the older person to effect change by understanding the processes of change (problem identification, evaluation, delineation of options, alternative strategies, cognitive dissonance, coping skills), and the contexts precipitating change (loss, widowhood, leisure time, stereotyping, underassessment of self, processes of aging).

As yet, few educators have actually translated into practice what we currently know about adult learning—for example, its plasticity, its continuity, its shift from content to process, and the expansion of its base to include affective and emotional as well as cognitive factors. Few have translated these parameters of adult learning into something usable for the practitioner designing educational programs for adults. Birren and Woodruff (1973) emphasize training teachers in lifespan development to effect attitude changes toward aging early in life; age integration of classes and training in lifespan development at the elementary, secondary, and undergraduate levels; organizing classes by interest groups instead of age groups; and encouraging affective and motivational experience rather than simply the development of cognitive skills in the classroom.

Gounard and Hulicka (1977) apply what is known about the effects of both cognitive and noncognitive factors on adult learning (see also Arenberg and Robertson-Tchabo, 1977; Woodruff and Walsh, 1975) to developing a variety of teaching and learning techniques designed to compensate for the negative effects these factors have on performance. Knox (1977) makes similar recommendations: using intentional learning activities to cope with life crises and adjustment, making role models with desired competence more available, and creating a setting in which adults feel free to explore their own educational objectives. He advocates linking organized knowledge and personal experiences as one way by which to foster a more positive outlook toward learning. Other methods for adult higher educators to facilitate growth include: (1) emphasizing abilities and life experiences; (2) acknowledging several distinct motivational typologies among adult learners; (3) clarifying the structural aspects of what is being taught; (4) making the learning experience salient in the older person's life; (5) pacing learning individually; (6) using varied learning resources like books, tapes, films, or experts; and (7) providing immediate reinforcements and feedback about the kinds of changes resulting from any kind of educational activity.

Higher-education researchers can investigate ways of: (1) improving instructional techniques to bring learning closer to home; (2) exploring new careers for older workers; (3) retraining older teachers to meet new community educational needs; (4) using retired professors in the design and conduct of older-adult education programs; and (5) creating older-adult peer teacher corps in higher education to provide counsel and to design meaningful curricula for older adults.

In these ways a positive learning environment would be created in higher education for lifelong learning. It might happen that some of the self-developmental orientation of the older adult educational endeavor might spill over to humanize the entire higher education milieu. Despite constriction, condescension, and negative expectation of ability with age applied by others in the higher education community, the Evening College Movement has flourished because it considers its clientele as part of a joint learning process. It has provided content relevent to the learner while emphasizing meaningfulness and self-development. The rest of us in higher education have something to learn from this experience.

Notes

1. Cox, J. W. Remarks to the State Board for Higher Education conference on continuing education. Annapolis, Md. January 19, 1978.

2. Christoffel, P. *The older adult and federal programs for life-long learning.* December 1977 (mimeograph).

3. Peters, D. L. *The decision to intervene: Early childhood education.* Paper presented at the Conference on Applied Human Development: Issues in Intervention. Pennsylvania State University, 1973.

4. Driver, J. D., & Ansello, E. F. *Personality differences in the elderly as a function of type and length of residence.* Paper presented at the 21st Annual Meeting of the Southeastern Psychological Association, Atlanta, March 1975.

References

Ahammer, I. M., & Baltes, P. B. Objective versus perceived age differences in personality: How do adolescents, adults, and older people view themselves and others? *Journal of Gerontology,* 1972, 27, 46–51.

Arenberg, D., & Robertson-Tchabo, E. Learning and aging. In J. E. Birren & K. W. Schaie (Eds.), *Handbook of the psychology of aging.* New York: Van Nostrand Reinhold, 1977.

Baltes, P. B. and Labouvie, G. V. Adult development of intellectual performance: Description, explanation, and modification. In C. Eisdorfer & M. P. Lawton (Eds.), *The psychology of adult development and aging.* Washington, D.C.: American Psychological Association, 1973.

Birren, J. E., & Woodruff, D. Human development over the life span through education. In P. B. Baltes & K. W. Schaie (Eds.), *Life-span developmental psychology: Personality and socialization.* New York: Academic Press, 1973.

Bortner, R. W. Systems implications of improvements in adult learning. In D. F. Hultsch & R. W. Bortner (Eds.), *Interventions in learning: The individual and society.* A monograph in the Continuing Explorations: Papers in Continuing Education Series. Pennsylvania State University, 1974.

Botwinick, J. *Aging and behavior.* New York: Springer, 1973.

Brubaker, T. H., & Powers, E. A. The stereotype of "old": A review and alternative approach. *Journal of Gerontology,* 1976, *31,* 441–447.

Canestrari, R. E. Teaching adults: Some practical perspectives. In D. F. Hultsch & R. W. Bortner (Eds.), *Interventions in learning: The individual and society.* A monograph in the Continuing Explorations: Papers in Continuing Education Series. Pennsylvania State University, 1974.

Clark, M. The anthropology of aging: A new era for study of culture and personality. In B. L. Neugarten (Ed.), *Middle age and aging.* Chicago: University of Chicago Press, 1968.

Clark, M., & Anderson, B. *Culture and aging: An anthropological study of older Americans.* Springfield, Ill.: Charles C. Thomas, 1967.

Cohen, D. An exposition of the concept of lifelong self-education. *Educational Gerontology,* 1977, *2,* 157–162.

Daniel, D. E., Templin, R. G., & Shearon, R. W. The value orientations of older adults toward education. *Educational Gerontology,* 1977, *2,* 33–42.

Furry, C. A., & Baltes, P. B. The effect of age differences in ability-extraneous performance variables on the assessment of intelligence in children, adults, and the elderly. *Journal of Gerontology,* 1973, *28,* 73–80.

Goulet, L. R. New directions for research on aging and retention. *Journal of Gerontology,* 1972, *27,* 52–60.

Gounard, B. R., & Hulicka, I. M. Maximizing learning efficiency in later life: A cognitive problem-solving approach. *Educational Gerontology,* 1977, *2,* 417–427.

Graney, M. J., & Hays, W. C. Senior students: Higher education after age 62. *Educational Gerontology,* 1976, *1,* 343–359.

Horn, J. L. Organization of data on life-span development of human abilities. In L. R. Goulet & P. B. Baltes (Eds.), *Life-span developmental psychology: Theory and research.* New York: Academic Press, 1970.

Horn, J. L. Human abilities: A review of the research and theory in the early 1970s. *Annual Review of Psychology,* 1976, *27,* 437–486.

Howell, S. C. Familiarity and complexity in perceptual recognition. *Journal of Gerontology,* 1972, *27,* 364–371.

Hoyer, W. J., Labouvie, G. V., & Baltes, P. B. Modification of response speed deficits and intellectual performance in the elderly. *Human Development*, 1973, *16*, 233–243.

Hulicka, I. M. Age changes and age differences in memory functioning: Proposals for research. *Gerontologist*, 1967, *7*, 45–52.

Hultsch, D. F. Adult age differences in the organizations of free recall. *Developmental Psychology*, 1969, *1*, 673.

Hultsch, D. F. Why are we trying to teach adults? In D. F. Hultsch & R. W. Bortner (Eds.), *Interventions in learning: The individual and society*. A monograph in the Continuing Explorations: Papers in Continuing Education Series. Pennsylvania State University, 1974.

Hultsch, D. F. Changing perspectives on basic research in adult learning and memory. *Educational Gerontology*, 1977, *2*, 367–382.

Hultsch, D. F., & Bortner, R. W. (Eds.). *Interventions in learning: The individual and society*. A monograph in the Continuing Explorations: Papers in Continuing Education Series. Pennsylvania State University, 1974.

Knox, A. B. *Adult development and learning*. San Francisco: Jossey-Bass, 1977.

Labouvie-Vief, G. W. Toward optimizing cognitive competence in later life. *Educational Gerontology*, 1976, *1*, 75–92.

Lindsey, R. Model California college system troubled by dropping enrollment. *The New York Times*, May 29, 1978, p. 1.

Looft, W. R. Socialization and personality throughout the life span: An examination of contemporary psychological approaches. In P. B. Baltes & K. W. Schaie (Eds.), *Life-span developmental psychology: Personality and socialization*. New York: Academic Press, 1973.

March, G. B., Hooper, J. O., & Baum, J. Life-span education and the older adult: Living is learning. *Educational Gerontology*, 1977, *2*, 163–172.

Meichenbaum, D. Self-instructional strategy training. A cognitive prosthesis for the aged. *Human Development*, 1974, *17*, 273–280.

Meyer, S. L. Andragogy and the adult learner. *Educational Gerontology*, 1977, *2*, 115–122.

Monge, R. H. What are we trying to teach adults? In D. F. Hultsch & R. W. Bortner (Eds.), *Intervention in learning: The individual and society*. A monograph in the Continuing Explorations: Papers in Continuing Education Series. Pennsylvania State University, 1974.

Reese, H., & Overton, W. Models of development and theories of development. In L. R. Goulet & P. B. Baltes (Eds.), *Life-span developmental psychology: Theory and research*. New York: Academic Press, 1970.

Schaie, K. W. Methodological problems in descriptive developmental research on adulthood and aging. In J. R. Nesselroade & H. Reese (Eds.), *Life-span developmental psychology: Methodological issues*. New York: Academic Press, 1973.

Schaie, K. W., & Gribbin, K. Adult development and aging. *Annual Review of Psychology*, 1975, *26*, 65–96.

Wass, H., & West, C. A. A humanistic approach to the education of older persons. *Educational Gerontology*, 1977, *2*, 407–416.

Withall, J. Adult learners and goals for change: A learning rationale, value system, and instructional conditions hypothesized to enhance the learning of older adults. In D. F. Hultsch & R. W. Bortner (Eds.), *Interventions in learning: The individual and society.* A monograph in the Continuing Explorations: Papers in Continuing Education Series. Pennsylvania State University, 1974.

Wittels, I. Age and stimulus meaningfulness in paired-associate learning. *Journal of Gerontology*, 1972, *27*, 372–375.

Woodruff, D., & Walsh, D. Research in adult learning: The individual. *Gerontologist*, 1975, *15*, 424–430.

What If the Consumer Holds Us Accountable?

Selma Zarakov
Palomar College

Consumers of education in junior and community colleges come under two categories: the traditional student, who arrives at this educational marketplace directly from high school, and the nontraditional student, who, except for being older, is difficult to characterize. For example, the 1977–1982 California Community College Five Year Plan describes some of the nontraditional students as physically, economically, socially, and culturally disadvantaged. Specific accounting includes reentry women, minorities, inmates, and the elderly. In addition, the ranks of nontraditional education consumers are supplemented by retired military personnel and by graduates of various levels of higher education who are seeking updated vocational certificates for licensing requirements. The California Community College Five Year Plan reports that, although these students are described as nontraditional, a term implying a deviation from the norm, they are in reality the majority of junior and community college enrollments.

Now engaged in direct service to large numbers of older students, the junior and community college must be aware of the characteristics of its older consumers and of the image it is projecting to them. Whereas the traditional younger enrollees are often dependent, one generation removed from the taxpayer, nontraditional older students purchase their own education directly through taxes or fees. Typically, the traditional younger student spends no more than two years at the junior or community college before transferring or earning a degree or certificate. The older student does not follow this pattern, but returns year after year to choose eclectically from among academic, vocational, personal growth, recreation, and retirement classes. Community service programs, or noncredit classes, contain large numbers of nontraditional students.

Older students tend to participate selectively in junior and community college education. They choose coursework for its quality and relevance and decide on an institution for its efficiency of operation, student services, educational philosophy, and faculty attitudes—more than for its "name." Self-supporting and long experienced at managing a budget amidst inflation and rising costs, older students most likely have a "consumer" orientation to education. We must be aware that the nontraditional, older student, who is knowledgeable about the deflated value of his earnings, will critically appraise the value he receives for his tax dollar at the community college.

From a consumer frame of reference, however, we see that too frequently junior and community colleges have done little to attract or accommodate the older student. The shortcomings are numerous, though the saliency of each requires further research. For example, presbyopia or blurred vision is common after age 40. When preparing college catalogs, brochures, and forms, junior and community colleges do not seem to consider this condition. Application forms are particularly notorious. Likewise, most health services at the colleges do not include glaucoma testing or diabetes and blood pressure screening, which are common medical procedures elsewhere for people over 35.

Tutoring and learning centers at junior and community colleges are primarily first-career oriented. Older audiences need career change advice, vocational supplement jobs, and classes in preparation for leisure and retirement.

Night classes pose special problems for older students. The time needed for adult eyes to adjust from bright light to dark increases with age. It may be that older people attending night classes and leaving bright classrooms for the subdued lighting of walkways and parking areas will be more subject to accident. Older people also seem more vulnerable to attack, and good security measures are important for people on campus after dark.

Obviously, the relative importance of each of these factors needs to be researched as it relates to junior and community college participation by older students. Colleges can attempt to identify in the present system some of the deterrents to enrollment and continued attendance by nontraditional students. We can facilitate the processes of applying, registering, enrolling, and scheduling classes. Expanding curriculum is not the only response toward expanding audiences.

Improvement in publicity is fundamental. Unfortunately, our traditional methods of advertising, publicizing, and operating can discourage the nontraditional audience from entering our doors. Many adults living within a few miles of community colleges are unaware of the classes, programs, and activities available for them, in part because junior and community colleges still promote themselves in a style aimed at high-school graduates.

What of the youth-oriented format of our institutions? Community colleges have already made many changes in response to the attendance of nontraditional students: evening and weekend classes, short-term classes, an increase in noncredit classes, extended degrees, an increase in the number of classes challenged by more experienced students, and extended off-campus activities. Nevertheless, the formats for registering and for advertising college activities are essentially youth-oriented in that they address high-school students already acquainted with the purpose of the community college and its procedures.

The explanations of programs and activities in the catalog are directed toward the high-school student. The introductions of catalogs typically describe sports activities, health services, and advice appropriate to recent high school graduates. Our physical education departments include classes for all age students, but our athletic programs and competitions are segregated for the young.

Fundamental changes are called for in college procedures. Perhaps two separate application forms are necessary. It is an affront to an older student who is coming to the junior or community college solely to take a single course in ceramics to be faced with a four-page application designed for high-school students. Questions about which parent the student is living with, the student's major subject area, academic records from previous schools, and peripheral information regarding student activities and honors are at best irrelevant and can be threatening to older students. Questions on mother's maiden name, father's occupation, source of financial support, athletic achievements, transcript and grade-point average, all schools attended since eighth grade, extracurricular activities, and previous academic history may reinforce the nontraditional older students' feeling that the campus is off limits to mature students and that they are out of place.

Our data banks probably contain much erroneous information supplied by impatient students of all ages, who are anxious to fill in the blanks and get to class. If this information is indeed necessary to the planners of higher education overall, and to those in higher education increasingly likely to have older students, I suggest that we accommodate our forms to the realities of the students.

Older student consumers are already challenging the educational system. It is in our own best interest to anticipate consumer concerns. Their impact on junior and community college education is going to grow. At least 15 percent of Americans are over 60 years old; of those over age 60, at least 60 percent of the men and 70 percent of the women have not completed high school. Yet, higher education is the next step and the only avenue for some of them.

The new adult market can fill empty seats, but first educators must make efforts to attract that audience. The need is there. With dynamic changes in fields of expertise, those who have vocations and professions must keep their education current. This trend to upgrade professional information indicates an increase in the education market. Retired people are discovering courses ranging from "Money Management and Pensions" to "Analyzing Society through Film." Since older students often view the dynamics of society from their own cohort center of reference, this new interaction of young and old may increase understanding in both directions and may bring older students into the current mainstream of activity.

Orienting more toward an older consumer audience may produce awkward periods of adjustment. Besides the previously mentioned sensitivites to value and the inappropriateness of some practices and procedures, other problems may present themselves. One is the lack of understanding among the faculty of the needs and motivations of nontraditional older students. Older students may initially say, "I can't do this," perhaps reflecting a belief that they are too old to learn. An uninterested faculty only fosters these feelings. The greater use of emeritus professors might ease this problem in that they are likely to be more sensitive to the issues of older students. Similarly, greater participation by older students in student government may also effect change.

Some major changes in higher education during the last ten years do address the special learning needs of older adults. Credit for life experience, independent study, off-campus locations, and other flexibilities have benefited these students. Some institutions, however, remain untouched by these innovations, or they segregate older-adult programs so that older adults do not become a part of main campus activities.

With the increasing numbers of older students, particularly those over age 60, it would seem advisable for us in higher education to consult with the emerging field of gerontology for information about personality, needs, and learning characteristics of older persons. With traditional student numbers on the decline, the junior and community college sectors must adapt to a new nontraditional audience with concern for both the producer and the consumer. If they do not, they may find themselves out of business.

Education for the Aging:
A Model for Developing Institutions

David Demko
Delta College

In education, the first step toward service to the older population may necessarily be something other than developing special programs for older people. The first step should be to facilitate the participation process, that is, to determine what obstacles keep older adults away from existing services and to develop a comprehensive strategy to remove these obstacles. This approach will help ensure that efforts to serve the elderly become an integrated part of the college mission. Special programs may be developed later.

This paper considers the following questions: Are the adult programs of one educational institution appropriate for another institution? Who are the elderly? What are their individual and group needs? What is the role of higher education in meeting those needs? For instance, what kinds of activities are appropriate for education providers? What should be the domain of other service providers in recreation, social service, and health?

The field of educational gerontology is rapidly expanding in content and complexity. Whereas a number of independently successful programs exist, it becomes difficult to predict success when programs are replicated in new locations and when overall efforts within the field appear to be fragmented. Therefore, this paper addresses some obvious issues and some obvious questions related to developing institutions (colleges and universities developing new programs in gerontology).

The first issue is called getting beyond the cliché. Developing institutions must recognize that "senior awareness" is not a passing fancy but a trend that is here to stay. Our efforts must not be perceived just as offering something nice for older folks to do. This increasing awareness should be perceived for what it is—a wave of the future that promises to increasingly influence all service providers. Churches can expect to serve older members; social workers can expect to interface with older clients; educators can expect to serve older learners; and the marketplace will no doubt continue to gear up to older consumer groups. Therefore, in the developing institution we must first recognize the legitimacy of the area.

The second issue is the isolationist philosophy. The most frequent comment from developing institutions is: We need a program for older people. We need to ask ourselves, Is what we already offer so irrelevant that it is in no way meaningful to older people? It is important to avoid any philosophy that might isolate the older population from existing service efforts.

This leads to the third issue, the program trap. To skirt this trap, we first review what services are currently provided and how these services are provided. Second, we ask ourselves why older adults do not participate in these programs. In other words, we identify the barriers preventing participation and develop strategies for removing them.

Therefore, education might serve the aging by not developing a program; this may come later. By addressing these issues during the initial stages of development, we begin to ensure that services to the older population will become natural and logical extensions of the college mission.

Basic Questions and Basic Concepts

Service providers have entered the field of aging so rapidly that they tend to overlook the full development of such basic questions as: What's the first step? What needs exist? How might educators respond? For instance, we should ask ourselves whether the older-adult programs of one community college are appropriate for another college or whether we are comparing apples and oranges in sharing information. If we succeed, do we know why? There can be no real answers to these questions until service providers define some basic concepts.

Facilitating Participation

The senior citizen is a myth that we have created, and service providers frequently oversimplify their definition of this complex target population. The question has traditionally been, Should a community college have a senior citizens program? The question we most need to ask is, Why don't older adults participate in education in the first place? Specifically, the need is to identify barriers and remove them.

An aspect of this approach distinguishes it from traditional approaches. Rather than focusing on specific types of programs, the approach should be a strategy of access—a way to facilitate the participation process itself. The end result of a plan to remove these barriers to participation is not a senior citizen program but an overall, comprehensive strategy for increasing the access of older adults to higher education.

It takes energy to overcome barriers, and the older consumer may doubt whether the service is worth it. Barriers are external (environmental) and internal (motivational). To remove external barriers we need strategies that create the opportunity for involvement; to remove internal barriers, strategies that develop motivation for involvement. There are five specific barriers.

The Economic Barrier   Most retirees' incomes are fixed, but inflation is not. As the cost of living rises, greater proportions of their incomes must be spent on the basic necessities of food, shelter, and clothing. This results in strict limitations on opportunities for personal growth and socializing which generally isolate the older individual.

Removing the economic barrier calls for establishing a tuition policy that provides for complete, partial, or sliding-scale reduction of tuition for older learners. A new tuition policy can be implemented in several ways. Reduced fees on a "space available" basis is an option for institutions concerned about free-tuition students competing with full-time students for classroom seats. Another possibility is a revolving fund. Fees paid by older students are partially or totally placed in a grant fund that, in turn, is made available to subsidize the education of older students who cannot afford to pay tuition.

The Geographical Barrier   Mobility often presents problems for older adults, limiting their opportunities for involvement. The cost of gasoline and car maintenance, increasing loss of physical function, and decline in sensory acuity not only limit older adults' actual ability to transport themselves from one place to another, but also significantly affect their perception of personal mobility. Minor obstacles may appear to be major, thereby making short distances appear long and routine directions complex. Mobility has special significance for the older woman. Two-thirds of the older population are women, and seven-tenths of all older women are widows. A widow is often left with an automobile whose maintenance was always the husband's job. Her use of the car may, therefore, decline, and mobility may become an increasingly complex obstacle.

Removing the geographical barrier calls for decentralizing the college's existing service delivery system to include off-campus sites in areas with high concentrations of elderly people. In many communities a network of neighborhood facilities serves the elderly; for example, nutrition sites, social service centers, recreation clubs, church affiliated senior centers, high-rise apartment complexes, and nursing homes. The length of the list generally depends on the size and elderly population of the geographic area. Most important, these facilities are accessible to various groups of older adults. Local resources that can help identify these facilities include city and county councils on aging, YWCA and YMCA, church organizations, libraries, area agencies on aging, metropolitan housing authorities, and community service directories. The first step then is to identify geographic areas of large elderly population. The most current census data are a good tool for accomplishing this. Next, compare how well the existing service delivery system of the college reaches those areas. Then try to use existing neighborhood facilities to fill gaps in the delivery system.

The Psychological Barrier Traditional youth-oriented concepts of education make it difficult for older adults to relate to the services of higher education. This may explain why needs assessments conducted by colleges may yield data that indicate a low interest in education among the older population. Education is generally perceived as a "life stage" that one enters, passes through, and exits at some point with no thought of returning.

Removing the psychological barrier calls for emphasis on eliminating older adults' perception of education as they experienced it in their youth. Educational programs such as course offerings and community services should be practical and informative so that older learners can apply the information to their day-to-day living situation. Programs should use informal group discussion techniques to allow the older learner to participate not only as a receiver of information but also as a provider of information, sharing meaningful life experiences. Programs of flexible length allow the older learner to sample coursework before making a commitment for an entire semester. Weekend programs and short-term residential institutes have proved quite popular as a sampling tool for the older population. Programs should also provide for flexibility in the grading system to allow initial participation at low risk. Grading may be unimportant to older learners, whose educational goals are often personal rather than career oriented.

The Sociological Barrier "Too old to learn" and "you can't teach an old dog new tricks" are only two of the many negative remarks we are likely to hear about the older learner. Moral support for returning adults is often lacking since family and friends view such participation as impossible and inappropriate for older adults. Circumstances such as retirement and widowhood, besides our youth-oriented society, tend to isolate the older adult from the mainstream of life. Therefore, older adults who choose to participate in formal educational settings are highly visible and may feel out of place when they first return to higher education.

Removing the sociological barrier involves developing an awareness of the extensive negativism about later adulthood and human aging. Stereotypes are held by young and old alike. Social isolation of the elderly also tends to perpetuate the misconceptions of aging because people lack a positive, firsthand interaction with the aged and the experience of aging. Therefore, emphasis must be placed on creating opportunities that make older-adult participation in higher education visible and normal. Furthermore, efforts to inform service providers and the general public about the normal processes of human aging should portray the personal growth as well as the losses of aging. This can be accomplished through effective inservice training for service providers, forums on aging for the public, and mass media publicity about existing educational activities involving older adults. Increased visibility of older learners will create an atmosphere that enhances their acceptability within an educational setting.

The Educational Barrier   The delivery system in higher education is usually predicated on the model developed for learners 18 to 25 years old. Although this barrier relates to the psychological barrier, it involves more. For example, educational institutions are geared to degree-granting goals, to delivery of services within fixed times, and to serving clients whose major life activity is the pursuit of academic coursework.

Removing the educational barrier involves the concepts that education must provide lifelong service and the opportunity for flexible participation and that educators must account for prior nonacademic learning experiences. Services must also be adaptable to the special needs and life styles of older adults. These concepts are not new, and they basically involve three components of education: course content, delivery system, and instructional technique.

By varying these three components, traditional services can be adapted to meet a variety of needs of special target groups. Various models are available. Continuing education units involve innovative course content, delivery system, and accreditation, although instructional technique may vary or remain the same as in traditional offerings. Credit by examination involves innovative delivery system and instructional technique for established course content. Home study programs involve an innovative delivery system and instructional technique for established course content. The model of experiential learning involves innovative instructional technique, but the course content and delivery system remain the same.

This incomplete list provides another framework for adapting education to special groups through the manipulation of the three basic component variables. It is important to note that the programs listed are not mutually exclusive. By applying this framework to educational services for older adults, we can begin to appreciate the variety of service possibilities that exist only in the area of course offerings.

The removal of barriers to better serve the older population has a major consequence for education. Such an approach requires service providers to attend to the participation process and to develop ways to facilitate it. Otherwise they may become initially and exclusively involved in attempting to develop a "senior citizen" program based on a somewhat global definition of what is actually a complex target population. By removing barriers, we can integrate the elderly as a natural and logical extension of the college mission.

Building a Program

Once we have begun to facilitate participation in existing services, the next step is to build a program based on needs. Traditional attempts at needs assessment have relied heavily on surveys, which tend to yield incomplete, if not confusing, results. The usual response to need surveys is: We (the older adults) do not want or need educational services. However, the high degree of participation by older adults in programs with which they are familiar and comfortable refutes the survey data. Therefore, we might assume that need surveys are not always effective when administered to adults who have a traditional concept of education. Need surveys alone, therefore, may not produce accurate results. An alternative source for determining need might be the existing body of literature pertaining to more or less universal conditions and circumstances associated with the normal process of aging. Several current models provide examples of needs of the older population, and the application of these models may begin to bridge the gap between theory and practice.

Life Cycle Perspective By using admittedly arbitrary age groupings within the older population, we can identify "clusterings" of circumstances that are somewhat consistent with each age grouping. From an amended version of Robert Benedict's *Life Cycle Perspective* (Manney, 1975) we find the following groups and circumstances. Individuals between 40 and 50 years of age may be faced with the task of developing new ways to relate within the family unit even when it is dispersed. Between 50 and 65 years of age older persons may face retirement, departure of children, onset of chronic health problems, and role changes. Those between 65 and 75 years of age may face mandatory retirement, fixed income, widowhood, death of friends, loss of coworkers, decline in sensory acuity, relocation, and setting new goals. Those between 76 and 85 years of age may face chronic problems as well as loss of strength. From 86 to death older persons may face critical income problems and dependence.

Although the above circumstances represent "threads" running through late adulthood rather than "life stages," they help us appreciate the diversity within the older population. Many more subgroups could surely be identified if one chose to use variables other than chronological age. The significance of this for higher education is that each subgroup has distinctly different program needs. The "senior citizen" is not a single or simple entity.

Adaptive Tasks According to the Clark-Anderson model (Manney, 1975), the older adult must accomplish five adaptive tasks to adjust to age. Briefly, the individual must admit that aging involves limitation, change physical activities and social roles, find new ways to fulfill needs, develop new criteria for self-evaluation, and establish new values and goals for life.

The need model identifies several areas where the older learner may require information and new skills. There is no reason why higher education could not design learning experiences to meet these needs.

Need Areas McClusky (1975) discusses a range of need areas from survival, through maintenance, to personal growth and beyond. These need areas are: (1) coping—the necessity for older adults to become able to cope independently with the life situation as well as relate meaningfully to others; (2) expressive—the need to engage in activities for the sake of activity itself; (3)

contributive—the desire of older adults to be useful and of service to others; (4) influence—the need of older adults to exert influence on the circumstances of living and the world around them; (5) transcendence—the need to achieve a sense of fulfillment accompanying a process by which older adults become less and less physical beings and more and more spiritual.

The major focus of existing community service programs appears to be meeting expressive needs. This focus not only circumvents coping needs, but also tends to neglect the other need areas.

Developmental Tasks Havighurst (1972) describes the developmental tasks of later maturity as: (1) disengaging from some of the active roles of middle age while leaving open the decision to engage or reengage in other roles such as those of grandparent, citizen, association member, and friend; (2) adjusting to a retirement income; (3) adjusting to decreasing physical strength and health; (4) dealing with bereavement and possibly living alone; (5) maintaining contact with grown children while remaining independent; and (6) developing interests and nurturing relationships with others outside of the family that help maintain self-esteem.

The application of these well-known needs models in educational programs for the older population could serve to develop a common grid within which community colleges could communicate programming ideas revolving around accepted need concepts. As a supplement or alternative to the needs survey, these need models could serve as a basis for designing "sampler" programs, which could serve as a point of entry for older adults by introducing them to higher education.

The Appropriate Role for Educators

With the increased awareness of older people, with the tremendous amount of programming activity in the field of aging, and with the diversity and complexity of agencies and funding sources in the field of aging, the various service models—recreation, health, social service, education—can readily become confused.

What is the appropriate role for education in providing services to the older population? Service providers in education need to ask this question because the continuance of an initial programming effort depends upon how well that service fits the mission of the college. If the program is not sanctioned as an educational service, it may eventually be discontinued.

A college might develop on-campus meal programs, information and referral, senior recreation centers, or outreach. But can these activities be sustained within higher education? What should educational service providers be doing, and what things should be the domain of other service models?

Today, the field of education for older adults is in a developmental stage. At this point service providers might adopt a limiting, albeit coherent role, which could later be expanded as the field grows. The educational model might be as follows. Education involves providing information, which includes the communication of skills, facts, and ideas. As service providers in education we should ask ourselves, What are the skills, facts, and ideas required by the various subgroups of the older population in order for the individuals within those groups to solve their own problems, make their own decisions, and adjust to their own aging process? Through the clarification of the educational model, the interplay with other service models will be less confusing.

Summary

The first step toward service to the older population may not necessarily require the development of a special program for older people. The first step should be to facilitate participation by determining what obstacles keep older adults away from existing services and developing a comprehensive strategy to remove them. This approach will help ensure that efforts to serve the elderly become an integral and integrated part of the college mission. Development of specialized programs may come later. And when they do, the needs models might well serve as a developmental guide.

Since the field of aging is at a developmental stage, much is being done. But educational service providers need to stop a minute and clarify their concepts of the older population. Who are the elderly? What needs do they have? What must our role be? With the use of universal concepts of target groups, needs, and roles by educational service providers, then information sharing among schools will become more meaningful. What one college develops will have meaning to another because each school will be cognizant of where a particular programming effort fits into the total strategy. Only then can education experience a cumulative growth in the field by building on success and understanding failure.

The purpose of encouraging developing institutions to look beyond the mere creation of courses and services for older adults is to acknowledge the underlying rationale of education for the later years. The key aspect is not what we offer, but why it is offered, and the potential impact that education has on the adult's journey into continued self-development in the later years.

References

Havighurst, R. *Developmental tasks and education.* New York: David McKay, 1972.

Manney, J. *Aging in American society.* Institute of Gerontology, University of Michigan-Wayne State University, Ann Arbor, 1975.

McClusky, H. *Education for the aging.* Institute of Gerontology, University of Michigan-Wayne State University, Ann Arbor, 1975 (manuscript).

Drama and the Problems of Aging

Michael D. Patrick
University of Missouri-Rolla

Although the University of Missouri-Rolla (UMR) has no drama department, it is aware of the strong interest in live drama in south-central Missouri. Because of this interest, the UMR Department of Humanities decided to experiment with drama as an extension activity to involve humanists with the general community. The basic idea was to produce a series of plays on an important humanistic theme and follow each performance with a panel of professional humanists in literature, philosophy, psychology, sociology, and history, who would engage the audience in discussing the drama in terms of social issues. Because the area in which UMR is located has a large population of older people, the social issue chosen was aging and all of its problems.

Four objectives were established for the program: (1) to demonstrate that good drama could be produced in small communities without major financial resources and without major theatrical facilities; (2) to make the general public aware of the problems; (3) to provide audiences and professional humanists with a common reference point for discussing the problems of aging; and (4) to give older people a forum where their problems could be presented in drama before an audience of all ages.

The clientele for this program was the general public of south-central Missouri. Because the United States Geological Survey, the Bureau of Mines, Fort Leonard Wood, the Missouri Geological Survey, and numerous other state and local government agencies are located in the area, the population includes a large number of professional people who work for these agencies or are retired from them. Besides, since the area is primarily rural with only small urban centers, the population also includes many retired farmers and small-business managers.

The first step in the planning was to write a proposal and submit it to the University of Missouri's Older Missourians Program Committee. After this proposal was funded in the amount of $2,800, the process began of contacting actors and technical crews to produce the drama, arranging for professional humanists to appear as panelists for each performance, and scheduling performances in the area.

In the course of the experiment, the humanities department presented four plays on 20 occasions in five towns and used two theatre groups—the Rolla Civic Theatre and the UMR Theatre Guild—to produce the plays. The first drama in the series was a simple one-act play involving five characters, no set, and a limited number of props. This play, *A Choice to Make* by Nora Stirling, is from the Plays for Living Series, which have no royalty fee. The play was easily transported and was performed for various groups including church groups and the general public in surrounding communities. Other performances were conducted in Rolla before groups of retired people, professional workers in gerontology, and residents of retirement homes. Each performance was followed by a panel discussion conducted by professional humanists including the director of the Rolla Senior Citizens Home and a psychiatrist.

The second play, *Chest Pains*, was more experimental. It was chosen to explore how serious drama on the problems of aging would be received in the area. Playwright Frank Levering, who was then at Harvard University, agreed to come to Rolla for the performances of his play. He, along with the director of the play, a professional social worker, and the chairman of the UMR Department of Humanities, formed a panel to discuss the controversial nature of the drama, including the language and the nature of the illness of the elderly man.

The third and fourth plays, *Whisper in My Good Ear* and *Save Me a Place in Forest Lawn*, were presented at the Rolla Senior Center, the Soldiers Home in St. James, the John Knox Retirement Village in St. Roberts, and the Rolla Community Hall. Again, following each performance, a panel of professional humanists interacted with the audience.

The experiment demonstrated that good drama could be produced in small towns at a minimal cost. The panel discussions demonstrated that the viewers of these plays were eager to exchange ideas with professional people in the humanities and gerontology. There seems to be little doubt among those who participated in the series—the actors, the technical crews, the professional humanists and gerontologists—that other communities can adapt the experience of this project to their own needs.

However, there were many problems. Without a permanent group of actors and technicians, each production meant starting anew with inexperienced people. In some ways this was beneficial because it extended the reach of the project into the community by forcing us to recruit many amateurs. But it also caused problems because a great deal of time was spent in trying to find a group of people to work together. The solution to this problem, though, was to rely on the director of each play to provide the organization each production needed. The limited facilities and equipment available presented another problem. Keeping the sets, props, and lights as simple as possible helped, and proved beneficial in many ways. The lack of equipment prompted the director to improvise more, the audience to use its imagination more, and the actors to develop their characterizations further.

Another kind of problem with the productions involved the audience. Although the plays were performed for a wide variety of audiences, ranging from small church groups through residents in retirement homes to large audiences drawn from the general public, the audiences had one thing in common. In general, since all these audiences were unaccustomed to viewing contemporary drama, the language of the plays and the prostate illness in *Chest Pains* caused some negative reactions. One member of the audience protested so strongly about this play that she wrote the governor of the state of Missouri. Another couple talked with the director afterward and called the language and the whole premise of the play vulgar. We thought that we had solved the problem by having the playwright himself discuss the play after each performance, but obviously his explanations of his motives for using certain profane and vulgar expressions were not satisfactory to everyone.

However, this problem does not necessarily indicate failure. It indicates that even though the impact was too painful in its graphic realism for some members of the audience, the play made an impact and caused people to think.

Invariably, after each performance, an older member of the audience would remark to one of the actors or the director that the play was not meant for older people—it was meant for younger people to show them what growing old is like. This remark is really a compliment to the actors and production staff because it reflects the older person's recognition of the realism of the production.

Still, most people who commented on the productions found them both entertaining and thought provoking. Many actually enjoyed the panel discussions following each performance more than the plays themselves, but most members of the audience found that the plays and the discussions complemented each other.

The series gave many people with limited opportunities and backgrounds an experience in live theatre. Often people will say that they have seen a play when they have actually seen a film or a television tape. Television and motion pictures have vast dramatic possibilities, but they cannot compete with the unlimited dramatic possibilities of live theatre. First, live theatre is life-size. The actors are there—not bigger than life, as in motion pictures, nor smaller than life, as in television. Second, each performance is a unique event in itself. Each night of performance the actors will act the play differently, and each night the audience will react to that performance differently. Third, while the play is going on, the audience forms a unique community participating in a unique event. In this community experience, the individuals of the audience form a common bond through which they can discuss their own lives and communicate their reactions to those who have shared the performance with them. Finally, community theatre enables the audience to share with the actors ideas and emotions that have been developed in the play. In the University of Missouri-Rolla experiment, each performance of the play was followed by an open discussion in which professional humanists, the director, and the cast shared their ideas with the audience. Through such factors, live theatre continues to be a living experience to all who participate in it.

A Selected Bibliography of Plays with Gerontological Themes

At a Beetle's Pace. Louis E. Catron. One male, one female. The problems of old age are given a fresh examination in this play, which takes place in some vague future where science has created a "utopia" that prevents people from every getting older and makes death almost unknown. (Royalty, $10–$15.)

Bright and Glorious. Phillis Coate Stratford. Two males, five females. Mrs. Eberts, a woman of 78 who has been seriously ill, wishes to give her granddaughter, Nancy, a quiet and commonplace way of looking on death. (Royalty, $5.)

Brighten Every Corner. A drama. George Herman. Six males, eight females. Sister Mary Martha, 72, of the Order of Our Lady of Peace, has died at the motherhouse of the Order in Little Rome, Iowa. Of no great social importance, her death received no more than a few lines in the evening papers, but this notification of her passing stirs the memory of people throughout the United States, from a state legislator to a quiet laborer who once tried to kill her. (Royalty, $5.)

Chest Pains. Frank Levering. Three males, four females. A man recovering from prostate surgery helps a young man overcome his psychological fears. (Royalty can be negotiated with Frank Levering, Orchard Gap, Virginia.)

A Choice to Make. Nora Stirling. Two males, four females. Edna, a lonely widow, learns that she can have a life of her own when her son moves away to a better job. (No royalty.)

Couplings and Groupings. Megan Terry. A collection of interviews that may be used as playlets, sketches, monologues, and so forth. (Single copy, $1.45. Royalty, $10 for the long sketches, $5 for the short ones.)

The Day It Rained Forever. A comedy. Ray Bradbury. Three males, one female. Three old men are rocking away their lives on the porch of an empty hotel in a desert miles from nowhere. Today is the one day of the year it has always rained, so it is one of unusual expectation for them. But as evening descends, the rain does not come. One man goes in to lie down and die, and another prepares to pack and leave. At this point they hear a heaving and puffing old car, which finally sighs and expires outside their door. From it emerges a "dandy large woman" and harp.

She not only revitalizes the old fellows; when she plays the harp, the rain comes in earnest. (Royalty, $10.)

An Evening of One-Act Stagers for Golden Agers. Albert M. Brown. The author, a member of the Academy of Certified Social Workers (ACSW), has written more than 50 plays for children and young adults in past years while working in settlement houses and camps. In recent years, however, as executive director of a housing project for elderly, his experience with "golden agers" (or senior citizens) has resulted in these six one-act plays. They do not require a great deal of "action." They could even be "acted out" as readings in the event that some elderly people may have some difficulty learning lines from memory. (Single copy, $2. Royalty, $5 each performance of each play, or $25 for all six, even when the plays are performed for charity or when no admission is charged.)

The Garden. A drama. Edward Pomerantz. Three males, four females. Story revolves around an old man who lives with his son and daughter-in-law and their two children. The old man lives in their house a total stranger; his only diversion is his garden. (Royalty, $5.)

George's Room. Alun Owen. One male, one female. A widow, not so old as to be unattractive, is persuaded to rent her late husband's room to a lodger who promises to be congenial. (Single copy, $1. Royalty, $5.)

The Gloaming, Oh My Darling. Megan Terry. Four males, six females. Two old crones in a sanitarium make their day with fantasies. The dead husband of one of them is nearby, but the other proclaims her marriage to him. (In *Viet Rock: Four Plays by Megan Terry.* New York: Touchstone Books, 1967. $2.95. Royalty, $10.)

The Hebrew Lesson. Wolf Mankowitz. Four males, one female. A young man with gun dashes into a room where an old Jew is studying. The sanctuary turns out to be a synagogue, and the Jew, a member of a race that has long been hunted and on the run, can sympathize with the youth. They exchange some Gaelic phrases, and then share a little Hebrew together. And this is what saves the youth when the Black and Tans storm and search the synagogue. (Royalty, $10.)

Lights, Camera, Action. A comedy suite. Robert Patrick. Two males, two females. A "suite" of three "mini-plays," which created a new dramatic form when performed at the Caffe Cino in 1967. *Lights:* An art-gallery opening brings a confrontation between an older woman and her gauche young protégé. *Camera:* Computer-matched over long-distance television, a boy and girl encounter a technological and temperamental contretemps. *Action:* An older and a younger writer write one another's lives, each unaware that they are living a cliché. (In Patrick, R. *Cheap Theatricks.* New York: Winter House, 1972. $3.95 Royalty, $10 per play, $30 for the suite.)

Lots of Old People Are Really Good for Something. A comedy. E. P. Conkle. One male, four females. Four young girls discover that old people can really be good for something. (Royalty, $5.)

A Mask for the Dead. A drama. Lillian Lipman. Two males, one female. The confrontation is between a widower and his married daughter, and the climax comes when she waits up for him one night to tell him that he must stop seeing his woman friend. (Single copy, $1. Royalty, $5.)

Nellie Was a Lady. A comedy. John Kirkpatrick. Two males, five females. Nellie is a retired school teacher living with her niece and the niece's friend. (Royalty, $5.)

Now We Are Free. A drama. James Lineberger. Two males, two females, extras. Estelle, an emancipated spinster, has assembled a traveling troupe dedicated to the eradication of guilt through vicarious suffering. (Royalty, $5.)

Porch. A drama. Jeffrey Sweet. Two males, one female. Amy's father is about to undergo surgery; Amy visits him for the first time since a bitter fight years before. (In *Best Short Plays of 1976.* Radnor, Pa.: Chilton Book Co., 1976. Royalty, $10.)

Saturday at the Cohens. A comedy-drama. Merle Claflin. Three males, five females. Morey Cohen's old mother and father now live with him—to the dismay of his wife, Sheila. Son Arnold brings his girlfriend, Linda Rosen, home for lunch. Linda, daughter of a rabbi, is very religious, but Arnold is not. Morey's old parents save the day when it seems the proposed marriage may dissolve over the religious conflict. (Royalty, $5.)

Save Me a Place in Forest Lawn. Lorees Yerby. Two females. Clara and Gertrude reveal secrets about their dead husbands and themselves. (Royalty, $10.)

Short Plays for the Long Living. Roger N. Cornish and John M. Orlock. Bare stage with props. Each of the six short plays requires a cast of two people, who share a dramatic experience for their fellows—an experience that touches the long living. These commissioned plays have varied uses: as discussion aids, as ways to flex unused muscles, as variations on improvisational work, or merely as reading for the joy of reading. *Running Away from Home:* A live-in father seeks independence from his overprotective daughter. *The Close-Down Set-Up of Emma:* An unmarried couple decides to move to a shared residence. *Autumn Drive:* A demanding husband teaches a nonchalant wife to drive. *Mrs. Lazer's Caller:* A widow finally accepts a date. *Meals on Wheels:* A lonely lady entices compassion and understanding from a delivery man. *Frosting:* Two men discuss the impending change when a wife graduates from college. A detailed introduction for performer and worker with elderly included. (Single copy, $2. Royalty, $5 each play.)

Steinway Grand. A drama. Ferenc Karinthy. One male, one female. The woman advertises a grand piano for sale, and the man calls to inquire about it. But on his second call, we begin to sense something is wrong with his inquiry; he is not really interested in the piano at all. In the third call, we suspect a swindle or a joke. His fourth call the widow allows to go unanswered. And now the full truth is out: The "buyer" is really a lonely man at the verge of despair. (Single copy, $1. Royalty, $10.)

The Suicide. A drama. Mario Fratti. One male, two females. A young married couple sit up waiting for her mother, who lives with them. They become overwhelmed with guilt as time passes, and they dwell on their shabby treatment of the old women. (In *The New Theatre of Europe, Volume II.* New York: Dell, 1965. Single copy, $2.25. Royalty, $10.)

Three by Two. Three one-act plays. Rena and Stanley Waxman. One male and two females for each play. *Please Call Me Sol* deals humorously with an elderly couple, a widow and a widower, who have some awkward and anxious moments as they seek a new life together in a second marriage. *A Table for Two* is a comedy about a couple that faces a moment of significant change when their last child flies off to college and leaves them. *Welcome Home* makes you laugh, but it hurts to see two people claw away at each other in a marriage that was not made in heaven. (Single copy, $2. Royalty, $5 each play.)

Three on a Bench. A comedy. Doris Estrade. Two males, two females. Mrs. Moore, a lonely widow, amuses herself by observing couples that come into the park and by helping them. (Royalty, $5.)

Uncle Bob's Bride. A comedy. Isla Paschal Richardson. One male, seven females. Uncle Bob's three nieces are bored with their country home. Uncle Bob will arrive with his bride and is sending an interior decorator. The girls declare war, resenting the sudden marriage of their bachelor guardian. (Budget play.)

The Way Out. A drama. John Kelly. Three males, one female. Trapps Donovan, an old trapper, sits in his lonely cabin in the Yukon mountains, talking to his bird, Timothy. (Single copy, $1. Royalty, $5.)

What Did You Say "What" For? A drama. James Paul Dey. One male, one female. The play has no real story or plot line, and a park bench is its only set. It involves a rather "mad" lady's attempts at conversation with a simple, unsuspecting little man. Beneath the bizarre dialogue and lunatic fun is indeed a level of human isolation crying out for a sympathetic ear. (Single copy, $1. Royalty, $10.)

Whisper into My Good Ear. William Hanley. Two males. Charlie, in his lonely old age, decides to commit suicide, and his best friend, Max, tries to persuade him not to. (Royalty, $10.)

Will Someone Please Tell Me What's Going on Here? A comedy. Jim Lee. One male, three females. The story involves Harold and Lucille, a bored, middle-aged couple; Florence, the spinster who lives next door; and Officer Buckley, a perpetually confused policeman. (Royalty, $10.)

References

Guide Books on Play Production

Guide to play production. New York: R. R. Bowker, 1975.

The theatre student series (13 volumes). New York: Richard Rosen Press, 1971.

Play Catalogs

Dramatists Play Services, Inc., 440 Park Avenue South, New York, N.Y. 10016.

Samuel French, 25 West 45 Street, New York, N.Y. 10036 (published annu-
    ally).
Pioneer Drama Service, 2172 Colorado Boulevard, Denver, Colo. 80220.
Theatre House, Inc., 400 West Third Street, Covington, Ky. 41011.